The World Food Problem

Tackling the Causes of Undernutrition in the Third World

SECOND EDITION

Phillips Foster
Howard D. Leathers

LYNNE
RIENNER
PUBLISHERS

BOULDER
LONDON

Published in the United States of America in 1999 by
Lynne Rienner Publishers, Inc.
1800 30th Street, Boulder, Colorado 80301

and in the United Kingdom by
Lynne Rienner Publishers, Inc.
3 Henrietta Street, Covent Garden, London WC2E 8LU

Library of Congress Cataloging-in-Publication Data
Foster, Phillips
    The world food problem : tackling the causes of undernutrition in
        the Third World / by Phillips Foster and Howard D. Leathers. — 2nd
    ed.
        Includes bibliographical references and index.
        ISBN 1-55587-703-6 (pbk. : alk. paper)
        1. Food supply—Developing countries. 2. Poor—Developing
countries—Nutrition. 3. Malnutrition—Developing countries.
4. Food supply—Government policy—Developing countries.
5. Nutrition policy—Developing countries. 6. Food supply—
Developing countries—International cooperation. I. Leathers,
Howard D. II. Title.
HD9018.D44F68   1998
363.8"09172'4—dc21   98-24979
                                                                 CIP

British Cataloguing in Publication Data
A Cataloguing in Publication record for this book
is available from the British Library.

Printed and bound in the United States of America

        The paper used in this publication meets the requirements
 ∞   of the American National Standard for Permanence of
        Paper for Printed Library Materials Z39.48-1984.

    5 4 3 2

☐ Contents

The World
Food Problem

☐ Foreword

Food is emotional, political, life-determining. Naturally, it fills the cultural outlook and colors of life for the half-billion rich people of the world. But the quest for food and the worry as to how that quest will fare bear with terrible immediacy on well over 1 billion people, the hungry and undernourished. It is central to the worries of another billion or two who are at risk of falling into the ranks of the hungry or who, having only recently reasonably ensured their departure from those ranks, remember hunger all too well.

Many rich countries of the world, as this book makes clear, are only a generation or two away from where much of the world is still mired. And in many countries, Finland and Japan, for example, the remembrance of hunger in war is still in the minds of senior political leaders and affects their approach to many issues of our international world.

The centrality of food is perhaps best marked by noting that for about 2 billion people, it is the direct employment in food and agricultural production, or the indirect employment created by expenditures of those who directly labor in agriculture, that determines their income—how much money they have to devote to food consumption. And it is the price of food that is the dominating determinant of what that money is worth. Or, to offer a numerical example, in rural India the proportion of the rural population in poverty so severe that they are undernourished and hungry fluctuates between 40 and 60 percent, depending on the weather and its effects on food production and food prices. No wonder so many of the poor are fatalistic and do not believe they have significant control of their lives.

Truly important, emotional, political subjects carry with them the controversy and irrationality that impedes progress. This is particularly true of food, the world food problem, and the remedies proffered. It applies to

ix

people of good will, dedicated to helping the hungry and the malnourished, as well as to the opportunists who also flock to misery.

Phillips Foster and Howard D. Leathers give us facts about the world food problem—an extraordinary array of facts, all important to understanding the issues. And because food touches so much, these facts cover a wide range of knowledge, about food directly and about the broad processes of development, growth, and distribution that largely determine access to food. But the myriad of facts we are given are built around a conceptual framework that selects the facts to be presented and weaves them into a coherent story, leading us to usable, applicable conclusions.

The conclusions that come out of this vast, complex story are just that: vast and complex. Many of the fortunate in the world who are driven to help those less fortunate owe it to the hungry and malnourished to read this book, to understand the processes which in a generation can abolish hunger and undernutrition, but which cannot so operate if quick fixes are pursued. The title of this book tells us that it deals with a problem, and the subtitle that it tackles the causes. This is not a book of quick fixes and treatment of symptoms.

I have emphasized the immensity of the food problem. The authors document that. It is important to do so and to grasp the immensity. If the problem is modest in extent, then it is reasonable to think that modest redistribution of food and income will solve the problem: perhaps only redistribution within poor countries. And perhaps we can diffuse our focus to related problems. But if the problem is immense, redistribution has to move to the point at which it hurts in the rich countries as well, and even that is not enough. Incomes must be raised, growth and development must occur. Trade-offs must be faced.

Our guides take us through these issues step by step. And they lead us to a terribly important and central conclusion. Yes, in one sense there is enough food in the world for everyone. But to get adequate purchasing power into the hands of the billions of poor, they must be made more productive, and because they are so much either directly or indirectly in the food and agriculture sector, we must wrestle with the food production problem. Thus, food production is central to the solution of the world food problem, but as much or more from an income generation and employment point of view as from a consumption point of view. Or to use the jargon of the day, most of the hungry get their "entitlement" to food by producing food. This issue requires facts, analysis, and synthesis. We get these in full measure.

I would like to close this foreword on a personal note. In laboriously building the International Food Policy Research Institute to its premier status, I was driven by the importance of facts as the basis for finding causes and then solutions to the world's problems and by the recognition that facts in our complex world are hard to come by. Thus the institute was built on the pursuit of facts in the context of a strategic vision. But weaving those facts into the policy determination fabric is in itself an immense task. Nothing could more delight and excite me than to see that work, and of course that of many others as well, woven so skillfully and thoughtfully and to such good effect as in this book by Phillips Foster and Howard D. Leathers.

But if the subject is so important and complex, why have we not had this book before? Perhaps because the emotion of the subject is so great that it required time for unearthing the facts, and the maturing process of the decade—plus of continual effort, dedication, and interaction that have gone into it. It is now for the rest of us to avoid disappointment by reading, absorbing, and acting, each in our own way.

John W. Mellor

☐ Preface

Since the first edition of this book was published in 1992, the world has changed along with our knowledge and understanding of the world food problem. Some significant developments have occurred, including:

- The Sixth World Food Survey has been published, presenting new detailed information about the extent and geographical contours of the problem.
- The World Food Summit of 1996 provided an international forum for analysis and discussion of the problem.
- Serious studies of the future of the world food problem have been undertaken and published by the Food and Agriculture Organization of the United Nations, the World Bank, the International Food Policy Research Institute, and the WorldWatch Institute.
- The interaction of agricultural production and environmental quality has become a subject of great concern and interest among analysts and policymakers.
- The breakup of the Soviet bloc and the end of the Cold War have coincided with a more widespread adoption of market-oriented policies, with less reliance on government intervention in markets.

Despite these changes, the principal messages of the first edition remain as valid today as they were then. Hunger, or undernutrition, remains a problem for hundreds of millions of people in developing countries. Poverty, income inequalities, population growth, and illness continue to be important causes of undernutrition. While continuing to emphasize these causes, the current edition puts slightly more emphasis than did the first edition on increasing agricultural production as a way of reducing the extent of undernutrition.

■ THE PLAN OF THE BOOK

We begin with an emphasis on definitions and facts. As the material develops, our emphasis changes to behavioral models of society (e.g., economic, demographic) and how these models relate to undernutrition. In the last section, we discuss how these models can be applied in evaluating nutrition policy alternatives.

In Part 1, malnutrition is identified as a leading killer throughout the world, with undernutrition in the developing world the main nutrition problem. Before considering the causes of undernutrition and policy alternatives to alleviate it, we examine the facts and provide answers to questions such as: What is malnutrition? How do we measure it? Who is malnourished? What are the trends?

In Part 2, we look at the main causes of undernutrition—the vehicles by which undernutrition is delivered to families—and attribute these causes mainly to economic, demographic, agronomic, and health variables. A number of models are introduced to help in understanding how these variables "deliver" or cause undernutrition.

In Part 3, we explore applications of the above-mentioned models as tools for the formulation and evaluation of public policy alternatives of interest to nutrition planners. It ends with a set of recommendations on how to achieve policy reform and speculations about the future.

We have integrated knowledge from a number of disciplines, taking as a central premise, well articulated by Beatrice Rogers (1988b), that "the solution to the world hunger problem will be achieved only through the integration of knowledge from the whole range of relevant scientific disciplines." Thus we have drawn on the fields of nutrition science, economics, demography, biology, chemistry, health science, geography, agronomy, history, anthropology, philosophy, and public policy analysis.

To a large extent, this book is data driven. From the opening chapter, in which we present the Carl Mabbs-Zeno famine figures, through the data on malnutrition in Part 1, and the numbers on elasticity and population in Part 2, to the future projections about production, consumption, and prices in the last chapter, the text is supplemented with illustrative tables, figures, and boxes.

* * *

In addition to the many people whose assistance was acknowledged in the first edition, the second edition owes a debt of gratitude to the students and teaching assistants of AREC 365 at the University of Maryland, College Park, and to our colleagues John Moore and Leslie Whittington for insight and recommendations.

Finally, we thank our wives and children for their support and understanding in this undertaking.

Phillips Foster
Howard D. Leathers

□ 1

Introduction

Hunger. It was prevalent everywhere. Hunger was pushed out of the tall houses, in the wretched clothing that hung upon poles and lines; Hunger was patched into them with straw and rag and wood and paper; Hunger was repeated in every fragment of the small modicum of firewood that the man sawed off; Hunger stared down from the smokeless chimneys, and started up from the filthy street that had no offal, among its refuse, of anything to eat. Hunger was the inscription on the baker's shelves, written in every small loaf of his scanty stock of bad bread; at the sausage-shop, in every dead-dog preparation that was offered for sale. Hunger rattled its dry bones among the roasting chestnuts in the turned cylinder; Hunger was shred into atomies in every farthing porringer of husky chips of potato, fried with some reluctant drops of oil.
—Charles Dickens, *A Tale of Two Cities*

■ HUNGER KILLS

A newspaper headline on starvation may conjure up in your mind the image of an emaciated infant, the victim of an Ethiopian famine. And if you are a history buff, words like Bengal or Ukraine may spring up. Despite huge relief efforts from Europe and North America, some 300,000 people died of hunger-related causes during the Ethiopian famine of 1983–1985 (Hancock 1985). News photographs and television images of rural Ethiopian families migrating in search of food, of babies with bloated bellies and spindly arms and legs, and with bodies too weak to sit up, have filled our consciousness with the horror of hunger. The 1990s have provided horror stories of their own: Famine in North Korea reached such an acute stage by late 1997 that there were reports of people eating grass and tree bark. Worldwide, one estimate puts deaths from starvation during the

1

1990s at from 100,000 to 200,000 per year (Kates 1997). Another study estimates that as many as 576,000 Iraqi children have died since the end of the Gulf War due to food shortages resulting from economic sanctions against the country (Zaidi & Fawzi 1995).

Yet these horrors pale beside the figures from a long list of 148 earlier famines compiled by Carl Mabbs-Zeno of the United States Department of Agriculture (USDA). In the past it was not unusual for major famines to wipe out people by the millions (see Tables 1.1–1.3). The Ukrainian famine of 1921–1922 may have taken 9 million lives, and the infamous Bengal famine of 1770 claimed perhaps 10 million.

The drama of famine involves not only hunger and death but enormous disruptions in the social fabric of the community. Normal social relationships are strained, families disintegrate, and the better-off may take advantage of the situation to exploit the worse-off (see Box 1.1).

Although the drama of famine tends to capture our attention, most hunger-related deaths do not occur in famines. They happen daily—quietly, largely unchronicled—all around the world. Figures vary, but one conservative estimate, using data provided by the World Health Organization (WHO) of the United Nations (UN), is that some 8 million children die annually from hunger. This amounts to one death every four seconds. Another way to put this number into perspective is to imagine the newspaper coverage that would occur if a 747 jet crashed, killing all 220 children on board; the deaths attributable to hunger are equivalent to 100 of these jet crashes every day (Food for the Hungry Homepage 1998).

The Food and Agriculture Organization (FAO) of the UN estimates that the number of chronically undernourished people in the developing world dropped slightly from 900 million people in 1969–1971 to 800 million in 1988–1990. When expressed as a percentage of the population, the drop is more dramatic: The 800 million was 35 percent of the population of developing countries from 1969 to 1971; the 900 million was 20 percent of the population of developing countries from 1988 to 1991 (see FAO WFS technical background document 1, 1996). The Bread for the World Institute (1997) estimates that the comparable figure for 1997 is 841 million. Based on these numbers, and taking into account that there are some hungry people in the developed world, we can conclude that 14–17 percent of the world's population suffers from chronic hunger.

Of course, as the numbers above make clear, not all the hungry die from hunger. What happens when you die from hunger? Describing famine-related death, an anonymous author writing for *Time* magazine put it eloquently and succinctly:

> The victim of starvation burns up his own body fats, muscles, and tissues for fuel. His body quite literally consumes itself and deteriorates rapidly.

Table 1.1 **Largest Famines in Europe**

Area Affected	Date	Excess Deaths (in thousands)	Area Affected	Date
Ukraine	1946–47	2,000	England	1321
Greece	1941–43	400	England, Ireland	1314
Lower Volga	1932–34	5,000	England, Scotland	
Ukraine[a]	1921–22	3,000	Ireland	1302
		9,000	England	1294
Eastern Urals	1911–12	8,000	England	1257–59
Ukraine	1905–06		England	1235
Western Plains, Russia	1897–98		Russia	1230–31
Volga Valley	1891–93		Ireland	1227
Ireland	1845–50	1,500	Novgorod, Russia	1215
Russia	1833–34		England, France	1193–96
Ireland	1822		England, Wales	1183
Poland	1770		England	1124
Bohemia	1770		Ireland	1116
Scotland	1766		England	1093
England	1740–41		Rostor-Volyn', Russia	1070–71
France	1661		England	1069
Ireland	1650–51		England	1042–48
Moscow	1601–03	500	Suzdal, Russia	1024
England	1594–95		England	1004–05
Ireland	1588–89		England	976
England, Ireland	1586		Bolobereg	971
Hungary	1586		England, Wales, Scotland	954–58
England	1549		Scotland	936–39
England	1527		England	310
England	1521		Scotland	306
Hungary	1505		Scotland	228
Ireland	1497		Ireland	192
Ireland	1447		Rome	185
England	1437–39		Italian Peninsula	79–88
Ireland	1410		England	54
England	1392–93		Rome	23
England	1353		Rome	AD 6
Europe[b]	1346–50	40,000	Rome	385 BC
England, Scotland[c]	1341–42		Rome	436 BC

Source: Mabbs-Zeno 1987.
Notes: a. Estimates from two different sources.
b. Most deaths not due to malnutrition.
c. No record of excess deaths exists prior to this date.

The kidneys, liver, and endocrine system often cease to function properly. A shortage of carbohydrates, which play a vital role in brain chemistry, affects the mind. Lassitude and confusion set in, so that starvation victims often seem unaware of their plight. The body's defenses drop; disease kills most famine victims before they have time to starve to death. An individual begins to starve when he has lost about a third of his normal body weight. Once this loss exceeds 40 percent, death is almost inevitable.

Table 1.2   **Largest Famines in India and Bangladesh Since 1700**

Area Affected	Date	Excess Deaths (in thousands)
Bangladesh	1974	1,000
Bengal	1943	1,500–3,000
Punjab, Central Provinces	1899–1900	2,500
Bengal, Bombay, Central Provinces	1885–97	5,000
Orissa, Ganjam	1888–89	1,500
Madras, Bombay, Hyderabad	1876–78	5,000–8,000
Punjab, Deccan	1868–70	2,500
Orissa, Hyderabad[a]	1865–67	1,900
		10,000
Madras, Deccam	1853–55	
North	1837–38	800
Southeast	1833–34	
Madras	1832–33	
Sind, Rajasthan, Madras	1812–13	1,500
West	1802–03	
Bombay, Hyderabad	1790–93	
Mahratta	1787	
Bihar, Madras, Mysore	1781–83	
Afgot, Chingleput, Madras	1780–82	
Bengal, Bihar	1770	10,000
Chingleput	1733	
Madurai	1709–21	
Decca	1702–04	2,000

Source: Mabbs-Zeno 1987.
Note: a. Estimates from two different sources.

Table 1.3   **Largest Famines in China Since 1800**

Area Affected	Date	Excess Deaths (in thousands)
China	1958–60	30,000
Honan	1941	3,000
Northwest	1929–32	5,000
Central	1925	
North	1920–21	500
North	1892–94	
Honan	1887–89	2,000
North	1876–79	10,000
China	1846–49	5,000
China	1810–11	20,000

Source: Mabbs-Zeno 1987.

Whereas adult males do die of hunger during a famine, the majority of deaths, whether from famine or from chronic undernutrition, occur among preschoolers. Pregnant and lactating women are also at substantial risk,

Box 1.1 Peasant Perceptions of Famine

Izzedin I. Imam

The structure of relationships in the village community prevents the hardships of famine from being borne equitably by all its members. These relationships allow those who occupy positions of influence and wealth further to widen the gap between themselves and those in a dependent situation. For example, once a natural calamity triggers expectation of a food shortage, the large landowners begin to divert food supplies into storage and wait for the prices to rise—thus turning adversity into their opportunity.

But the landless have no such option. Futhermore, the drop in production also reduces the demand for their labor—the only resource they possess. Wage rates fall and the wage laborers find themselves at the mercy of those who can offer work or who have cash to offer in return for their few possessions.

In such a situation, often the only recourse is to start selling off the only possessions the household may have. Generally, the landless pawn their goods to money lenders, a term generally applied to anyone with surplus assets, such as the landowners. The hope is always that one day the loan will be repaid and the object recovered. But this virtually never happens. The interest charged on the loan is usually so crippling that the debtor has next to no chance of being able to repay the principal in the time allotted and the object passes into the possession of the money lender.

Pawning usually begins with those items which are expendable, such as ornaments or jewelry. Eventually as the desperate need for cash to buy food increases, every household item, including utensils, may be pawned or sold at any available price.

As a last resort the household head may leave his family and set off to an uncertain destination in hope of finding employment. Some of those who migrate return periodically to give any earnings to their families. But anxieties over whether those who migrate will return grow with time, as commonly they do not. The wives left behind may take up employment doing chores in the richer households, living off the leftovers of the rich family's meals. One woman in Rowmari who could no longer stand the cries of her hungry children hung herself—leaving them behind with no one to care for them. A case was reported from Melanda, Jamalpur, of a woman who was said to have sold her four children and turned to begging.

Source: Extracted from Imam 1979.

although less so than children. Children suffer malnutrition in a multitude of ways. They may be crippled by vitamin D deficiency (rickets), blinded by vitamin A deficiency (xerophthalmia), or stunted by lack of protein (kwashiorkor), for instance. But the most common form of child undernutrition results simply from a lack of sufficient calories, with disease and death too often the result.

To visualize the most common scenario, played out again and again in the Third World, picture a loving but poorly educated, poverty-stricken mother with several children. Food is scarce. Her youngest child has not been growing for months because of undernourishment and the baby's resistance to disease has fallen to a very low level. He drinks from the family's supply of unclean water; the older members of his family can handle the microorganisms in the water, but he develops diarrhea. He loses interest in eating. He seems more willing to take liquids, so the mother removes solids from his diet. Because he is unable to obtain sufficient nourishment from the liquids to conquer his illness, his diarrhea continues. Finally, in a desperate but seemingly logical attempt to stop the diarrhea, his mother removes the liquids. Although the child by now is feverish, limiting liquids accelerates the baby's loss of fluids. Severe dehydration follows, with death not far behind.

■ FACTORS INFLUENCING FOOD SUPPLY AND DEMAND IN THE FUTURE

As we look to the future, the quality of life worldwide will depend on whether the world's food supply will grow faster or slower than the world's food demand. If food supplies grow faster than demand, almost certainly the average quality of life in the world will improve. If supply outpaces demand, food prices will fall; this will make it easier for poor people to afford an adequate diet; for rich people, it will free income to spend on other goods and services. Similarly, if demand grows faster than supply, average quality of life will likely deteriorate.

In analyzing future prospects for food supply and demand, the four critical factors, which we refer to as the "four Ps," are

- Population
- Prosperity
- Pollution or environmental quality
- Productivity in agriculture

The impact of *population* growth on food demand is obvious. More mouths to feed means more demand for food. The question of whether food production can grow as fast as population is posed by Thomas Malthus in his "Essay on the Principle of Population" (Malthus 1890).

Widespread economic *prosperity* means that more people can afford adequate diets, and that they are more likely to have access to health care, a sanitary water supply, and education. Prosperity as measured by income per capita also affects food demand. As people reach higher income levels, they tend to buy more food in a wider variety, including meat and animal products. Therefore, 6 billion relatively affluent people require significantly more agricultural production than do 6 billion relatively poor people.

Pollution (or environmental quality) and the availability of land and water resources needed for agricultural production are critical to the future. To what extent can we expand the area devoted to agricultural production? Will soil erosion or water pollution leave us with less arable or irrigable land? Will there be global climate changes that influence agricultural production?

Agricultural *productivity* measures our ability to increase food production without increasing the amount of agricultural land. No matter what happens to environmental quality and land and water resources, the future food supply will continue to grow if productivity increases fast enough. Productivity per acre can increase provided farmers apply more fertilizer, or use more labor or other inputs per acre. Productivity per acre can also increase through new technology (such as new seed varieties).

These four factors interact with each other in complex ways:

- As population grows, urban and industrial water users compete with agriculture for scarce water.
- Population growth slows as people become more prosperous.
- As agricultural productivity increases, economic prosperity improves for the entire economy.
- Increased use of agricultural chemicals may improve productivity while harming the environment.

The above discussion suggests some of the ways that government policies can influence the long-term food supply-and-demand situation. However, the complexity of interactions illustrates how difficult deciding among various policy alternatives can be. Appropriate policy changes are the subject of the last part of this book. The discussion of policy alternatives in this chapter will give only a brief introduction to this important topic.

■ THE MAIN NUTRITION POLICY ALTERNATIVES

When you stop to think about it, food raises some of the most important emotional associations in our culture. What a positive association most people have of a mother feeding her baby. Or consider the food associations with some of our important festivals and rituals—Thanksgiving, Christmas, Passover, Communion. And what would a birthday party or a wedding reception be without a cake? The immediacy and presence of the nutrition problem and its involvment with the particular human suffering that is connected with such emotion-laden facets of our lives make the hunger problem cry out for a solution—and not only a solution, but a solution *soon*.

☐ Treating Symptoms

Our immediate reaction to hunger tends to be one of charity. If people are hungry, why not feed them? And so we develop a multitude of charitable programs. In high-income countries churches set up soup kitchens, rock music groups perform special concerts, and governments install food-stamp plans. The international aid community makes surplus food available to food-deficit areas through Food for Peace (U.S. government–sponsored) and the World Food Program of the UN.

With severely limited budgets for out-and-out charity, Third World governments have set up food-rationing schemes and placed ceiling prices on basic foods. They have forcibly procured food from farms at below-market prices and resold it to consumers at below-market prices in government "fair-price" shops. In an attempt to make food more readily available to their consumers, Third World governments control the movement of food from one region of the country to another and limit the export of food grains.

Both industrial and Third World governments attempt to improve nutrition (through food fortification programs) by adding, for example, vitamins and minerals to white bread.

All these urgent and timely programs intervene somehow in the food-marketing system and attempt to redistribute food among households to reduce hunger. As such, they can be called *nutrition intervention programs*. When nutrition intervention programs provide needy people with food purchased in the marketplace, charitable donors, or taxpayers in general, pick up the tab. But many intervention programs lower the cost of food for the needy in other ways. Governments, for instance, may pass laws setting food-price ceilings, or they may subsidize food consumption by procuring food from farmers by way of police power, and then redistributing it to the nonfarm population. In these cases, resource holders in agriculture (landowners, farm managers, farm workers) provide the food subsidy.

But whether paid for by charitable organizations, taxpayers, or the farmers themselves, nutrition intervention programs do not treat the *causes* of hunger. If we make an analogy to medical science, we might say that nutrition intervention is more concerned with treating the *symptoms* of hunger than its causes.

☐ Treating Causes

Treating the causes of hunger is a slower, more complex task than the activities just described. As the international aid community and Third World countries work together in treating the causes of hunger, a number of avenues open to them (discussed in some detail in Part 3 of this book). In this section we provide only a preview of these avenues.

Programs and policies to subsidize food production (rather than food consumption) attempt to lower the cost of food in the marketplace through increasing the quantity offered for sale. Food production subsidies, including public investment in agriculture, take many forms, such as sponsoring agricultural research and development programs, financing rural education programs, or providing farmers with low-cost irrigation water. (See Box 20.3 for a discussion of the way the word *subsidy* is used in this book.)

Most Third World countries have embarked on programs to reduce their birth rates in the hope of reducing the pressures of population on food supplies. Public health programs (e.g., supplying cities with cleaner drinking water) improve nutrition as healthier people make more-efficient use of the food they consume. Improving employment opportunities for the poor and taxing the rich (to provide social programs such as education) is a way of improving the lot of those who might otherwise go hungry.

■ A NUTRITION POLICY DILEMMA

Treating the causes of hunger is a complex undertaking because the causes themselves are many and complicated. Later in this book we devote several chapters to understanding the causes of hunger, but in summary here we state simply that the main causes can be grouped under three headings: (1) economic; (2) demographic; and (3) health. Particular economic, demographic, and health situations result in malnutrition in families or family members. We call these variables the *nutrition impact vehicles,* because it is through them that malnutrition is delivered.

The particular economic, demographic, and health situation found in any one country or region can be traced to the particular policies, programs, or projects (or lack of them) that have been promulgated by that country's or region's leaders throughout its history. For instance, the lack of a supply of clean drinking water in a particular city can be attributed to past policies, programs, or projects; or, if you prefer, to the *lack* of appropriate policies, programs, or projects. The presence of a largely illiterate (and therefore underproductive) farm population can be attributed to the educational policies and programs of the country or region.

In any case, if we are to treat the causes of malnutrition, we must adjust the public policies, programs, or projects of a given country or region so that the nutrition impact vehicles no longer combine to deliver malnutrition. International aid donors and recipient countries have been working together over the years to improve standards of living, including nutritional standards, of people in the Third World. Many of their efforts have focused on changing the economic, demographic, and health situations for the better.

The magnitude of nonmilitary international aid is shown in Tables 1.4 and 1.5. Major aid recipients are among those countries with lower per capita incomes, although the data clearly show here that aid-flows are influenced by geopolitical as well as humanitarian considerations. On the right-hand side of Table 1.4, for instance, notice that Israel and the Palestine Administrative Area are credited with respectively $273 and $144 per capita per year of international aid, yet the Central African Republic received only about $52 per capita, and Bangladesh and Ethiopia did not even appear in the top 25 per capita recipients. The World Bank estimates the following as 1994 per capita incomes in these countries: Israel, $14,530; Central African Republic, $370; Bangladesh, $220; and Ethiopia, $100.

Notice also that donor countries provide substantially different proportions of the gross national product (GNP) for aid (Table 1.5). For instance, although Japan and the United States provided the largest amounts

Table 1.4   Ranking of 25 Major Recipients of Aid, 1991–1996

	By Average Annual Receipts (in millions of U.S. dollars)			By Average Annual Receipts per Capita[a] (in U.S. dollars)	
1	Egypt	2,993	1	Israel	272.78
2	China	2,953	2	Nicaragua	157.81
3	India	2,107	3	Palestinian Adm. Areas	144.37
4	Indonesia	1,688	4	Guinea-Bissau	125.08
5	Bangladesh	1,565	5	Gabon	123.13
6	Israel	1,479	6	Jordan	121.38
7	Philippines	1,180	7	Mauritania	114.37
8	Mozambique	1,163	8	Zambia	111.56
9	Pakistan	1,115	9	Nambia	110.90
10	Ex-Yugoslavian States	1,042	10	Bolivia	90.44
11	Ethiopia	1,031	11	Papua New Guinea	88.36
12	Zambia	1,026	12	Congo	85.16
13	Tanzania	1,020	13	Senegal	76.42
14	Cote d'Ivoire	988	14	Albania	75.63
15	Kenya	789	15	Botswana	74.66
16	Morocco	778	16	Cote d'Ivoire	71.71
17	Thailand	730	17	Gambia	70.87
18	Uganda	712	18	Mozambique	70.00
19	Nicaragua	674	19	Rwanda	68.28
20	Ghana	661	20	Mongolia	64.46
21	Bolivia	655	21	Honduras	63.09
22	Sri Lanka	639	22	Lesotho	62.69
23	Vietnam	621	23	El Salvador	60.61
24	Senegal	619	24	Guinea	59.31
25	Cameroon	561	25	Cent. Afr. Rep.	52.80

Source: OECD/DAC Statistical Reporting Service:
http://www.oecd.org/dac/htm/dacstats.htm
Note: a. Average annual aid receipts divided by 1993 population. Includes only countries with 1993 populations of 1 million or greater.

Table 1.5   Ranking of the 21 Largest Donors of Aid, 1991–1996

	Ranked by Total Overseas Development Assistance (ODA) (annual average for years 1991–1996)				Ranked by ODA as a % of GNP (annual average ODA divided by 1995 GNP)	
		$ million	% of total			% of GNP
1	Japan	11,755	20.1	1	Sweden	0.943
2	United States	9,961	17.0	2	Denmark	0.937
3	France	7,989	13.6	3	Norway	0.877
4	Germany	7,228	12.3	4	Netherlands	0.754
5	United Kingdom	3,160	5.4	5	France	0.551
6	Italy	2,876	4.9	6	Finland	0.478
7	Netherlands	2,797	4.8	7	Canada	0.396
8	Canada	2,272	3.9	8	Belgium	0.345
9	Sweden	1,978	3.4	9	Switzerland	0.343
10	Denmark	1,462	2.5	10	Luxembourg	0.332
11	Spain	1,331	2.3	11	Germany	0.321
12	Norway	1,193	2.0	12	Australia	0.317
13	Australia	1,071	1.8	13	United Kingdom	0.289
14	Switzerland	981	1.7	14	Austria	0.279
15	Belgium	864	1.5	15	Italy	0.264
16	Austria	604	1.0	16	Portugal	0.261
17	Finland	503	0.9	17	Spain	0.250
18	Portugal	252	0.4	18	Japan	0.237
19	Ireland	111	0.2	19	Ireland	0.210
20	New Zealand	108	0.2	20	New Zealand	0.210
21	Luxembourg	56	0.1	21	United States	0.140

Source: OECD/DAC Statistical Reporting Service:
http://www.oecd.org/dac/htm/dacstats.htm

of aid in 1996, they were far down the list in terms of percentage of GNP allocated to aid. The $55 billion that the aid donors provided to Third World countries in 1996 financed a range of programs from food donations to assistance in agricultural research.

Resources are scarce, and competition for charitable funds, international donor assistance, and Third World government expenditures is keen. But for those who want to spend more resources on reducing hunger, one of the toughest decisions is how to allocate expenditures between direct food assistance (nutrition intervention), which helps alleviate suffering sooner (treating symptoms), and programs to adjust the nutrition impact vehicles (treating causes) so that, later, they deliver less malnutrition. A difficult trade-off results because spending more resources on nutrition intervention leaves fewer resources for adjusting the nutrition impact vehicles.

Those with a short, or present, time orientation tend to emphasize treating symptoms. Because the priority of any government is to stay in power, politicians tend to be present time–oriented. By contrast, academics and government technocrats tend to see the big picture; they are more fu-ture time–oriented, and therefore more likely to favor treating causes. Most people would prefer both to feed the hungry today and to end hunger tomorrow. But resources are limited and choices must be made. Figure 1.1 organizes the main points of the dilemma we have been discussing.

Figure 1.1   A Nutrition Policy Dilemma

**Policies, Programs, Projects
(or lack of them)**

**Causes of Malnutrition
(Nutrition Impact vehicles -- Economic, Health, Demographic)**

Malnutrition

Alternatives:	• Treat symptoms (nutrition intervention)	• Treat causes (adjust nutrition impact vehicles)
Trade-off:	• More resources to treating symptoms • Fewer resources left for treating causes	• More resources to treating causes • Fewer resources left for treating symptoms
What mix to use?	• Present Time Orientation: Emphasize treating symptoms	Future Time Orientation: Emphasize treating causes

■ PART 1

MALNUTRITION: WHAT ARE THE FACTS?

Malnutrition is a leading killer. In high-income countries one variant of malnutrition—overnutrition—is the main nutritional problem. In the Third World another variant—undernutrition—is the main problem. The problem of Third World undernutrition is exacerbated by secondary malnutrition—malnutrition stemming from causes such as disease.

Before considering the causes of undernutrition, and policy alternatives to alleviate it, we must examine the facts and provide answers to these questions: What is malnutrition? What are its effects? How do we measure it? Who is malnourished? What are the trends?

☐ 2

Malnutrition Defined

One common definition of malnutrition is "overconsumption or underconsumption of any essential nutrient." This chapter will be devoted to exploring this definition.

■ FOUR TYPES OF MALNUTRITION

The internationally famous nutritionist Jean Mayer (1976) identifies four types of malnutrition: (1) overnutrition; (2) secondary malnutrition; (3) dietary deficiency or micronutrient malnutrition; (4) protein-calorie malnutrition.

☐ Overnutrition

When a person consumes too many calories, the resulting condition is called *overnutrition*. Overnutrition is the most common nutritional problem in high-income countries such as the United States, although high-income people in low-income countries also suffer from this type of malnutrition. The diet of the world's high-income people is usually overladen with calories, saturated fats, salt, and sugar. Their diet-related illnesses include obesity, diabetes, hypertension, and atherosclerosis.

☐ Secondary Malnutrition

When a person has a condition or illness that prevents proper digestion or absorbtion of food, that person suffers what is called *secondary malnutrition*. (It is called "secondary" because it does not result directly from the nature of the diet, as do the other types of malnutrition, which are termed *primary.*) Common causes of secondary malnutrition are diarrhea, respiratory illnesses, measles, and intestinal parasites. The following mechanisms cause secondary malnutrition:

- *Loss of appetite (anorexia).*
- *Alteration of the normal metabolism:* For example, when the body shifts some of its attention to fighting infection. Among other things, production of disease-fighting white blood corpuscles may be increased and body temperature may be raised.
- *Prevention of nutrient absorption:* For instance, diarrheal infections irritate the lining of the gastrointestinal tract, creating difficulty in absorbing nutrients and at the same time causing it to shed contents before full digestion has had time to occur.
- *Diversion of nutrients to the parasitic agents themselves:* Parasites such as hookworms, tapeworms, and schistosome worms rob the body of nutrients it would otherwise retain (Briscoe 1979; Martorell 1980).

Public health measures such as providing sanitary human waste disposal and clean water are especially important in reducing secondary malnutrition. Secondary malnutrition often accompanies and exacerbates other types of undernutrition.

☐ Dietary Deficiency or Micronutrient Malnutrition

A diet lacking sufficient amounts of one or more essential micronutrients such as a vitamin or a mineral results in dietary deficiency. Although a deficiency of any micronutrient can become a serious problem, most nutritionists are primarily concerned about deficiencies in vitamin A, iodine, and iron.

Vitamin A. Deficiency of vitamin A can cause xerophthalmia, or night blindness. It is also associated with increased mortality from respiratory and gastrointestinal disease. One study suggested that vitamin A supplements could reduce deaths of children between six months and five years by 23 percent. Recent research suggests that vitamin A plays a role in maintaining the immune system and in fighting cancer.

Iodine. Iodine deficiency causes goiter and leads to a reduction in mental abilities. Babies born to iodine-deficient mothers can suffer from "cretinism," which can cause children to become slow learners. One study indicates that even mild iodine deficiency can reduce intelligence quotients (IQ) by 10–15 points. Iodine deficiency is the greatest single cause of preventable brain damage and mental retardation. WHO estimates that one-third of the world's people live in "iodine-deficiency environments."

Iron. Iron deficiency, or anemia, causes reduced capacity to work, diminished ability to learn, increased susceptibility to infection, and greater risk of death during pregnancy and childbirth. More than 40 pecent of people in developing countries are estimated to suffer from iron deficiency.

Other micronutrients. Recently, nutritionists have become concerned about zinc deficiencies. Zinc now appears to be effective in increasing the growth of very young children; it also reduces the incidence of diarrhea and assists in absorption of other micronutrients. Other diseases caused by micronutrient deficiencies include rickets (soft bones), caused by vitamin D deficiency; scurvy, caused by vitamin C deficiency; and beri-beri and pellagra, caused by deficiencies in B-vitamins. Recent research (Tang et al. 1993) indicates that the risk of contracting acquired immunodeficiency syndrome (AIDS) is substantially lower among men who consumed very high levels of niacin (a B-vitamin), vitamin A, and vitamin C.

When compared with underconsumption of protein or calories, the problem of underconsumption of micronutrients appears relatively easy to solve. The missing elements are inexpensive, and programs to provide them are relatively easy to initiate. In the United States, "iodized" salt (salt to which iodine has been added) protects us from iodine deficiency, specially fortified milk provides vitamin A (and vitamin D), and iron pills (or multiple vitamins with iron) are a common source of iron. Examples of successful interventions in the developing world are as follows:

- In Guatemala, dietary anemia was greatly reduced in a rural community after the inhibitants were persuaded to substitute iron cooking pots for aluminum pots.
- Also in Guatemala, fortification of sugar with vitamin A has been effective, and experiments are now under way to fortify sugar with iron.
- In Brazil, a school's drinking water was fortified with iron, creating a noticeable improvement in students' iron levels at a cost of about 15 cents per student per year.
- In China, iodine deficiency was treated by dripping potassium iodate solution into the water of an irrigation canal. The amount of iodine excretion by people in the area increased two-and-a-half times.

Other interventions to improve micronutrient malnutrition include making vitamin pills available to the population and cultivating plants that contain one or more micronutrients. The World Bank (1994) estimated in 1994 that it would cost about $3 per year to meet a person's entire needs for vitamin A, iron, and iodine. By comparison, an anti-oxidant formula of vitamin E, beta-carotene, and vitamin C may cost $60 per person per year.

Despite the apparent easy solution to these vitamin and mineral deficiencies, the problems have remained surprisingly persistent. In the mid-1990s, the World Bank launched a "Micronutrient Initiative" to reduce these types of deficiencies. This remains an important policy because of the huge impact on public health that relatively small expenditures can have. As we shall see in the next chapter, the health impacts of micronutrient deficiencies are significant. However, the solutions to these deficiencies are more likely to come from fortification programs such as those described above, and less likely to come from additional food consumption and production.

☐ **Protein-Calorie Malnutrition**

The underconsumption of calories or protein—known as *protein-calorie malnutrition* (PCM) or *protein-energy malnutrition* (PEM)—is a problem that can only be solved by increasing the amount of food that an individual eats. A person suffering from PCM is short of the protein or calories needed for normal growth, health, and activity. PCM hardly ever occurs in families with enough income to satisfy their basic needs for food, shelter, clothing, and heat; PCM is found predominantly in low-income countries where poverty is widespread.

In extreme forms, PCM manifests itself as the potentially fatal nutritional disorders known as kwashiorkor and marasmus (see Boxes 2.1 and 2.2). Kwashiorkor is most likely to be encountered among populations where the diet is heavily based on cassava (as in West Africa) or on plantains (as in parts of Latin America and southern Uganda). These particular plant foods are almost completely devoid of available protein, and children who are weaned on them are at high risk for severe protein deficiency. Marasmus is most likely to occur under conditions of extreme poverty in which children are weaned onto a gruel that contains modest amounts of protein, but where available food is nutritionally inadequate. Marasmus is thus more common among the poorest populations of the world, such as those of Ethiopia, Nepal, and Bangladesh. Without warmth, loving care, and expert medical attention, children with marasmus or kwashiorkor may quickly die.

■ **CALORIES AND PROTEIN**

Because PCM is a major source of nutrition-related disease, and because reducing PCM requires increasing food consumption, much of this book will focus on PCM. These two elements—calories and protein—are both derived from food and are both necessary for growth, health, activity, and

Box 2.1 Kwashiorkor

Eleanor Whitney and Eva Hamilton

The word kwashiorkor originally meant "the evil spirit which infects the first child when the second child is born." It is easy to see how this superstitious belief arose among those Ghanaians who named the disease. When a mother who has been nursing her first child bears a second child, she weans the first and puts the second on the breast. The first child soon begins to sicken and die, just as if an evil spirit had accompanied the new baby into the world and set out to destroy the older child. What actually happens, of course, is that protein deficiency follows soon after weaning, for while breast milk provides these children with sufficient protein, they are generally weaned to a protein-poor gruel.

Millions of children in the world are affected by kwashiorkor. It typically sets in around the age of two. By the time children with kwashiorkor are four, their growth is stunted; they are no taller than they were at two. Their hair has lost its color; their skin is patchy and scaly, sometimes with ulcers or open sores which fail to heal. Their bellies are swollen with edema; they sicken easily, and are weak, fretful, and apathetic.

The swollen belly of the kwashiorkor child is due to edema; blood protein is so low that fluid leaks out into the body. Since the child is too weak to stand much of the time, the fluid seeks the lowest available space—in this case the belly. The picture of such a child is one of skinny arms and legs and a greatly swollen belly. On first glance you might think the child is fat, but if the fluid could be drawn off, his true condition would be revealed: he is actually a wasted skeleton, just skin and bones.

The body follows a priority system when there is not enough protein supplied to meet all its needs. It abandons its less vital systems first. When it cannot obtain amino acids enough from dietary sources, the body switches to a metabolism of wasting, and begins to digest its own protein tissues in order to supply the amino acids needed to build the most vital internal proteins and keep itself alive. Hair and skin pigments (which are made from amino acids) are dispensable and are not manufactured. The skin needs less integrity in a life-and-death situation than the heart, so its maintenance ceases and skin sores fail to heal. Many of the antibodies are also degraded in order that their amino acids may be used as building blocks for heart and lung and brain tissue. Children with a lowered supply of antibodies cannot resist infection and readily contract dysentery, a disease of the digestive tract. Dysentery causes diarrhea, leading to rapid loss of those nutrients—including amino acids—which these children may be receiving in food. Thus dysentery worsens the protein deficiency, and the protein deficiency in turn increases the likelihood of a second or third or tenth attack of dysentery.

The water loss in diarrhea increases losses of the water-soluble B vitamins and vitamin C. The children's inability to manufacture protein carriers for the fat-soluble vitamins makes them deficient in vitamins A and D as well. Their inability to manufacture protein carriers for fat often leaves them with fat accumulated in the liver tissue, from which it would normally be carried away. As the liver clogs with fat, its cells become unable to carry out their other normal functions, and gradually they atrophy and die.

Source: Reprinted from *Understanding Nutrition* by Whitney, Hamilton & Rolfes, copyright 1990 by West Publishing Company. Used by permission of Wadsworth Publishing Company.

Box 2.2 Marasmus

Eleanor Whitney and Eva Hamilton

When children are almost totally deprived of food, they cannot obtain the energy necessary to maintain their body systems, much less that necessary for growth. Marasmus, a wasting disease, results. Invariably, protein deficiency occurs with this condition, as available protein is used not to build body protein but to supply energy (which takes priority). As a result, the marasmic child has many, though not all, of the same symptoms as the child with kwashiorkor.

Marasmic children are wizened little old people in appearance, just skin and bones. They are often sick because their resistance to disease is low. Their hearts are weak, and all their muscles are wasted. Their metabolism is slow. They have little or no fat under their skin to insulate against cold. Their body temperatures may be subnormal. The experience of hospital workers with victims of this disease is that their primary need is to be wrapped up and kept warm. They need love, since they have often been deprived of maternal attention as well as food.

Unlike the kwashiorkor child, who is fed milk until weaning, the marasmic child may have been neglected from early infancy. The disease occurs most commonly in children from six to eighteen months of age in all the overpopulated city slums of the world. Since the brain normally grows to almost its full adult size within the first two years of life, marasmus impairs brain development and so may have a permanent effect on learning ability.

Marasmus also occurs in adults in countries where calorie deficiency is prevalent.

Source: Reprinted by permission from *Understanding Nutrition* by Whitney, Hamilton & Rolfes, copyright 1990 by West Publishing Company. Used by permission of Wadsworth Publishing Company.

survival. But their nutritional roles are different. More important, calories and proteins are derived from foods in different ways, and a diet must be carefully planned if it is to be adequate in both.

☐ **Nutritional Role of Calories and Proteins**

Calories are a measure of the energy contained in food (see Box 2.3). The body gets energy from carbohydrates (e.g., sugar and starch) and fats (e.g., corn oil and butter). Calories are used by the body to provide energy needed for

- The "involuntary functions" such as breathing, blood circulation, digestion, and maintaining muscle tone and body temperature

---

Box 2.3 Calories and Kilocalories

In physics, chemistry, and engineering, a calorie is the amount of heat energy required at sea level to raise the temperature of one gram of water one degree centigrade. A kilocalorie (abbreviated Kcal) is the energy it takes at sea level to raise the temperature of 1,000 grams of water (a kilogram—also a liter) one degree centigrade.

Nutritionists always quote their data in kilocalories, but unfortunately commonly shorten the word to Calories. Usually people capitalize the word Calorie when intending to indicate a kilocalorie as distinguished from calorie. But the convention is not always observed. At any rate, when you are reading nutrition literature and see the word *calorie* (note the lower case c), it is safe to assume that it means kilocalorie.

There is another thing to bear in mind when comparing nutritional calories to those in the physical sciences. The energy value of foods found in the standard handbooks, such as *Agricultural Handbook* no. 8, represents the energy available after deductions have been made for losses in digestion and metabolism. The system for determining these energy values was developed through the classic investigations of W. O. Atwater and his associates at the Connecticut Agricultural Experiment Station.

For more information on this subject, consult U.S. Dept. of Agriculture 1963.

- Physical activity
- Mental activity
- Fighting disease
- Growth

The human body makes the millions of different proteins that it needs from some 20 amino acids, which are the building blocks of the body's proteins. Proteins function in ways other than providing a source of calories:

- They are necessary for building the cells that make up muscles, membranes, cartilage, and hair.
- They carry oxygen around our bodies.
- They carry nutrients into and out of cells and help assimilate food.
- They contribute to the development of antibodies that fight disease.
- They work as enzymes that speed up the digestive process.

Simple organisms such as yeasts and algae can synthesize almost all of the amino acids they need. But humans cannot synthesize some amino acids; we make insufficient quantities of others for our requirements. To live, therefore, we must consume enough *essential amino acids* (those which the body cannot produce in sufficient quantities). Of the approximately 20 amino acids needed, nine are essential. Because the body cannot manufacture them, we must consume them as part of our diets. Proteins containing these amino acids are found in egg white and milk—two examples of dietary proteins that contain all the essential amino acids; thus these foods are referred to as sources of *complete proteins*.

Not all foods that contain protein are sources of complete proteins. Protein molecules in food are composed of fixed proportions of amino acids. A balanced protein is one in which the essential amino acids appear in the same ratio to each other as the body needs them for constructing its protein molecules. (This ratio is shown in Table 2.1, and lists the recommended daily allowances [RDA] for a healthy adult male.)

If you consume more amino acids than you need, your body cannot use them for making proteins; instead, it burns the amino acids for energy. If you consume less of an amino acid than you need, a portion of other amino acids goes to waste for want of the "matching" part needed to manufacture protein molecules. Whitney and Hamilton (1977:92) provide a delightful analogy:

> Suppose that a signmaker plans to make 100 identical signs, each saying LEFT TURN ONLY. He needs 200 L's, 200 N's, 200 T's and 100 each of the other letters. If he has only 20 L's, he can make only 10 signs, even if all the other letters are available in unlimited quantities. The L's limit the number of signs that can be made. The quality of dietary protein depends first on whether or not the protein supplies all the essential amino acids, and second on the extent to which it supplies them in the relative proportions needed.

You can get balanced protein from animal products like meat, milk, eggs, and cheese, but not from isolated grain or vegetable products. You can, however, get balanced protein by combining different *types* of grains and vegetable products (see Figure 2.1). Consuming a certain quantity of beans provides you with more than your needs for the amino acid lysine, but leaves you short on methionin and cystine. Consuming a certain quantity

Table 2.1   Balanced Protein for a Healthy Adult Male, NAS Standard

Essential Amino Acid	RDA (in milligrams)
Phenylalanine	1,100
Tyrosine	1,100
Methionine	1,100
Cystine	1,100
Leucine	1,000
Lysine	800
Valine	800
Isoleucine	700
Threonine	500
Tryptophan	250

Figure 2.1 Protein Complementarity Between a Cereal and a Pulse

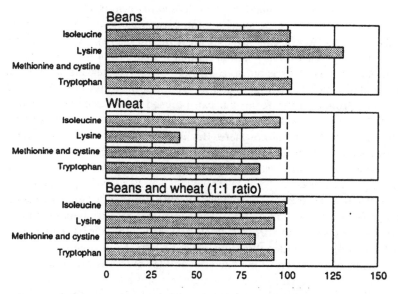

of wheat leaves you short of all the amino acids, especially lysine. A 50-50 mix of beans and wheat provides a reasonably balanced mix.

☐ The Chemical Process of Producing Dietary Calories and Protein

The energy that our bodies use comes from the sun; but our bodies cannot absorb solar energy directly and use it for physical growth and activity. The chemical process by which plants transform solar energy into a form of energy (in plants) that can be absorbed by humans or animals is known as *photosynthesis:* Carbon dioxide plus water plus radiant energy from the sun yields (in the presence of chlorophyll) a carbohydrate plus oxygen plus water. Written as a chemical equation:

$$\text{Chlorophyll}$$
$$6CO_2 + 12H_2O + \text{Light energy} \rightarrow C_6H_{12}O_6 + 6\,O_2 + 6\,H_2O$$

Using enzymes, a plant can rearrange the carbon, hydrogen, and oxygen atoms of the carbohydrate, or sugar ($C_6H_{12}O_6$), as shown in the above equation, to form starch or fat.

The conversion of sugar to starch is energy-efficient: Practically all the energy in the original sugar can be released in burning the starch made from it. The conversion of sugar to fat, however, is about 77 percent energy-efficient; so we can say that most of the energy in the original sugar can be released in burning the fat that is made from it.

Making amino acids is not so easy. Like carbohydrates and fat, amino acids contain carbon, hydrogen, and oxygen, but they also contain nitrogen, and nitrogen in the form that can be used to build amino acids is scarce. In the process of photosynthesis, plants can use carbon dioxide (CO_2) straight from the atmosphere. But in making amino acids, nitrogen cannot be used as N_2, the form in which it is found in the atmosphere. It has to be converted to more complex forms, such as ammonia (NH_3), before the plant can use it.

Converting atmospheric nitrogen to usable nitrogen is called *nitrogen fixation*. It can be done in a commercial fertilizer plant, where energy is combined with some raw organic stock such as naptha. Or it can be done by nature, which provides three other ways of fixing nitrogen: (1) lightning storms; (2) nitrogen-fixing bacteria; and (3) blue-green algae. By and large, the nitrogen fixed by blue-green algae is not available to plants useful to man. Leguminous plants, such as beans, peas, and alfalfa, provide a suitable environment on their roots for nitrogen-fixing bacteria and thus have an extra boost of nitrogen available. (For more on legumes, see Box 2.4.)

The fixed nitrogen taken up by plants becomes available in the food chain to make amino acids, and ultimately, proteins. Plants and animals must spend energy (use up sugar) to synthesize amino acids. They spend still more energy to recombine these amino acids into enormous molecules of protein. As a result, the energy available from burning a protein is substantially less than the energy used to produce that protein. By contrast, the amount of energy released in the burning of a carbohydrate or fat is closer to the amount of energy it took to make it in the first place.

☐ Protein: More Expensive than Carbohydrate or Fat

The chemistry involved in producing calories and proteins helps explain why proteins are scarce relative to carbohydrates and fats. The relative scarcity implies that putting adequate protein into our diets is going to be more expensive than consuming adequate calories. And, generally speaking, we do pay a premium for protein-rich foods. For instance, you probably know that hamburger is a richer source of protein than rice and that hamburger costs more per pound than rice (and you can get about twice as many calories from a pound of rice as you can from a pound of hamburger).

Box 2.4 Types of Edible Seeds

Most of the calories consumed in the world come from edible seeds. Even in high-income countries where livestock products are so important in the diet, the livestock themselves eat substantial quantities of these edible seeds.

There are two kinds of edible seeds: cereals and pulses. Cereals are characterized by one seed leaf (the seed does not split easily), pulses by two seed leaves (the seed splits easily). Cereals, also called grains, come from grasses, while pulses come from legumes. In general the cheapest calories are available through the cereals. The cheapest fats are from the pulses or palms like the coconut. The cheapest proteins are often from the pulses, with soybeans being the prizewinner for lowest cost. In the Third World, corn (i.e., maize) sometimes competes with the pulses for the lowest-cost protein.

The major edible seeds, together with their percentage of protein content, are:

Cereals		Pulses	
Rice	6.7	Beans, white	22.3
Corn (Maize)	7.8	Peas, dry	24.2
Millet	9.9	Lentils	24.7
Sorghum	11.0	Peanuts	26.0
Wheat, hard		Soybeans	34.1
red winter	12.3		

You notice that the protein content of the cereals is in all cases under 14 percent, while the pulses provide protein content of over 20 percent.

The coconut palm is more similar to a grass than to a legume and its protein content reflects this fact. The protein content of dried coconut meat is 7.2 percent. Dried coconut meat is about 4 percent water. The dried cereals in our list generally run from 10 to 14 percent water, by weight.

Finding the cheapest sources of protein, carbohydrates, and fats is of critical concern to the poorest people in the world. Table 2.2 shows the retail prices and nutrient values of foods in the Philippines in 1984; this allows us to consider the costs and nutritional values of a variety of diets in a low-income country. From the table we can see that the cheapest source of calories is corn grits, the cheapest source of protein is soybeans, and the cheapest source of fat is coconut. On a per gram basis, the cheapest protein is over six times more expensive than the cheapest calories. A similar calculation for Indonesia in 1978 found the cheapest protein over 12 times more expensive than the cheapest carbohydrate (Indonesia, Diro Pusat Statik 1981; Indonesia Oleh Direktorat Gizi Departemen Kesehatan R. I. 1979).

Table 2.2 Relative Importance of Foods in the Diet, and Retail Peso Price of Nutrients, Philippines, 1984

	1 Kcal Available for Consumption per Capita per Day 1981	2 Percentage of Calories in Diet	3 Price per 100 g as Purchased	4 Kilocalories per 100 g Edible Portion	5 Price per 1,000 Kcal	6 Protein per 100 g Edible Portion	7 Price per 100 g Protein	8 Fat per 100 g Edible Portion	9 Price per 100 g Fat
Cereals	1465.3	56.6							
Rice, milled, ordinary	981.1	37.9	.463	363	1.27	6.7	6.91	0.4	115
Corn, grits, white	368.8	14.2	.405	362	1.1	8.7	4.66	0.8	50
Wheat flour	98.6	3.8	.752	364	2.06	10.5	7.16	1.0	75
Others	16.8	.6							
Starchy Roots and Tubers	199.4	7.6							
Sweet potato	61.9	2.4	.304	119	2.52	.97	31.34	.35	87
Cassava, white sweet	128.1	4.9	.241	108	2.23	.44	54.77	.15	161
White potato (Irish)	1.2	—	.875	64	13.67	2.0	43.75	.08	1094
Gabi (taro)	3.4	.1	.554	86	6.44	1.8	30.77	.15	369
Other roots	3.0	.1							
Cassava flour and starch	1.8	.1							
Sugars and Syrups	258.0	9.9							
Centrifugal sugar, white	222.5	8.5	.751	387	1.94	0	—	0	—
Banochs and muscovado	4.0	.2		376		0.2		0.4	
Others	31.5	1.2							
Pulses and Nuts	34.2	1.3							
Peanuts, shelled	4.7	.2	1.807	564*	3.20	26.0*	6.95	47.5*	4
Mongo, green	9.7	.3	1.392	354	3.93	24.4	5.70	1.0	139
Other dried beans except soy	1.8	.1							
Soybeans and products	1.9	.1	1.148	403*	2.84	34.1*	3.37	17.7*	6
Coconut for food	11.8	.5							
Mature coconut in shell	8.6	.3	.215	169	1.27	2.1	10.24	14.5	1
Young coconut in shell	3.2	.1							
Other nuts, unshelled	0.3								
Other pulses and nuts	4.0	—							
Vegetables	33.8	1.3							
Cabbage	10.6	.4	.958	18	53.32	1.1	87.09	.24	399
Yardlong beans, green (sitao)	9.4	3.6	.640	33	19.39	2.9	22.07	.18	355
Tomatoes	2.5	.1	.747	27	27.69	.89	83.93	.29	258
Others	11.0	.4							

Table 2.2 Continued

	1 Kcal Available for Consumption per Capita per Day 1981	2 Percentage of Calories in Diet	3 Price per 100 g Purchased	4 Kilocalories per 100 g Edible Portion	5 Price per 1,000 Kcal	6 Protein per 100 g Edible Portion	7 Price per 100 g Protein	8 Fat per 100 g Edible Portion	9 Price per 100 g Fat
Fruits	168.0	6.5							
Banana (latundan)	110.3	4.2	.825	69	11.95	.87	94.83	.21	393
Calamansi	2.2	.1	.933	12	82.28	.15	622	.38	245
Other vitamin C–rich fruits	19.3	.7							
Other fresh fruits	35.8	1.4							
Meat									
Beef (rump)	8.8	.3	3.939	110	35.80	20.7	19.03	2.4	164
Pork (ham)	110.6	4.3	3.288	281	11.70	14.8	22.22	24.2	14
Poultry (broiler)	13.1	.5	2.349	81	29.00	14.4	16.31	2.2	107
Milk and Milk Products	27.1	1.0							
Fresh milk	.4	0		64		3.3		3.6	
Powdered and other dry	7.2	.3		476		24.1		22.5	
Dry skimmed milk	18.0	.7	3.523	363*	9.70	35.9*	9.81	.8*	440
Eggs	20.4	.8							
Chicken	16.4	.6	2.460	143	17.20	10.8	22.78	9.5	26
Duck	4.0	.2	2.860	156	18.33	10.1	28.31	10.9	26
Fish	74.3	2.9							
Milkfish	54.8	2.1	1.269	90	14.10	12.5	10.15	4.0	32
Small shrimps (susha)	10.5	.4	2.842	60	41.36	11.8	24.08	.49	580
Mollusk	7.1	.3							
Fats and Oils	103.3	4.0							
Vegetable (coconut)	91.8	3.5	1.541	883	1.74	.02	99.1	2	
Butter (commercial)	3.6	.1		720		.5		81.6	
Butter (homemade)	7.1	.3							
Miscellaneous	55.7								
Beer and other alcohol	22.9	.9							
Total	2,590.7								

Sources: Nutrients per 100 grams: Food Composition Tables, Food and Nutrition Research Institute, February 1980, except cereals and items marked*, for which see Food Composition Table for Use in East Asia, FAO, USDHEW, 1972. Relative importance in the diet: NEDA Food Balance Series Number 8, Food Balance Sheet for the Philippines CY 1977 to CY 1981, pp. 58–62. Prices: white sugar, National Sugar Trading Corporation; wheat flour, NFA, July 1, 1984, retail price; coconut oil and coconut for food, United Coconut Association of the Philippines; powdered milk, Pampanga Market, May 1985, deflated by estimate to July 1984; soybeans, U.S. wholesale price 1984/85 times 2.5; all others, Bureau of Agricultural Economics, average retail price, Philippines, 1984.

Because your body receives calories from carboydrates, proteins, and fats, it makes sense to compare the costs of calories from the various foods. For the Philippines, cereals and coconut oil win hands-down in this contest. With the average diet, Filipinos eat 56.8 percent of their calories as cereals. Despite their low-cost protein, pulses do not figure much in the average diet—probably because their calories are too expensive. Filipinos have evidently found, over the generations, that if they buy enough (inexpensive) calories as rice or maize, they consume enough protein. But they have also discovered that it does not work the other way around. If you buy enough (of the most inexpensive) protein, you do not get enough calories; in this sense, rice and corn are a more economical diet than are soybeans. Table 2.3 presents a low-cost diet that was designed so that its cost is about half that of the average diet.

☐ **Which Is the Bigger Problem:**
   Protein Deficiency or Calorie Deficiency?

Because protein is more expensive than carbohydrates, the question arises: Should we show more concern about the protein intake of poor people than we do about their calorie intake? Until the 1970s, nutritionists believed that protein was the central concern.

No doubt, protein deficiency can and does occur. However, the experience of the past 30 years demonstrates that calorie deficiency is a more widespread problem. For example, a study of 15,000 Indian preschool children in the 1960s found that 35 percent showed evidence of both calorie and protein deficiency, 57 percent showed evidence of calorie deficiency but not protein deficiency, but virtually none showed evidence of protein deficiency without an accompanying calorie deficiency.

Recent numbers on food's availability also indicate that calorie deficiency is likely to present a bigger problem than protein deficiency. FAO numbers for 1995 show that in sub–Saharan Africa, food available per capita would provide 2,144 calories per day (less than the 2,350 calorie-per-day number that reflects an average of calorie-recommended dietary intake for adult men and adult women) but would provide 51.6 grams of protein (above the 50 grams per day that is an average of the recommended dietary allowances [RDAs] for adult men and adult women). Similarly, numbers from the FAO's Sixth World Food Survey for 1990–1992 show that among the least developed countries, food supplies provide 50 grams of protein per capita per day, but only 2,040 calories per capita per day.

Nevin Scrimshaw, a world-famous advocate of the importance of protein in the diet, puts it like this: "It is true that adult protein needs are met by most traditional developing country diets when they are consumed in sufficient quantity to meet normal energy needs" (Scrimshaw 1988).

Table 2.3   Average Diet and Inexpensive Diet for the Philippines: Nutritional Value and Cost

Daily Grams of	In Average Diet	In Cheap Diet
Cereals (rice)	400	140
Starch (cassava)	185	170
Sugar	65	10
Coconut	15	10
Pulse (mongo)	5	200
Fruit-Vegetables (banana)	335	50
Meat-Dairy-Fish (dry skim milk)	77	0
Fats-Oils (vegetable oil)	15	5
Calories/day	2,590	1,534
Grams of protein/day	60	60
Cost/day (pesos)	$P8.37	$P4.43

■ HOW MUCH OF A NUTRIENT IS ENOUGH?

Before describing what can happen when a person does not get enough of a nutrient, we need to explore what "enough" means. Of course, no single standard applies to everyone. Each person is different. Growing children have different nutritional needs than mature adults. Men have different nutritional needs than women. Active people have different nutritional needs than sedentary people. And some people are just different for unexplainable reasons. For example, we all know someone who can eat and eat yet never gain weight; that person has a *higher metabolism,* or a higher daily need for calories than the rest of us.

These differences are reflected in the RDA, the most commonly used standard for nutrient sufficiency. Table 2.4 shows RDAs for 17 different age-sex groups for calories, protein, and 17 vitamins and minerals. How these recommendations are designed is shown in Figure 2.2. The normal (bell-shaped) shows the distribution of people in a certain group (say men between the ages of 19 and 22) according to how much of a certain nutrient (say calories) each person needs. Some men in this age group need few calories (near point A); some need a lot of calories (near point G). On the curve, point D is the mean (or average) requirement. The degree to which the bell curve is spread out around the mean is measured by a statistic called the *standard deviation* (SD)—a large standard deviation means that the curve is a relatively flat spread-out bell; a small standard deviation means a tall, skinny bell. An intake level at point F is calculated by taking the standard deviation, multiplying it by two, and adding the result to the mean. Statisticians have shown that point F calculated in this way will show the following characteristics: Nearly all (97.5 percent) of the people in the group will have a requirement that is less than F; only 2.5 percent of the population will have a requirement greater than F. The RDA for a nutrient in a given age-sex group is set at point F by adding two standard deviations to the mean requirement for the group.

In the United States, food labels report the extent to which a food meets the *Reference Daily Intake* (RDI), which is calculated from RDAs but which does not reflect different levels for different age-sex groups. The RDAs are currently (in 1998) under review by the National Academy of Sciences, and a revision is expected out in the next year. The revision will contain recommendations for additional nutrients, will revise the recommended levels for others (for example, new RDAs for calcium will be higher than those shown in Table 2.4), and will list a maximum recommended intake for certain nutrients.

Figure 2.2   **Distribution of Nutrient Requirements in a Typical Population of Healthy Individuals**

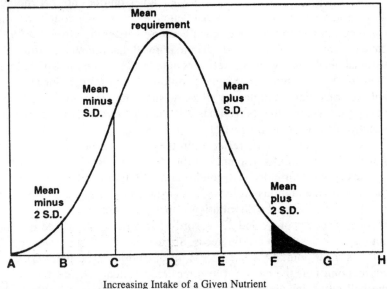

Increasing Intake of a Given Nutrient

Source: From "The Requirements of Human Nutrition," by Nevin S. Scrimshaw and Vernon R. Young. Copyright © 1976 by Scientific American, Inc. All rights reserved.
Note: The curve is bell-shaped.

Table 2.4 Recommended Daily Dietary Allowances, NAS, 1974[a]

Age (years)	Weight (kg)	Weight (lbs)	Height (cm)	Height (in)	Energy (kcal)[b]	Protein (g)	Vitamin A Activity (RE)[c]	Vitamin A Activity (IU)	Vitamin D (IU)	Vitamin E Activity (IU)	Ascorbic Acid (mg)	Folacin (ug)	Niacin (mg)	Riboflavin (mg)	Thiamin (mg)	Vitamin B6 (mg)	Vitamin B12 (ug)	Calcium (mg)	Phosphorus (ng)	Iodine (ug)	Iron (mg)	Magnesium (mg)	Zinc (mg)
Infants																							
0.0–0.5	6	14	60	24	kgx117	kgx2.2	420[d]	1,400	400	4	35	50	5	0.4	0.3	0.3	0.3	360	240	35	10	60	3
0.5–1.0	9	20	71	28	kgx108	kgx2.0	400	2,000	400	5	35	50	8	0.6	0.5	0.4	0.3	540	400	45	15	70	5
Children																							
1–3	13	28	86	34	1,300	23	400	2,000	400	7	40	100	9	0.8	0.7	0.6	1.0	800	800	60	15	150	10
4–6	20	44	110	44	1,800	30	500	2,500	400	9	40	200	12	1.1	0.9	0.9	1.5	800	800	80	10	200	10
7–10	30	66	135	54	2,400	36	700	3,300	400	10	40	300	16	1.2	1.2	1.2	2.0	800	800	110	10	250	10
Males																							
11–14	44	97	158	63	2,800	44	1,000	5,000	400	12	45	400	18	1.5	1.4	1.6	3.0	1,200	1,200	130	18	350	15
15–18	61	134	172	69	3,000	54	1,000	5,000	400	15	45	400	20	1.8	1.5	2.0	3.0	1,200	1,200	150	18	400	15
19–22	67	147	172	69	3,000	54	1,000	5,000	400	15	45	400	20	1.8	1.5	2.0	3.0	800	800	140	10	350	15
23–50	70	154	172	69	2,700	56	1,000	5,000		15	45	400	18	1.6	1.4	2.0	3.0	800	800	110	10	350	15
51+	70	154	172	69	2,400	56	1,000	5,000		15	45	400	16	1.5	1.2	2.0	3.0	800	800	110	10	350	15
Females																							
11–14	44	97	155	62	2,400	44	800	4,000	400	12	45	400	16	1.3	1.2	1.6	3.0	1,200	1,200	115	18	300	15
15–18	54	119	162	65	2,100	48	800	4,000	400	12	45	400	14	1.4	1.1	2.0	3.0	1,200	1,200	115	18	300	15
19–22	58	128	162	65	2,100	46	800	4,000	400	12	45	400	14	1.4	1.1	2.0	3.0	800	800	100	18	300	15
23–50	58	128	162	65	2,000	46	800	4,000		12	45	400	13	1.2	1.0	2.0	3.0	800	800	100	18	300	15
51+	58	128	162	65	1,800	46	800	4,000		12	45	400	12	1.1	1.0	2.0	3.0	800	800	80	10	300	15
Pregnant					+300	+30	1,000	5,000	400	15	60	800	+2	+0.3	+0.3	2.5	4.0	1,200	1,200	125	18+	450	20
Lactating					+500	+20	1,200	6,000	400	15	80	600	+4	+0.5	+0.3	2.5	4.0	1,200	1,200	150	18	450	25

Notes: a. The allowances are intended to provide for individual variations among most persons as they live in the United States under usual environmental stresses. Diets should be based on a variety of common foods in order to provide other nutrients for which human requirements have been less well defined.

b. Kilojoules (kJ) = 4.2 X kcal.

c. Retinol equivalents.

d. Assumed to be all as retinol in milk during the first six months of life. All subsequent intakes are assumed to be half as retinol and half as B-carotene when calculated from international units. As retinol equivalents, three-fourths are as retinol and one-fourth as B-carotene.

Source: U.S. National Academy of Sciences 1974:129.

☐ 3

Impacts of Undernutrition

In the last chapter, we focused on underconsumption of calories, protein, and micronutrients as the most serious types of malnutrition. In this chapter, we describe some of the impacts of these types of undernutrition on physical and mental health. How can you tell when someone is undernourished? What are the symptoms? Or, if you wish, what are the observable impacts of underconsumption of calories, protein, or micronutrients?

■ REFERENCE GROUPS

Because calories and protein are necessary for the growth of the human body, the most obvious physical manifestations of undernutrition are in the individual's size. A person's size can only be evaluated by comparing it to the sizes of other people (the *reference population*). These comparisons lead to statements like "Tommy is shorter than average," meaning that "Tommy is shorter than the average person in the reference population." Or we might say, "Adele is in the ninety-fifth percentile of height," meaning "95 percent of people in the reference population are shorter than Adele."

☐ Defining an Appropriate Reference Group

The purpose of a reference population is to provide a standard against which the growth and maturation of particular individuals can be judged. By observing how much one person deviates from others of a similar status (age and sex, for example), we can draw inferences about the subject's nutritional status.

Similarly, whenever you try to guess someone's age, you use (as at least some of your clues) the person's body size and configuration. That is, your life experience teaches you what to expect in the way of variations in height, weight, and even fatness, as people grow and develop, and from this (and other clues, such as amount of gray hair and wrinkled skin) you deduce age.

In setting up a reference population, it is important to control for as many variables as possible that might influence the observed variables. For example, if an individual is much shorter than the reference group, we don't learn much if the individual is four years old and the reference group is composed of teenagers. Therefore, reference groups are chosen so that we can compare persons of approximately the same age and sex.

□ Nature vs. Nurture, or Heredity vs. Environment

In addition, we can expect variations in populations of different countries, or in people of different ethnic backgrounds. Figure 3.1 shows variations of body weights in seven Latin American countries and the United States. Boys in all eight countries start life with similar weights, but by adulthood, we see considerable variation among countries.

Figure 3.1   Median Male Weight-for-Age in Seven Latin American Countries and the United States

Weight in kilograms

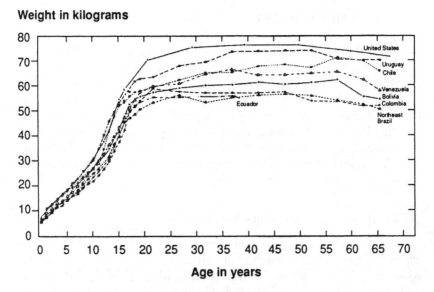

Source: Adapted from U.S. White House, President's Science Advisory Committee 1967:37.

In Figure 3.2, the height of the U.S. population is contrasted with that of an Indian village (Bagbana) surveyed by Foster in 1981 (unpublished data). The U.S. data here and elsewhere in the chapter are from a survey by the U.S. National Center for Health Statistics (NCHS) (U.S. Department

Figure 3.2   NCHS (U.S.) Median Height-for-Age vs. Median Height-for-Age, Bagbana Village, India

Male

Height in centimeters

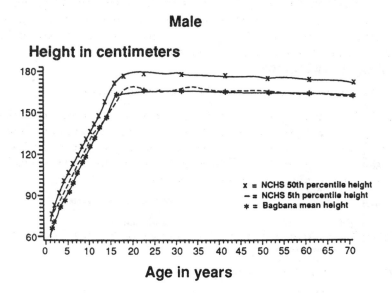

x = NCHS 50th percentile height
— = NCHS 5th percentile height
* = Bagbana mean height

Age in years

Female

Height in centimeters

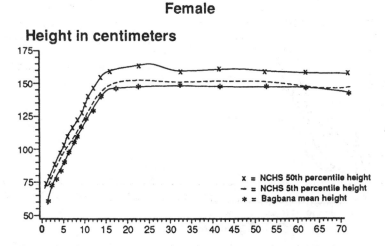

x = NCHS 50th percentile height
— = NCHS 5th percentile height
* = Bagbana mean height

Source: Adapted from Dever 1983:71.

of Health and Human Services 1981). Both males and females in the village are at about the fifth percentile of height observed in the United States.

In Figure 3.3, the weights of Bagbana villagers are compared to a U.S. reference population. The villagers are close to the U.S. population during the first couple of years of life, but the difference increases with age, especially for females. By age 70, the village females' weight is only

Figure 3.3   NCHS (U.S.) Median Weight-for-Age vs. Median Weight-for-Age, Bagbana Village, India

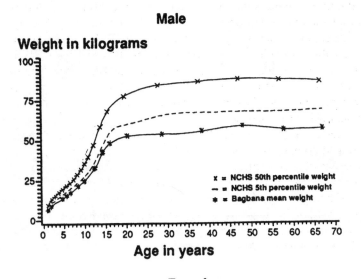

Male

Weight in kilograms

x = NCHS 50th percentile weight
— = NCHS 5th percentile weight
* = Bagbana mean weight

Age in years

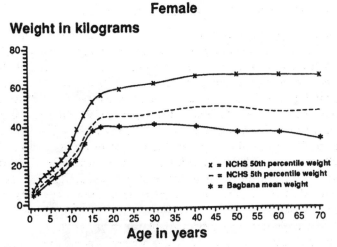

Female

Weight in kilograms

x = NCHS 50th percentile weight
— = NCHS 5th percentile weight
* = Bagbana mean weight

Age in years

Source: Adapted from Dever 1983:73.

slightly over 50 percent of weight of U.S. females of the same age. Are the Indian women underweight? Are the U.S. women overweight? Are the weight and height differences attributable to nutrition?

Even after differences in age, sex, and ethnic background have been controlled for, there will still be differences among individuals. Given variations among individuals within a population, to what extent are the variations in stature the result of differences in genetic potential, and to what extent do they arise from living conditions (including nutrition)?

Stephenson, Latham, and Jansen (1983:53) compared growth data from U.S. children, privileged African children, and underprivileged African children, and concluded that ethnic differences were less important than other factors as determinants of growth in children: "Poverty, poor food intakes, infectious and parasitic diseases and other environmental factors combine together to prevent children from realizing their growth potential. There are, of course, genetic influences which lead to differences of body size, and especially of stature, but it seems that in prepubertal children, heredity is a much less significant cause of below-average growth than are other factors."

Environmental influences are major determinants of the body-size characteristics of a population. This will provide a basis for *anthropometric measurement* of malnutrition discussed in the next chapter. But we must bear in mind that, especially for a particular individual, body size is the product of heredity and environment. Note also that, despite substantial genetic variation in height and weight within any population, the growth trajectories of infants and very young children are much more uniform than those of older children.

☐ Measuring Deviations from the Reference Population

The whole point of using a reference population is to decide whether an individual's height or weight is roughly "normal." If an individual's height or weight is below a certain amount (referred to as a *cut-off point*), then he or she may be presumed to have a nutritional problem. The three most commonly proposed candidates for cut-off points are each based on deviation from the *median score*. "Median" means that half the reference population is larger and half is smaller. Thus, if the median weight of a reference population is 90 pounds, then half the people in that group weigh more than 90 pounds, and half weigh less. The three candidates for cut-off points are: (1) percentile; (2) percentage of the median; and (3) standard deviation unit. For the purposes of explanation, we use weight as the variable being measured and compared to the reference population. The terms can also be applied to any other variable, such as height.

Percentile measures what percent of the reference population weighs less than the individual. Thus, if the individual's weight is at the "thirtieth percentile," this indicates that 30 percent of the reference population weighed less than the individual. The median weight is the fiftieth percentile.

We calculate percentage of the median by dividing the individual's weight by the median weight for the reference population. Thus, if the individual weighs 60 pounds, but the median weight in the reference group is 90 pounds, the individual is at 66 percent of the median (60/90 = 66 percent).

Standard deviation unit, or "Z-score," is a statistical measure of dispersion away from the mean. An observation that is two standard deviation units below the mean will be approximately on the second percentile—only 2 percent of the reference population will weigh less than this amount. For measures of height and weight, experience shows that two standard deviations below the mean is usually fairly close to 75 percent of the median. Experience also shows that the average weight (and height) of population groups is usually quite close to the median. Nutritionists commonly use the Z-score as a cut-off point for defining undernutrition (Krick 1988:326–328).

■ EFFECTS OF UNDERNUTRITION ON PHYSICAL GROWTH AND SIZE

If a person consumes insufficient calories or protein, that person's growth and size are likely to be affected. In considering this impact, we should discriminate between *acute undernutrition* and *chronic undernutrition*. Acute undernutrition is short-term, severely inadequate food intake, such as one might see during famine or war. The human body can recover from a relatively short bout of acute undernutrition; people who lose weight in a famine can gain it back when the famine ends. In some cases, children whose growth has slowed during a famine will regain their normal size when the famine ends. Chronic undernutrition refers to long-term inadequacy of protein and/or calories. Chronic undernutrition causes physical effects even when it is moderate. The physical effects of undernutrition include the following.

☐ Low Height-for-Age, or Stunting

An individual whose height is low for her age is said to be *stunted*. Such a person may have suffered from chronic undernutrition at some time during the growth years. Low height-for-age is a symptom of past undernutrition; the person may or may not be undernourished today. We find evidence of the link between nutrition and height in a variety of places.

In Figure 3.4, you see the heights at age seven of a national sample of British children born during a single week in 1958. Children were broken into five classes according to their fathers' occupations. Children of the upper classes were taller than those of the lower classes, and presumably differences in nutrition accounted for at least some of the height differences.

Figure 3.4   Height Differences Among British Children by Social Class of Father and Number of Children in Family

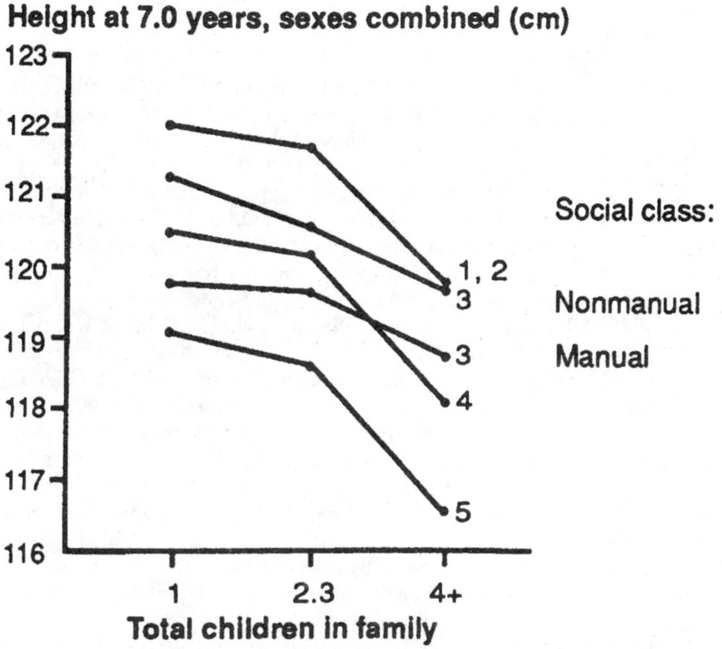

Height at 7.0 years, sexes combined (cm)

Social class:

1, 2   Nonmanual

3   Manual

Total children in family

Source: Adapted from Tanner 1977:347; data from Goldstein 1971.

During the period from 1889 to 1950, the populations of Northern Europe and North America were growing taller at the rate of approximately one centimeter per decade. The trend has stopped in most well-off sections of these countries, but continued in Japan into the 1970s (Tanner 1977:349). Similarly, in the Indian village of Bagbana, 61 percent of adult sons were taller by an average of 3.1 centimeters (1.25 inches) than their fathers. Presumably these secular trends in height of populations during the past one hundred years is largely the result of better health and nutrition.

As Box 3.1 shows, considerable empirical evidence exists of the positive relationship between protein consumption and the heights of humans.

The curves in the top part of Figure 3.5 show the usual reference population used for comparing the height of a girl under three years old. A 21-month-old girl who is 85 centimeters in length is on the fiftieth percentile—half the reference population is shorter than 85 centimeters and half is taller. If the girl is only 79 centimeters tall at 21 months, then more than 95 percent of the reference population are taller than the girl. Such a girl would have *low height-for-age,* or *stunting,* and thus would show this symptom of past undernutrition.

Box 3.1   Nutrition and Body Size

J. S. Weiner

In India the greater stature, stronger constitution, and superior physical resistance of the Sikhs of northern India, as compared to the Madrassi of the south, seem directly related to the high protein of the Sikh diet derived from meat, milk, and milk derivatives as compared to the vegetarian diet of the Madrassi. McCarrison fed rats on these two types of diet; those on the Sikh diet weighed an average of 225 [grams] compared to 155 g on the other. Of the two genetically similar populations of Hutu in Ruanda, studies by Hiernaux, those living in the more fertile and healthier regions were on average 7 [kilograms] heavier and had greater thigh- and chest-measurements.

In the studies of Boyd Orr and Gilks in East Africa, on the Kikuyu and the Masai tribes of Kenya, we are faced with the operation probably of both genetic and nutritional factors. The Kikuyu are farmers, living on a diet of cereals, tubers, and legumes; the Masai, on the other hand, are cattle-raisers, whose diet includes meat, milk, and ox-blood which they take from the animals. These two human groups, living side by side in the same natural environment and the same climate, differed markedly in their physical measurements. The Masai men were 7.5 [centimeters] taller and 10.25 kg heavier than their Kikuyu counterparts. This difference, in Boyd Orr and Gilks's opinion, is a direct result of their fundamentally different diets. The Masai, through an abundant use of food of animal origin, enjoy a diet balanced in proteins, while the Kikuyu live under conditions of permanent protein hunger.

De Castro observed something similar in the north-east of Brazil. In the littoral regions and in the dry backland area far from the coast the diet is high in proteins because the inhabitants live by fishing. In the backland also the protein intake is high, since it is a cattle-raising region with abundant production and consumption of meat, milk, and cheese. But in the jungle zone, where sugar-cane monoculture established itself and drove out all other food-producing activities, the diet is very poor, being based on cassava or manioc flour, the protein content of which is extremely low. These dietary differences, particularly of protein, would explain the differences in body-size among three human groups living within a fairly restricted geographical area.

Source: Weiner 1977:419–420. Reprinted by permission of Oxford University Press.

☐ Low Weight-for-Height, or Wasting

People who are currently undernourished are thin. In scientific jargon they exhibit *low weight-for-height,* or *wasting.* The curves in Figure 3.6 show the usual reference population against which the weights of young girls are compared to their heights. (Note that age is omitted in this comparison.) A girl who is 65 centimeters long and weighs seven kilograms is on the fiftieth percentile. That is, half the girls of her height weigh more than 7 kilos, and half weigh less. If a girl is 65 centimeters tall but weighs only

Figure 3.5   NCHS Percentiles of Girls' Height-for-Age and Weight-for Age, Birth to 36 Months

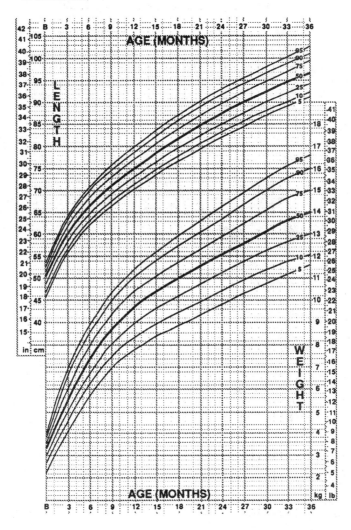

Source: Reprinted from U.S. Department of Health, Education and Welfare 1976.

6 kilos, then more than 95 percent of the reference population of this height weigh more than she does. Thus, she is said to have low weight-for-height, exhibiting a symptom of current undernutrition.

☐ **Low Weight-for-Age, or Underweight**

Low weight-for-age is a symptom of either past or present undernutrition. Individuals with low weight-for-age are referred to as *underweight*. Look

Figure 3.6   NCHS Percentiles of Girls' Weight-for-Height, Birth to 36 Months

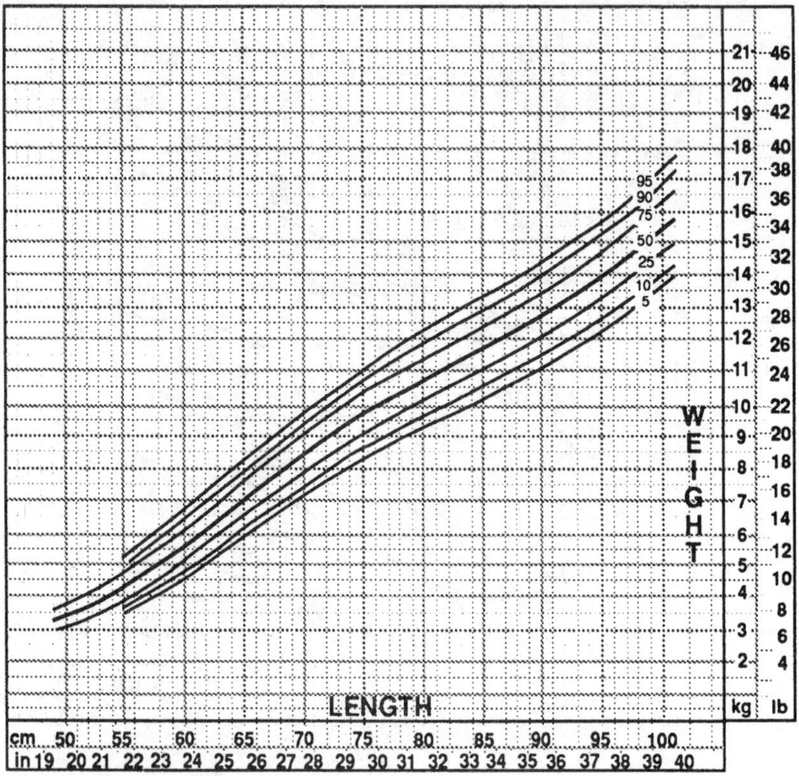

Source: Reprinted from U.S. Department of Health, Education and Welfare 1976.

at the curves in the bottom half of Figure 3.5. A 24-month-old girl who weighs 12 kilos is at the fiftieth percentile. If she weighs 9.8 kilos, more than 95 percent of the reference population weigh more than she does. At 9.8 kilos, she is 82 percent of the reference median.

☐ Age, Sex, and Fat

There is a marked tendency for the human body to add fat as it ages. In Table 3.1, you see how the percentage of the total body that is fat increases from early adulthood to old age. In past eons of human evolution, perhaps older people, no longer being involved in the hunt (men) or in childbearing (women), tended to be shortchanged on food during periods of hunger. Yet because older people could still be useful, there may have been survival value to the clan if the seniors retained fat reserves to tide them over seasons of short food supplies.

Table 3.1   NCHS Median Percentage of Total Body That Is Fat, Adult Males and Females by Age

Age	Males	Females
18–24	16	27
25–29	18	29
30–34	23	31
35–39	23	32
40–44	26	35
45–49	26	36
50–54	27	39
55–59	27	39
60–64	27	40
65–69	26	38
70–74	26	38

Source: Adapted from Frisancho 1989:Table IV.19, p. 57.

Note that throughout adulthood women, on the average, have a greater percentage of fat in their bodies than men. During pregnancy, women provide nutrients to the growing fetus, and during lactation (postpartum), food for the newborn. Throughout most of human evolution, it was probably difficult for a mother to consume as many calories as both she and her offspring needed during the last few months of pregnancy and the first few months of lactation. There was therefore survival value in the woman's being provided with a reserve supply of fat to tide her and the baby over during this critical period. At the same time, for the family as a whole there was probably survival value in the man's body being heavily muscular.

No single part of the body represents the fat content of the whole body. Even if you calculate total body density by weighing people and then comparing their weights to the weight of the water they displace when submerged in a tank, it is almost impossible to estimate accurately the percentage of the entire body that is fat. Nevertheless, the mid-upper arm is considered to be fairly representative of the body as a whole and is used as an indicator of nutritional status.

Figure 3.7 shows how the fat content of the mid-upper arm changes with age for U.S. males and females. If you compare the data in Figure 3.7 with that of Table 3.1, you will notice that the mid-upper arm tends to be fattier than the body as a whole.

In Figure 3.7, you see the tendency for fat percentage to fall after birth and then rise again in adulthood. Although born with a reserve fat supply ("baby fat"), humans, like other mammals, tend toward intense activity during their growing period. (See Figure 3.8 for a good illustration of spontaneous physical activity and calorie intake by rats during their growth phases.) What with the energy requirements of growth in addition to youthful physical activity, humans tend to reduce their fat reserves during their growth years, only to build them back up in adulthood.

Figure 3.7 Median Percentage of Mid-Upper Arm That Is Fat, by Age and Sex, U.S. Whites, 1971–1974

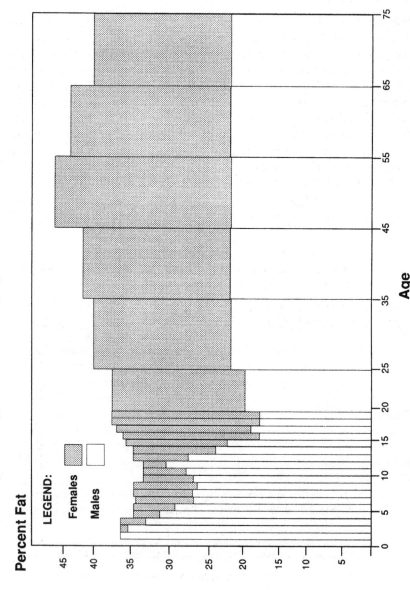

Source: Frisancho 1981:Table III.

■ UNDERNUTRITION, MENSTRUATION, AND BREAST-FEEDING

□ Delayed Age of Menarche

The female sex hormone, estrogen, is produced from cholesterol, a fat (Pike & Brown 1984:42). The fatter a woman is, the more estrogen she is likely to produce. An undernourished girl is likely to produce less estrogen than a well-nourished girl of the same age; therefore, the well-nourished girl is likely to begin menstruation at a younger age. Delayed age of menarche (age of first menstruation) is an indicator of low levels of calorie intake. Girls in the United States reach menarche earlier today than they did a century ago because they now produce a higher percentage of fat (and estrogen). Because vigorous exercise reduces body fat, well-fed young girls who are also athletes often reach menarche later in life than do their more sedentary counterparts.

Table 3.2 shows a geographic breakdown of menarche. Notice how much higher the age of menarche is in the Third World populations listed

Figure 3.8 Changes in Spontaneous Physical Activity and Caloric Intake in Male Rats During Growth

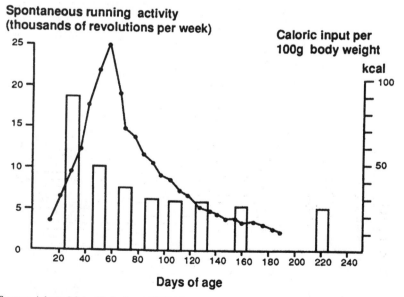

Source: Adapted from Parizokova 1977:16.

Note: The dots show running activity (measured on the left-hand scale), and the vertical bars show caloric intake per day per 100 grams of body weight (measured on the right-hand scale).

in the bottom half of the table than in the presumably better-nourished industrialized populations in the top half. Not all the advantages lie with the
well-nourished populations. Recent research suggests that women who
have fewer ovarian cycles (late menarche) are at reduced risk for breast
cancer. Evidence also exists that lean women are less inclined to cancer
because their lower levels of estrogen may reduce the growth of cells that
can start tumors.

☐ Breast-feeding as Birth Control

In the next section, we will review the importance of breast-feeding to
the health of infants. An additional benefit of breast-feeding is that it
postpones the recurrence of menstruation after childbirth. The same hormone (prolactin) that stimulates the production of breast milk also sup-
presses ovulation. In addition, the production of breast milk tends to use
up the body's supply of fat, reducing estrogen production and impeding
ovulation. The use of breast-feeding to postpone ovulatory cycles after
childbirth is referred to as the *Lactational Amenorrhea Method* of birth
control. The method is at least 98 percent effective if three conditions are
met: (1) the mother has not experienced the return of her menstrual periods; (2) the mother is fully or nearly fully breast-feeding; (3) the baby
is less than six months old. Studies in developing countries confirm the
effectiveness of breast-feeding as a birth control method: In Chile, only
one of 422 breast-feeding women became pregnant during the six months
after childbirth; in Pakistan, there was one pregnancy among 391 women;
in the Philippines, there were two pregnancies among 485. The experience

Table 3.2   Median Age of Menarche, by Location of Population Studied

Place	Median Age	Year of Observation
Santiago, Chile (middle class)	12.3	1971
Hong Kong (affluent)	12.5	1961–65
Madrid (affluent)	12.8	1968
United States, all	12.8	1960–70
Hong Kong (middle class)	12.8	1961–65
Sydney, Australia	13.0	1970
Hong Kong (lower class)	13.3	1961–65
India, all urban	13.7	1956–65
Baghdad (poor)	14.0	1969
India, all rural	14.4	1956–65
South Africa (Bantu, rural)	15.0	—
Rwanda (Tutsi)	16.5	1957–58
Rwanda (Hutu)	17.0	1957–58
New Guinea (Lumi)	18.4	1967

Source: Evelth & Tanner 1967:Table 15.

in Pakistan and the Philippines showed 98–99 percent effectiveness for a full year after childbirth among women meeting the first two of the above three conditions (Family Health International 1997). One study estimates that breast-feeding is by far the most widely used contraceptive method in India—six times more important than the birth control pill, four times more important than sterilizations and intrauterine devices (IUDs), and nearly twice as important as condoms (Gupta & Rohide 1993).

■ UNDERNUTRITION AND CHILD HEALTH

Undernutrition is an especially serious problem for infants and children because their immune systems are less fully developed than those of adults. Therefore they are more susceptible to diseases than are adults. Undernourished children are especially susceptible, because their bodies are already weakened.

☐ Mothers' Nutrition, Breast-feeding, and the Health of the Baby

Mothers who are undernourished during pregnancy are likely to give birth to babies with low birth weights. These babies start life malnourished and are significantly more likely to die in the first year of life; in fact, during the period shortly after birth, low-birth-weight babies die at a rate 40 times that of normal babies (Samuels 1986; Overpeck et al. 1992). Low birth weight for an infant indicates that the infant was malnourished in the womb or that the mother was malnourished during her own infancy, childhood, adolescence, and pregnancy. The malnourishment is typically due to underconsumption of calories and protein; however, it can also result from underconsumption of micronutrients such as iron (Levinger 1995).

If the baby is breast-fed, her health is significantly improved. Breast milk contains all the nutrients a child needs during the first months of life. Breast milk also helps the baby fight infection. In developing countries, breast-feeding contributes to infant health in two indirect ways. First, breast-feeding provides the baby with a guaranteed food supply; the infant does not have to compete with other family members for scarce food. Second, the breast-feeding assures that the baby will have a clean food supply; babies who do not breast-feed are exposed to diseases caused by unsanitary food and water. According to one estimate, 1.5 million children in the developing world die because they are not breast-fed (Grapentine 1998). Even women who are suffering from mild to moderate undernutrition are able to produce sufficient milk to feed their infants; severe undernutrition such as that resulting from a famine does compromise a woman's ability to produce breast milk (Prentice, Goldberg & Prentice).

Nutrition can also influence the mother-child AIDS transmission. A study in Malawi indicated that women with vitamin A deficiencies were more likely to pass on the HIV virus to their infants. Among pregnant women who were HIV-positive, the transmission rate for those with the highest vitamin A concentrations was 7 percent; for women with the lowest vitamin A concentrations that rate was 32 percent (Semba et al. 1994).

☐ **High Infant and Child Mortality Rates**

Death is the most dramatic of adverse effects of undernutrition. As mentioned in Chapter 1, deaths from acute undernutrition—such as those that occur in famines—are not nearly as big a worldwide tragedy as are deaths in which chronic undernutrition weakens the ability of people to resist diseases. This form of fatal undernutrition is an especially large problem among children.

Childhood mortality is a significant problem, as Figure 3.9 illustrates. More than 20 percent of the 52 million people who died in 1995 were between birth and five years old. Yet this age category accounts for about only 11 percent of the population. The only age category with more deaths is 75 and older. The death rate is especially high for Third World children. WHO reports: "Defined as the probability of dying by the age of five years, the global average in 1995 was 81.7 per 1000 live births; 8.5 in the industrialized world, 90.6 in the developing world and 155.5 in the least developed nations" (WHO 1996b).

Childhood diseases, to which undernutrition contributes through weakening the immune system, are major killers of children in developing countries (Dever 1983). Intestinal disorders that lead to diarrhea are the leading child killers in developing countries, but other diseases associated with malnutrition such as pneumonia, influenza, bronchitis, whooping cough, and measles are also important.

WHO reports that "Malnutrition has been found to underlie more than half of deaths among children in developing countries" (WHO 1997). One study of 53 developing countries estimated that 56 percent of child deaths are caused by the "potentiating effects of malnutrition in infectious disease." Eighty-three percent of the nutrition-related child deaths are caused by mild-to-moderate malnutrition; only 17 percent are caused by severe malnutrition (Pelletier et al. 1995). Recently, analysts of health policy have introduced a concept called Disability Adjusted Life Years (DALYs), which measures total amount of healthy life lost, whether from premature mortality or from temporary or permanent disability. A study for WHO

Figure 3.9   Death and Population in the World by Age, 1995

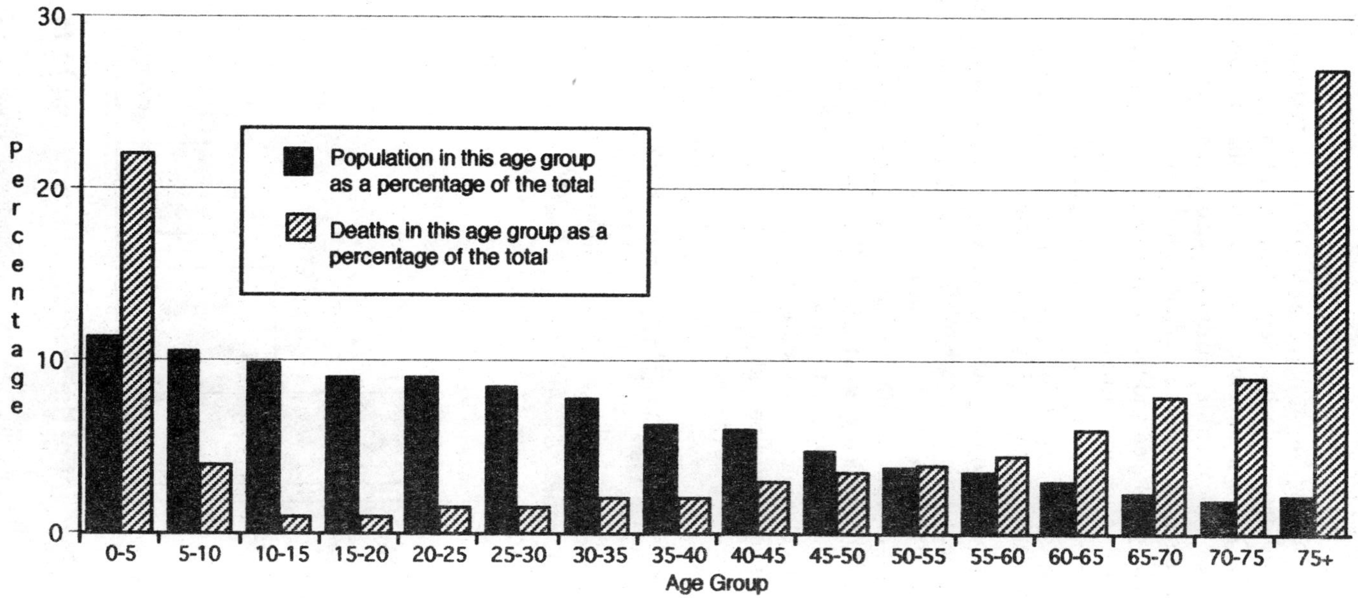

Legend:
- Population in this age group as a percentage of the total
- Deaths in this age group as a percentage of total

X-axis: Age Group (0-5, 5-10, 10-15, 15-20, 20-25, 25-30, 30-35, 35-40, 40-45, 45-50, 50-55, 55-60, 60-65, 65-70, 70-75, 75+)

Y-axis: Percentage (0, 10, 20, 30)

Source: UN, WHO, http://www.who.ch/whr/1997/fig13.gif

estimates that poor nutrition is responsible for 46 percent of life years (DALYs) lost to children (WHO 1996a).

Keilmann and McCord (1978) showed that infant mortality doubles with each 10 percent decline below 80 percent of the median weight-for-age. Figure 3.10 is a graphic representation of their results.

The risk of death from nutrition-related disease in the Third World decreases dramatically after the second year of life (Figure 3.11). Differences between the developed and the developing countries in death rates among children under five are startling and are dramatized by comparing the data for representative Third World countries (top six lines of Table 3.3) with representative developed countries (bottom four lines of the same table). Again, these differences are heavily related to differences in nutrition.

The emphasis in this section has been on deaths caused by disease related to undernutrition. Disease related to undernutrition is not always fatal, or course. WHO's World Health Report 1995 states: "As a result of iodine deficiency—a public health problem in 118 countries—at least 30,000 babies are stillborn each year and over 120,000 are born mentally retarded, physically stunted, deaf-mute or paralysed. A quarter of all children under age 5 in developing countries are at risk of vitamin A deficiency." Interactions between nutrition and health are discussed in Chapter 13.

**Figure 3.10 Mortality in Children Age 1–36 Months by Nutritional Status,
Punjab, India**

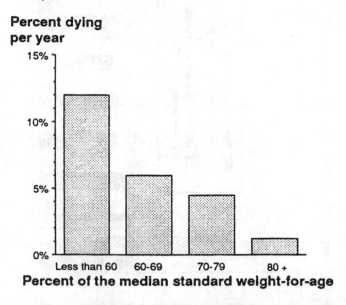

Source: Adapted from Galway et al. 1987:31. Data from Keilmann & McCord 1978.

Figure 3.11 Third World, Age-Specific Diarrheal Mortality Rates

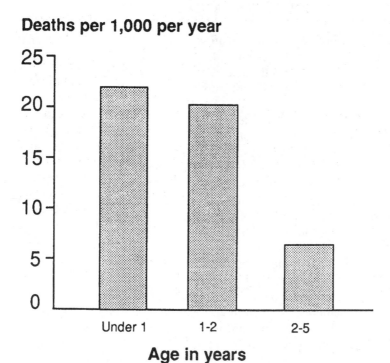

Source: Adapted from De Zoysa et al. 1985:9.

Table 3.3   Child Mortality Rates in Selected Countries, 1970

	Percentage in Age Group Who Die Each Year		Percentage That Die Before Fifth Birthday	Age at Which Same Percentage as in Column 3 Have Died in United States
	Under 1 (1)	1–4 (2)	(3)	
India	13.9	4.40	28.1	63
Pakistan	14.2	5.30	31.0	66
Egypt	11.7	3.93	24.8	61
Guinea	21.6	5.20	36.7	68
Cameroon	13.7	3.93	26.5	62
Guatemala	8.9	2.75	18.5	57
Taiwan	2.0	0.43	3.6	20
Japan	1.5	0.14	1.9	1
United States	2.1	0.10	2.5	5
Sweden	1.3	0.07	1.7	1

Source: Adapted from Latham 1984:56.

■ EFFECTS OF UNDERNUTRITION ON INTELLECT, EDUCATION, AND LEARNING

Ancel Keys, working with conscientious objectors during World War II, found that male adults subjected to diets leading to measurable undernutrition first experienced intellectual problems. Later, as their undernutrition continued, the men suffered problems with physical dexterity (Keys et al. 1950).

More recent research has tended to focus on the potential effect of childhood undernutrition on later intellectual development and achievement. If a mother suffers from undernutrition during pregnancy, her baby can suffer from reduced intellectual capacity and cognitive functioning. When malnourished women were given protein supplements during pregnancy, improvements in their children's cognitive functioning could be observed to age six or seven (Hicks et al. 1992). If pregnant women are given adequate calories and protein, the effects on their offspring can be sustained into adolescence and even young adulthood (Pollitt et al. 1993).

In the United States, low-birth-weight babies were found to have problems succeeding in school. They were more likely to need special education services, and they were more likely to repeat a grade (Levinger 1995).

Chronic malnutrition in children—especially during the first two or three years of life—can impair mental development directly (since brain development is negatively affected) and indirectly (because undernourished children are less active, and therefore their brains are less stimulated) (World Bank 1997).

In a study conducted in Hyderabad, India, children who had previously suffered from kwashiorkor scored an average of 35 points below their matched controls on IQ tests administered up to six years after their recovery. However, the authors note that it was difficult to determine "to what extent this is a result of the epidsode of kwashiorkor and to what extent it is due to other factors" (Champakam, Srikantia & Gopalan 1968).

Iodine deficiency is the most significant avoidable cause of mental retardation worldwide. An overview of 18 studies shows that iodine-deficient groups have IQ levels that are 13.5 points below those of non-iodine-deficient groups (Bleichrodt & Born 1994). To see how important a difference of this magnitude can be, consider that a person with an IQ of 100 is at the median score (half the population gets scores of less than 100, half greater than 100); a person with an IQ of 86.5 has a score higher than only about 20 percent of the population (and lower than 80 percent). Deficiencies in other micronutrients such as iron and vitamin A are also associated with impaired intellectual abilities (Levinger 1994).

Using the Bayley scales for cognitive skills, Gretl Pelto (1987), professor of nutritional science at the University of Connecticut, in a seven-year longitudinal study of nutrition and cognitive development among 78

Mexican preschool children, tested short-term memory, responsiveness to stimulus, attention and distractability, abstract categorization skills, and sedentary passivity. She found that children with little animal food in their diets were short in stature and delayed in cognitive development, and that delays in intellectual development resulted from nutritionally induced growth stunting.

Chavez and Martinez (1982) studied child development among poor Mexican peasant families. They set up a controlled experiment in which one set of families was given supplemental food for the child through three years of age, and for the mother while she was pregnant and lactating. The control group was a set of families matched to the treated group to have similar genetic and socioeconomic characteristics, but given no food supplements. Of the many tests for neurological maturation and mental performance given to each set of children, in virtually every instance—walking, control of bladder, and language development—the control children lagged behind the treated children. The better-nourished children were found to be more precocious in constructing three-word sentences (see Figure 3.12).

Chavez and Martinez stress that it is not possible, at this time, to determine the ultimate significance of the gap between the undernourished and better-nourished children; the undernourished children may catch up later in life. There is some evidence that intellectual impairment is (at least partially) reversible if nutrition is improved. Winick and colleagues (1973) tracked severely undernourished Korean orphans and found no signs of mental impairment years after their adoption by U.S. families.

Galler (1986), in a longitudinal study in Barbados, matched 183 children who had a history of PEM, or kwashiorkor, with 129 classmates without any such history but of similar age and sex, and from the same socioeconomic group. Both sets of children were followed from age five to 18 years. By sexual maturation, the previously undernourished children had essentially caught up with the matched group in terms of physical growth, but demonstrated small deficits in IQ throughout the growth period. The most striking difference between the groups was a fourfold increase in the frequency of attention deficit disorder (ADD) among the previously undernourished. This syndrome is characterized by decreased attention span, impaired memory, high distractability, restlessness, and disobedience, and was found to reduce educational progress among the previously undernourished children to a far greater extent than the slight deficit in IQ they experienced.

Recent studies in the Philippines and Kenya found a significant relationship between nutritional status and educational attainment as measured by test scores (Glewwe et al. 1996; Bhargava 1996). Other research shows that if children miss breakfast—if they fast for 16 hours or more—their school performances suffer. In particular, students suffer from poorer

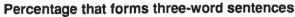

Figure 3.12 Age at Which Child Constructs First Three-Word Sentence,
Cumulative Percentage, Mexico

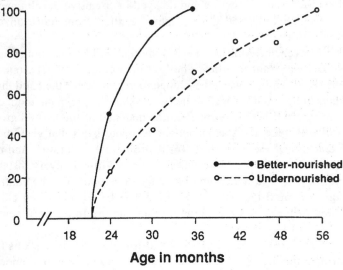

Source: Adapted from Chavez & Martinez 1982:90.

memory and ability to pay attention. World Bank nutrition specialist Alan
Berg (1973) points out that education also suffers from missed days of
school due to nutrition-related illnesses. He cites the case of four Latin
American countries where "illness caused children to miss more than 50
days of school a year."

■ EFFECTS OF UNDERNUTRITION
ON LABOR PRODUCTIVITY

Undernutrition can reduce productivity through work time lost to sickness,
lower productivity when working, and a decrease in the total number of
working years during a lifetime.

Nobel Prize–winning economist Robert Fogel has studied how nutrition has influenced economic productivity. Food shortages were so severe
in Europe in the eighteenth and early nineteenth centuries that "the bottom
20 percent subsisted on such poor diets that they were effectively excluded
from the labor force," being too weakened from hunger to work. Fogel estimates the improved nutrition accounts for 30 percent of the growth in income per capita in Britain between 1790 and 1980 (Fogel 1994).

A study of Chinese cotton-mill workers found that the women were able to do 14 percent more work for each one-gram increase in their hemoglobin—increases attained by giving the workers iron supplements (Li et al. 1994).

In a study of agricultural workers in Colombia and the United States, Spurr, Barac-Nieto, and Maksud (U.S. Department of State 1976) looked at the relationship between nutritional status and physical work capacity. They concluded that a high correlation exists between the two variables. Among undernourished Colombian sugar cane cutters, physical work capacity was reduced to the order of 50 percent.

As described earlier in the chapter, undernutrition during childhood results in stunting, or low height-for-age. Smaller adults are less productive workers in many jobs—they cannot lift and carry as much heavy weight, for example, as larger adults. The *1995 World Development Report* of the World Bank estimates that this stunting causes an economic loss of $8.7 billion per year worldwide. In addition, they find that an increase in a person's height by 1 percent is associated with an increase in that person's wages by 1.38 percent. Other work shows that wages are higher and unemployment rates are lower among men who are taller—evidence that nutritional status is reflected in the market's evaluation of the person's ability. (See Strauss and Thomas [1998] for a thorough review of related literature.)

☐ 4

Measuring Undernutrition

Because resources for coping with undernutrition are scarce and therefore need to be spent wisely, we must accurately identify and measure it.

■ MEASURING NUTRITIONAL STATUS OF THE INDIVIDUAL

Direct measures of nutritional status involve the direct examination of individuals. The common methods of direct assessment are clinical, biochemical, dietary, and anthropometric. Each method has shortcomings and each results in a somewhat different assessment of the nature and extent of nutritional disorders.

☐ Clinical Assessment

Clinical assessment of nutritional status relies on the examination of physical signs on the body that are symptomatic of nutritional disorders (Jelliffe 1966). Kwashiorkor, for instance, is accompanied by loss of pigment in the hair (it often turns reddish) and by edema (swelling) of the ankles. Using clinical observation (looking for a generalized swelling at the base of the neck above the collarbone), the Philippine nutrition survey found that the goiter rate in subjects nine years old and over was high—3.1 percent.

Correct identification of nutritional disorders using physical signs depends not only on the training and skill of the clinician but on how well the signs are manifested in the particular individual. Clinical signs are difficult to quantify and are usually obvious only in the advanced stage of the disease; for this reason, clinical assessment can be used in only the most severe and specific types of nutritional disorders.

☐ Biochemical Assessment

Biochemical assessment requires examination of body fluids such as blood or urine for the complex metabolic changes that accompany nutritional disorders. In the Philippine nutrition survey, over 14,000 blood samples were drawn and analyzed. From these samples and from using standards of the World Health Organization of the United Nations, 27 percent of the population were found to be anemic. The highest rates of anemia occurred in those under one year (51 percent) and in pregnant women (49 percent).

Biochemical tests provide an accurate indication of short-term nutritional problems, but their complexity and expense are an impediment to their widespread use in field surveys. Imagine the problems associated with persuading a sample of over 14,000 individuals living all over the Philippines to submit to having blood drawn—then transporting these samples to appropriate laboratory apparatus for analysis before they deteriorate in the heat!

☐ Dietary Assessment

Dietary surveys are often employed to assess nutritional status. Two approaches are used: (1) dietary recall, in which the subject is asked to remember what he or she ate, say during the past 24 hours or the past seven days; and (2) dietary record, in which someone records the amount of food consumed at mealtimes, often by weighing it. Both methods have their advantages and drawbacks.

Dietary recall has the advantage of researchers' being able to interview the subjects when they are not expecting to be surveyed; they are less likely to adjust their consumption because of the survey. Yet it is often difficult to remember exactly what you or members of your family ate during the past 24 hours, much less during the past week. And estimates of quantity consumed are particularly prone to error in recall surveys.

When keeping food records, especially if every portion of food must be weighed, the cook tends often to simplify the diet to make record-keeping easier (Quandt 1987). Subjects in the food record-keeping survey are especially likely to adjust their diets so that things will "look better" to the surveyor, especially if the surveyor is in the household for the sole purpose of making and recording the measurements.

In both types of surveys, measuring the quantity of food consumed by breast-fed babies presents difficulties. And in both cases, seasonal variation in consumption may confound the data unless appropriate adjustments are made. For instance, the Philippine survey was done from February through May, a time when access to the countryside is easier because of the relative absence of monsoon rains and typhoons. The retail price of tomatoes, for example, is typically 250 percent higher in November than it is in April. Similarly, the price of rice tends to be low during the survey period, while the price of corn tends to be high (Philippines Ministry of Agriculture 1981a, b). The unadjusted survey data thus sometimes overestimate annual consumption of tomatoes and rice, which are in abundant supply during the survey period, and to underestimate the consumption of corn.

In either case (dietary recall or record), results of the survey can be used to determine amounts of various nutrients consumed; these amounts can then be compared to a dietary standard appropriate to the particular country being observed, to determine nutritional status.

In the Philippine survey, food energy intake was 1,808 kilocalories per capita per day, which was 89 percent of the national target of 2,031. Protein intake was at 50.6 grams, or target level. Consumption steadily increased with increasing per capita income, especially for items such as refined sugar, soft drinks, cooking oil, pork, chicken, eggs, evaporated milk, and mangos. The proportion of the households found to have met a 100 percent adequacy level for various nutrients is given in Table 4.1.

Dietary assessment is useful in studies relating consumption and income, or in determining food allocation patterns within the family. But care must be taken in interpreting the results of such surveys. Food intake is not always a good index of nutritional status. For instance, secondary malnutrition can substantially degrade the nutritional status of an otherwise appropriately fed individual.

☐ Anthropometric Assessment

Anthropometry is the science of measuring the human body and its parts. As we saw in Chapter 3, human physical growth (increase in size) and development (differentiation) are both responsive to variations in calorie and protein intakes. Because of this, measurements of the human body, when compared to a reference standard, provide clues as to protein and calorie

Table 4.1   Households Meeting 100-Percent Adequacy Levels for Various Nutrients, Phillippines, 1982

Nutrient	Percentage of Households
Energy (calories)	32.9
Protein	46.0
Iron	35.5
Calcium	26.3
Thiamine	19.3
Riboflavin	8.1
Niacin	66.5
Ascorbic acid	35.2

Source: Philippines National Science and Technology Authority 1984.

nutrition. This is especially true during youth, when growth is so rapid, but to some extent also true during adulthood, when various dimensions change gradually with aging. Thus anthropometry can be used to suggest the protein and/or calorie nutritional status of adults as well as children. For instance, measurements showing adequate muscle but low fat suggest calorie deficiency; measurements showing inadequate muscle but adequate fat suggest protein deficiency. (The method of estimating fat content and, therefore by deduction, muscle content of the body was described in the previous chapter.)

We should note immediately that nutrition is not the only influence on bodily growth and development. Growth and development can also be affected by such variables as genetic disposition, health, hormonal abnormalities, or deficiencies in micronutrients (e.g., zinc deficiency is associated with poor growth). Because anthropometry does not provide particularly useful clues as to dietary deficiencies (micronutrient shortages), it is not normally used to measure them. Nevertheless, because nutritional status is by far the most common variable normally influencing bodily growth and development, and because deficiencies in calories and/or protein are by far the most important causes of subnormal growth and development in the Third World, anthropometry is generally assumed to provide strong clues as to protein and calorie nutrition in the Third World. In the Philippine National Nutrition Survey, for example, using a cut-off point of less than 85 percent of the standard weight-for-height, 10 percent of preschool children were found to be moderately to severely undernourished. Using an alternative anthropometric measure, the survey found less than 75 percent of standard weight-for-age: 27 percent of preschoolers were found to be moderately to severely undernourished.

In developed countries, anthropometry is used most often as a measure of overnutrition, which is the most common nutritional problem among high-income people. Adults who are trying to keep their weight down are using the anthropometric measure weight-for-height as a reference standard, although they seldom think of their activities in such technical terms. Using a body-mass index, which is determined by dividing weight in kilograms by height in centimeters squared, the NCHS found 8 percent of the adult men and 11 percent of the adult women in the United States to be severely overweight (U.S. Department of Health and Human Services 1987).

Low-income people in Third World countries are at risk for undernutrition (insufficient calories), which is commonly exacerbated by secondary malnutrition (e.g., a diarrheal infection that robs the body of nutrients). Anthropometric measures are useful in flagging this type of nutritional disorder, that is, some combination of undernutrition and secondary malnutrition. Because of the strong link between the two, undernutrition and secondary malnutrition are commonly grouped together and called, simply, *undernutrition*. And that is what we will do throughout the rest of this book.

Since 1966, when the WHO published a monograph by D. B. Jelliffe titled *The Assessment of the Nutritional Status of the Community*, which provided a set of standardized anthropometric measurements useful in nutritional assessment, anthropometry has become the most widely used tool in nutritional assessment. The most common measures used for anthropometric assessment of nutritional status are height, weight, and a combination of arm circumference and skin-fold thickness. They are usually used in conjunction with sex and age (as in weight-for-age or height-for-age) and sometimes in combination with each other (as in weight-for-height).

Low cost and a relatively high degree of accuracy combine to make this method so popular. Training time of field surveyors is cut to a minimum. The measurements are relatively easy to take, and the tools required are simple to use: scales, tape measures, measuring boards, skin-fold calipers. Intelligent amateurs can be trained in a matter of days to take accurate measurements. By contrast, training technicians to recognize and diagnose undernutrition from clinical symptoms can take weeks or months. (From the point of view of accuracy, age data may be the biggest problem in using anthropometry. Third World adults often have only a vague idea of how old they are, and illiterate mothers sometimes have difficulty telling the age of their children.) Capital requirements for anthropometry are minimal. Compared to the laboratory apparatus involved in biochemical analysis, anthropometric tools are inexpensive. And anthropometry measures the *results* of nutrition (the size and shape of the body) rather than nutritional inputs (as in dietary intake). Because of its quantitative nature, anthropometry can be used to judge varying degrees of undernutrition—not just its presence or absence. And by using a mix of anthropometric indices, researchers can make judgments about a nutritional disorder (protein or caloric) as well as the time dimension of the disorder (past or present).

One commonly quoted index of undernutrition, stated in terms of weight-for-age, uses a deviation of 25 percentage points or more below the reference standard (equal to or less than 75 percent of standard weight-for-age) as a definition of undernutrition. But that is not the only reasonable measure. For instance, WHO has recommended the use of weight-for-height and height-for-age, instead of the more popular weight-for-age measure.

Choosing a classification system for undernutrition involves selecting an appropriate anthropometric measure or measures in conjunction with an appropriate set of criteria (deviations from the reference standard) to identify undernutrition, or various levels of it. No matter which system is chosen, the aim is to flag those in most need of help, either because they are undernourished or because they are in danger of becoming so.

We will describe and briefly discuss four different but widely used classification systems: (1) Gómez weight-for-age; (2) Waterlow weight-for-height combined with height-for-age; (3) Shakir arm circumference; and (4) Body Mass Index.

Gómez weight-for-age. Gómez and his colleagues (1956) developed the first widely used method of classifying nutritional disorders on the basis of growth. They used percentage of the median weight-for-age of their reference population to classify nutritional status in children. Children greater than 90 percent of the median were called normal; those from 76 percent to 90 percent were called mildly malnourished; those from 61 percent to 75 percent, moderately malnourished; and those at 60 percent or below, severely malnourished. The last three categories are sometimes designated simply as first-, second-, and third-degree malnutrition, with no reference made to Gómez. In this case, third-degree means severely malnourished. Because preschool children, particularly weaning children, are the most-at-risk group for undernutrition, the nutrition classification systems have concentrated on this group. The Gómez system, or variations of it, has become the most widely used method of monitoring preschool children's growth in the Third World. It is sensitive to small changes in weight, and the only tool required is portable and widely available. It is usually a good indicator of present and/or past undernutrition, and is considered a valid measure during the preschool years.

Because Third World populations often track well below the European and U.S. data (review Figures 3.2 and 3.3), there is a strong motivation for Third World governments to build their own reference tables. Colombia, India, Brazil, and the Philippines have established their own reference populations. In Table 4.2, the Philippine and U.S. reference standards are compared. The Philippine data track the U.S. data for the first two years, but by the sixth birthday, the Philippine data have dropped to 90 percent of those for the United States. The Gómez-like cut-off point applied to the Philippine data and quoted earlier in this chapter—that is, that weight under 75 percent of (Philippine) standard weight-for-age put 27 percent of preschoolers in the moderately to severely undernourished category—is somewhat more forgiving than using Gómez cut-off points with the NCHS standards.

It is questionable how useful applying Gómez cut-off points to adult data is. In Figure 4.1, Bagbana villagers are tracked against the NCHS reference population. Examination of Figure 4.1 yields some interesting speculations: Middle-aged to older Indian villagers are mostly moderately to severely undernourished; middle-aged to older people in the United States are overweight; so optimal nutrition lies between that of the Indian village and that of the United States.

We see also in Figure 4.1 a phenomenon commonly found in low-income Third World populations; namely, that the indicated severe undernutrition rate (look at the line for severe undernutrition) tends to decline

Table 4.2   Philippine and U.S. Weight-for-Age Reference Standards for Preschool Children (in kilograms)

Age in Years	U.S. (median weight) Boys (1)	Girls (2)	Average (3)	Philippines (4)	Percentage That Column 4 Is of Column 3
1	11.7	10.7	11.2	11.2	100
2	13.5	12.7	13.1	13.1	100
3	15.4	14.7	15.0	14.7	98
4	17.6	16.7	17.2	16.1	94
5	19.4	19.0	19.2	17.8	92
6	22.0	21.3	21.6	19.4	90

Sources: U.S. Department of Health and Human Services 1987; Philippines National Science and Technology Authority 1984:218.

Figure 4.1   Gómez Classification by Age, Bagbana Village, 1981

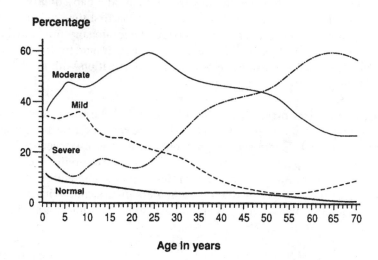

Source: Adapted from Dever 1983:88.

during the first six years of life. This is partly because, as the child grows up, he more easily commands his share of the family's food resources (weaning children are notoriously difficult to feed) and partly because the weakest individuals have already succumbed to malnutrition and disease. With their early deaths, the remaining population of older children "looks better."

Waterlow weight-for-height combined with height-for-age. Although the Gómez system is usually a good indicator of undernutrition, it may fail to flag as a problem an unusually tall child who is presently undernourished, and it may erroneously flag as a problem the unusually short child who is adequately nourished. To avoid these types of problems, Waterlow and colleagues (1977) developed a classification system that ingeniously, yet logically, combined height-for-age (which identifies past undernutrition) with weight-for-height (which identifies present undernutrition). The classification system is summarized in Table 4.3.

The beauty of this system is that it is likely to identify correctly individuals who are presently at risk for undernutrition and eliminate from present consideration those who merely have been undernourished in the past. A disadvantage is that it requires height (length) measurements in addition to age and weight data. Length is considerably more difficult to obtain than weight, especially from children under two. The operation requires a special board and two trained surveyors. While one holds the baby's legs straight and moves the baby's feet close against the footboard, the other moves the headboard against the top of the baby's head, taking care to hold the head in the prescribed position. Needless to say, when two strangers, no matter how gentle they try to be, hold a baby tightly in the prescribed position on this new contraption for the first time in her life, a certain amount of kicking and screaming, and occasionally urinating and defecating, can be expected. The exercise can be traumatic for all concerned. The results of using the Waterlow classification with the NCHS data in Bagbana are shown in Figure 4.2.

Shakir arm circumference. One of the more interesting features of child growth and development is that, while the body of a well-nourished child is gaining in length and weight from one to five or six years of age, his or her mid-upper arm circumference remains essentially the same! Using this observation, Shakir (1975) developed a screening device to identify severely undernourished preschoolers that is simplicity itself. It consists of a tape that is wrapped around the child's mid-upper arm, lightly

Table 4.3   Waterlow Weight-for-Height Combined with Height-for-Age

Height-for-Age	Weight-for-Height	Status
90% or better	80% or better	Normal
90% or better	Less than 80%	Wasted (current undernutrition)
Less than 90%	80% or better	Stunted (past undernutrition)
Less than 90%	Less than 80%	Wasted and stunted (both present and past undernutrition)

Note: The reference standard is the NCHS median.

Figure 4.2   Waterlow Nutritional Status Classifications, Bagbana Village, 1981

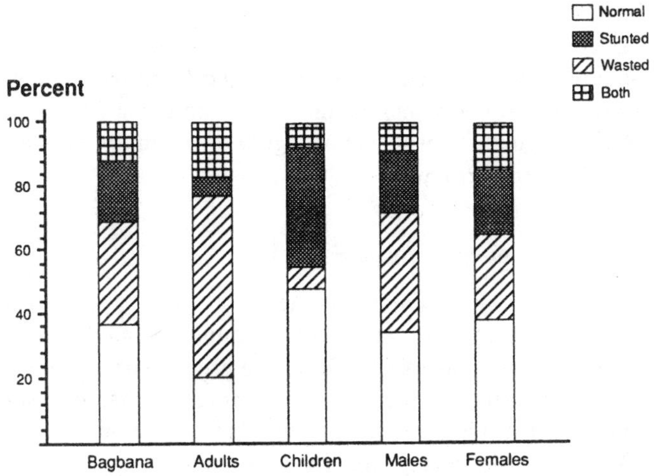

Source: Adapted from Dever 1983:90.

enough to not compress the skin but firmly enough to fit exactly. The reference standard used is 16.5 centimeters. A circumference of greater than 14 centimeters (85 percent of standard) is considered normal. Between 12.5 and 14 centimeters (76 percent to 85 percent of standard) is classed as undernutrition. Under 12.5 centimeters (less than 76 percent of standard) is classed as severe undernutrition. The tape is inexpensive and can be made by hand, if necessary. If the tape is coded with culturally appropriate colors (e.g., green, yellow, and red), even illiterate health workers can do the classification.

The accuracy of the system is good for severe cases and moderate for mild cases. Nevertheless, because of its simplicity and because it works on preschoolers without age data, it has become an important screening tool.

Body Mass Index. As a measure of undernutrition (or overnutrition) among adults, FAO and WHO now regard the Body Mass Index, or BMI, as the most suitable. BMI is calculated as weight in kilograms divided by the square of the height in meters. According to the FAO (Sixth World Food Survey 1996), a BMI below 18.5 is regarded as lower than normal and thus indicative of undernutrition. Twelve-and-a-half percent of adults in China and 48.6 percent in India have a BMI below this critical level. A person six feet tall with a BMI of 18.5 would weigh about 135 pounds. In the United States, the National Institutes of Health (NIH) puts the ideal ranges for BMI at from 21 to 23 for women and from 22 to 24 for men.

■ MEASURING NUTRITIONAL STATUS IN THE AGGREGATE

Above we discuss various ways to determine an individual's nutritional status. Policymakers also need to learn about the nutritional status of large groups. They need to know the extent of undernutrition in a continent or subcontinent, in a country, in a state or region of a country, or among some demographic or ethnic group.

□ Drawing Inferences from a Sample

Of course, if we can measure the nutritional status of a number of representative individuals in a country or in a group, we can draw inferences about the extent of malnutrition in the whole group. The science of statistics deals with the problem of how to determine the characteristics of an entire population (in this case, the extent of malnutrition in a country or among a group) by observing the characteristics of a sample from that group. So if we have anthropometric evidence categorizing (say) 11,000 children under the age of five in Nigeria, which tells us that 34 percent of these children are undernourished, this might allow us to deduce that 34 percent of all children in Nigeria are undernourished.

□ Mortality or Disease Rates

A second way of drawing inferences about the incidence of malnutrition in a country or other large group is to examine aggregate data about effects of malnutrition and to draw inferences from that data. For instance, low birth weights or high infant mortality rates in a country or region are assumed to indicate high rates of undernutrition. Aggregate data like this can provide a pretty good first approximation on where you are likely to find substantial numbers of undernourished people. Because undernutrition and poor health often occur together, aggregate data on morbidity can also provide indirect measures of the incidence of undernutrition in that country or region.

The Philippines does one of the most careful jobs of nutrition surveillance of any developing country. According to the 1982 Nationwide Nutrition Survey (Philippines National Science and Technology Authority 1984), 52 percent of the country's population was afflicted with roundworms (ascariasis). Hookworm infection was noted among 19 percent of the male population from 13 to 59 years of age. Of the 14,785 subjects examined, 69 percent were found to test positive for some kind of parasite. With morbidity data such as this, one could expect to find substantial rates of undernutrition in the Philippines.

High infant and child mortality rates or high morbidity rates are suggestive of high rates of undernutrition in a population. But these variables do not measure nutritional status directly. Rather, undernutrition is inferred from the nonnutritional aggregate data.

☐ Food Balance Sheets or Food Availability Measures

Another indirect approach to identifying regions or countries with nutritional problems is to look at food balance sheets. Table 4.4 is a simple food balance sheet for corn (maize) in Swaziland for the year 1987/88. Annual human consumption for one commodity such as corn is estimated by adding up beginning-of-the-year stocks, production, and imports, and subtracting from this total exports, amount used as livestock feed, amount used for seed, and end-of-the-year stocks.

Once human consumption is estimated for every food commodity in a country, the food consumed can be converted to calories and nutrients, and per capita consumption figures can then be derived. Table 4.5 is such a completed food balance sheet for India. If a country's per capita consumption turns out to be below amounts recommended by nutritionists, we have good cause to assume that a substantial block of its population is undernourished.

Measures derived from food balance sheets—in particular, calories per capita per day—have become perhaps the most widely used measures of malnutrition. The big advantage of such measures is that they are readily available from the UN's FAO for almost every country for a number of years or time periods. (See FAO's Sixth World Food Survey, 1996, or food balance sheets in FAOSTAT.)

However, the measures are not free of problems. We have emphasized that calories are not the sole nutrient of concern in identifying malnutrition. In addition, as noted in Chapter 2, not a single level of nutrient requirement applies to all people. And if we are looking at national data (for

Table 4.4   Annual Food Balance Sheet for Corn, Swaziland, 1987/88

Category	1,000 Tons
Beginning stocks (carryover from last year)	3
Production	88
Imports	54
Exports	5
Fed to livestock	37
Seed	3
Ending stocks (carryover into next year)	4
Human consumption	96

Source: U.S. Department of Agriculture 1988:40.

Table 4.5 Food Balance Sheet, India, Average 1984–1986 (Population = 684,534,000, Units = 1,000 Metric tons)

	Production	Imports	Stock Changes	Exports	Processed Trade (E-1)	Domestic Supply	Domestic Utilization — Feed	Seed	Manufacturer — Nonfood Use	Manufacturer — Use	Food Waste	Food	Kilograms/Year	Grams	Per Day — Calories	Per Day — Protein	Fat Grams
Grand total															2056	49.7	32.6
Vegetable products															1952	44.2	25.6
Animal products															104	5.5	7.0
Grand total exc. alcohol															2056	49.7	32.6
Cereals													183.3	502.2	1369	32.5	6.4
Wheat	34550	676	-1333	159	17	36383	415	2739			2771	30459	44.5	121.9	380	11.1	1.8
Paddy rice	74716	61	-6130		895	80012	299	4562	2		4450	70700	103.3	283.0	683	12.8	1.5
Barley	2020	2		16		2006	242	145	4		133	1482	2.2	5.9	14	.4	.1
Maize	6440	9	60			6389	122	444	52		798	4973	7.3	19.9	64	1.6	.6
Millet	9124		-329			9453	122	313			433	8585	12.5	34.4	107	3.1	1.2
Sorghum	11216	1	792			10425	135	381			728	9182	13.4	36.8	120	3.5	1.3
Cereals NES	52					1											
Prepared cereals NES		10			-1	62						61	.1	.2	1		
Roots and tubers													19.6	53.6	42	.6	.1
Cassava	5904					5904					403	5501	8.0	22.0	19	.1	
Potatoes	9353			17		9336		1412			1455	6468	9.5	25.9	18	.4	
Sweet potatoes	1491					1491					75	1416	2.1	5.7	5	.1	
Sugars and honey													20.2	55.3	186	.3	
Sugar cane	143670	6				143676	1580	9483		131886		727	1.1	2.9	1		
Raw sugar	5385		-931	2	286	6028				6		6022	8.8	24.1	86		
Noncentrifugal sugar	7910					7910	432			413		7065	10.3	28.3	99	.3	
Pulses													12.5	34.3	120	7.0	1.1
Dry beans	2561	48		1		2608	130	273			130	2073	3.0	8.3	28	1.8	.1
Dry peas	295					295	15	23			15	242	.4	1.0	3	.2	
Chick-peas	4474	3		1		4476	570	256			90	3561	5.2	14.3	52	2.8	.8

(continued)

Table 4.5 continued

	Production	Imports	Stock Changes	Exports	Processed Trade (E-1)	Domestic Supply	Feed	Seed	Nonfood Use	Manufacturer Use	Manufacturer Food Waste	Food	Kilograms/Year	Per Day Grams	Per Day Calories	Per Day Protein	Per Day Fat Grams
Pigeon peas	1867					1867	93	57			93	1624	2.4	6.5	22	1.3	.1
Lentils	408	15				423	21	28			21	353	.5	1.4	5	.3	
Pulses NES	901	2		1		902	45	99			45	713	1.0	2.9	10	.6	.1
Nuts and oilseeds													5.2	14.4	28	.7	2.4
Cashew nuts	183	34			134	83			37			46	.1	.2			
Almonds		4				4						4					
Walnuts	16					16						15		.1			
Soybeans	433					433		31	260		13	130	.2	.5	2	.2	.1
Groundnuts in shell	6009		303		47	5659		635	4501		322	200	.3	.8	3	.1	.2
Coconuts	4444				-62	4506			1606			2900	4.2	11.6	17	.2	1.5
Castor beans	220	1				221		5	210								
Sunflower seed	55					55			55								
Rapeseed	1845	24				1869		23	1759			87	.1	.3	2	.1	.2
Safflower seed	274					274		7	262		5						
Sesame seed	436		-20	9		447		10	317		10	111	.2	.4	3	.1	.2
Cottonseed	2621					2621	460	144	1492	393	131						
Linseed	411	1				412		28	310		8	66	.1	.3	1		.1
Oilseeds NES	131			6		125		8	89		3	26		.1	1		
Vegetables													58.6	160.4	37	2.3	.3
Cabbages	463					463					23	440	.6	1.8			
Tomatoes	743					743					74	669	1.0	2.7	1		
Cauliflower	650					650					32	617	.9	2.5			
Dry onions	2579			159		2420					129	2291	3.3	9.2	3		
Garlic	202			4		198					10	187	.3	.8	1	.1	
Green beans	41					41					4	37	.1	.1			
Green peas	253					253					25	228	.3	.9	1		
Fresh vegetables NES	35667			3		35664			143			35521	51.9	142.2	31	2.0	.3

(continued)

Table 4.5 continued

Fruit	Production	Imports	Stock Changes	Exports	Processed Trade (E-1)	Domestic Supply	Feed	Seed	Nonfood Use	Manufacturer Use	Food Waste	Food	Kilograms/Year	Grams	Per Day Calories	Protein	Fat Grams
Bananas	4535					4535					907	3628	23.1	63.4	29	.3	.2
Oranges	1153					1153					115	1038	5.3	14.5	9	.1	
Lemons and limes	485			1		484					49	436	1.5	4.2	1		
Grapefruit and pomelo	20					20					2	18	.6	1.7			
Citrus fruit NES	30					30					3	27		.1			
Apples	734			1		733					73	660	1.0	2.6	1		
Pears	64					64					6	57	.1	.2			
Apricots	15					15					1	13		.1			
Cherries	4					4						4					
Peaches and nectarines	15					15					1	13		.1			
Plums	28					28					3	25		.1			
Grapes	196	8			-26	230					21	209	.3	.8			
Figs	2				-1	3						3					
Mangoes	8365					8365				33	837	7495	10.9	30.0	13	.1	.1
Pineapples	548					548				55		493	.7	2.0	1		
Dates	34				34				1		34						
Papayas	262					262					39	222	.3	.9	2		
Fresh tropical fruit NES	1215			7		1208				24	182	1001	1.5	4.0	1		
Fresh fruit NES	493	3				496					50	446	.7	1.8			
Meat and Offals													1.3	3.7	6	.5	.4
Mutton and lamb	120			4		116						116	.2	.5	1	.1	.1
Goat meat	268					268						268	.4	1.1	2	.2	.1
Pig Meat	70					70						70	.1	.3	1	.1	.1
Chicken meat	111					111						111	.2	.4	1	.1	.1

(continued)

Table 4.5 continued

	Production	Imports	Stock Changes	Exports	Processed Trade (E-1)	Domestic Supply	Feed	Seed	Nonfood Use	Use	Food Waste	Food	Kilograms/Year	Grams	Calories	Protein	Fat Grams
									Domestic Utilization → **Manufacturer**					**Per Day**			
Eggs													.9	2.6	4	.3	.3
Hen eggs	733					733				18	73	642	.9	2.6	4	.3	.3
Fish and seafood													3.1	8.4	5	.9	.2
Freshwater diadrom	928					928						928	1.4	3.7	3	.4	.1
Demersal fish	449				1	448			47			401	.6	1.6	3	.2	
Pelagic fish	653				36	617	125					492	.7	2.0	1	.2	
Milk													38.2	104.7	66	3.8	3.6
Whole cow milk	13033				-44	13077					156	12921	18.9	51.7	31	1.5	1.7
Skim cow milk					-448	448						448	.6	1.8	1	.1	
Buffalo milk	17000					17000	4303				819	11878	17.4	47.5	32	2.1	1.7
Goat milk	923					923					11	912	1.3	3.7	2	.1	.1
Oils and fats													6.4	17.5	153		17.3
Vegetable oils and fats													5.3	14.7	130		14.7
Soybean oil	47	517				564						564	.8	2.2	20		2.2
Groundnut oil	1260	1		4		1257			32			1226	1.8	4.9	43		4.9
Coconut oil	189	23				212			35			177	.3	.7	6		.7
Palm oil		439				439			42			397	.6	1.6	14		1.6
Sunflower seed oil	16	1				17						17	.1	.1	1		.1
Rapeseed oil	580	136				716			3			713	1.0	2.9	25		2.9
Safflower oil	73					73						73	.1	.3	3		.3
Sesame seed oil	127					127			11			116	.2	.5	4		.5
Cottonseed oil	209	9				218						218	.3	.9	8	.	.9
Linseed oil	102	1				103			48			55	.1	.2	2		.2
Rice bran oil	109					109			11			98	.1	.4	3		.4

(continued)

Table 4.5 continued

					Processed		Domestic Utilization								Per Day		
	Production	Imports	Stock Changes	Exports	Trade (E-1)	Domestic Supply	Feed	Seed	Use	Nonfood Use	Manufacturer Food Waste	Food	Kilograms/Year	Grams	Calories	Protein	Fat Grams
Animal oils and fats																	
Tallow	10	31				41						41	1.0	2.8	24		2.7
Ghee of buffalo milk	515					515						515	.8	2.1	18		2.0
Butter of buffalo milk	124					124						124	.2	.5	4	.4	.4
Spices																	
Pepper, white/long/black	29		−1	22		8					1	6					
Anise, badian, fennel	20	1				21						20	.1	.1			
Pimento, allspice	529			6		523					26	496	1.2	3.4	10	.4	.2
Cloves, whole & stems		1				1						1					
Nutmeg, mace, cardamom	5					5					6	6					
Spices NES	415	2		87		330					8	321	.7	2.0	6	.2	.1
Stimulants																	
Green coffee	126			76	3	47					6	41	.5	1.3	4	.1	
Cocoa beans									1				.5	1.5	1	.1	
Tea	559			223		336					6	330	.1	.2	1	.1	
Areca nuts (betel)	185					185				179	6		.5	1.3	1		

Source: FAO 1991:158-159.

a population that includes infants, children, and adults) we see an especially wide variation in the nutritional requirements of the population. In addition, the information on food availability shows us only the average nutrient intake. Some people in the country or region consume less than the average, and some more than the average. So even if average caloric intake is greater than average caloric requirement, a country can still suffer significant undernutrition. Therefore, comparing caloric intake to caloric requirement does not always give an accurate view of the extent of undernutrition. For example, the FAO reports that during the 1990–1992 period, India and Senegal had virtually the same calories available per person per day (2,310 in India, 2,320 in Senegal). However, anthropometric data for the two countries in the late 1980s found that the percentage of children who are underweight was 63.9 percent in India and 21.6 percent in Senegal.

Aggregate food intake measures can also be used to estimate the percentage of a population that has inadequate food intake. FAO's Sixth World Food Survey uses the following method: Average caloric intake per capita is calculated from food balance sheets. An estimate of the statistical variance of caloric intake per capita is derived from studies of individuals. These two statistics (average and variance) give an estimate of the distribution of food intake: what percentage of the population has caloric intake below 2,000 calories per day; what percentage below 2,500, etc. Once a minimum food requirement is identified for the population, that distribution will then tell us what percentage of population intakes less than the minimum requirement. Minimum food requirements are identified for different age and sex classes (e.g., children under 10, males over 10, etc.). Minimum requirements are calculated in two ways. First, we can ask, "What level of calories would give a person of average height a minimally healthy weight?" A minimally healthy weight is determined as a BMI of 18.5. (See above discussion of BMI.) A second method is to determine the *basal metabolic rate* (BMR) for the population. The BMR shows the number of calories needed for survival when the body is at rest. The minimal food requirement is calculated by multiplying the BMR by a constant (1.56 is used in the Sixth World Food Survey).

Undernutrition:
Who, Where, When?

In the last chapter, we saw a number of ways to measure undernutrition. In addition, some measures are based on somewhat arbitrary cut-off points. Given this situation, we should not be surprised to find that estimates of undernutrition can only be approximations.

Nevertheless, we know enough about what we mean by undernutrition to put the severity of the problem into perspective. In this chapter we consider the following questions: How widespread is undernutrition? What kinds of people suffer from it? When do they suffer (or when have they suffered)? And where do they live?

■ GLOBAL TRENDS IN LONG-TERM PERSPECTIVE

Table 5.1 shows estimates of the number of people worldwide who are affected by undernutrition-associated conditions. In addition, as reported in Chapter 1, there are estimates that at least 8 million children die each year from malnutrition-related causes. Table 5.2 presents different estimates of the numbers of undernourished people around the world. Notice that, as the definition of *undernourished* tightens, the number of people identified as undernourished drops.

Over time, the number of undernourished people has declined. This is illustrated by Table 5.3. For the developing world as a whole, the number of undernourished people dropped from 918 million in the early 1970s to 906 million in the early 1980s to 841 million in the early 1990s. Expressed as a percentage of the population, the drop has been more dramatic; over one-third of the developing world's population was undernourished in the early 1970s; by the 1990s, the proportion had dropped to one-fifth. However, the

Table 5.1   World Population Affected by Malnutrition, WHO and FAO Data

Deficiency	Status	Population	Prevalence (millions)
Iodine	At-risk	Worldwide 1995	1,571
Iodine	Brain damage due to iodine deficiency	Worldwide 1995	43
Iodine	Goiter	Worldwide 1995	656
Vitamin A	At-risk	Worldwide, children under age 5, 1995	251
Vitamin A	Xerophthalmia in children under age 5	Worldwide, children under age 5, 1995	2.8
Iron	Iron deficient or anemic	Worldwide 1995	2,150
Energy	Inadequate food intake	Developing countries 1990-92	918
Protein and energy	Stunted	Developing countries, children under age 5, 1990–92	215

Source: Sixth World Food Survey, and WHO, UN, Micronutrient and Trace Element Deficiencies—General Information.

Table 5.2   Different Estimates of the Number of Malnourished People
              in Developing Countries

Source of Estimate	Time Period Covered	Definition of "Minimum Requirement"	Number of Malnourished People (millions)
Sixth World Food Survey (1996)	1969–71	1.55 BMR (males) 1.56 BMR (females)	918
World Bank (1986)	1980	90% of RDA	1045
ACC/SCN (1987)	1979–81	1.2 BMR	465
Sixth World Food Survey (1996)	1979–81	1.55 BMR (males) 1.56 BMR (females)	906
FAO (1992)	1979–81	1.54 BMR	843
FAO (1992)	1988–90	1.54 BMR	785
Sixth World Food Survey	1990–92	1.55 BMR (males) 1.56 BMR (females)	841

Source: 6th World Food Survey, and Uvin (1993).
Note: "BMR" is basal metabolic rate. "RDA" is recommended dietary allowance as calculated by FAO/WHO.

Table 5.3   Trends in Number and Percentage of People Undernourished,
              by Continental Area

Area	1969–71	1979–81	1990–92
	Number of Undernourished (millions)		
Sub-Saharan Africa	103	148	215
Near East and North Africa	48	27	37
East and Southeast Asia	476	379	269
South Asia	238	303	255
Latin America and Caribbean	53	48	64
All Developing Countries	918	906	841
	Proportion of the Population that is Undernourished (percent)		
Sub-Saharan Africa	38	41	43
Near East and North Africa	27	12	12
East and Southeast Asia	41	27	16
South Asia	33	34	22
Latin America and Caribbean	19	14	15
All developing countries	35	28	20

Source: Sixth World Food Survey.

declines have not been spread evenly throughout the developing world. Progress in Asia has been remarkable; the number of undernourished people has dropped by over 25 percent (nearly 200 million people) since the early 1970s, and the percentage of undernourished people has dropped from 38 percent to 18 percent. These declines offset worsening conditions

Figure 5.1 Index of World Food Production per Capita, 1961–1997

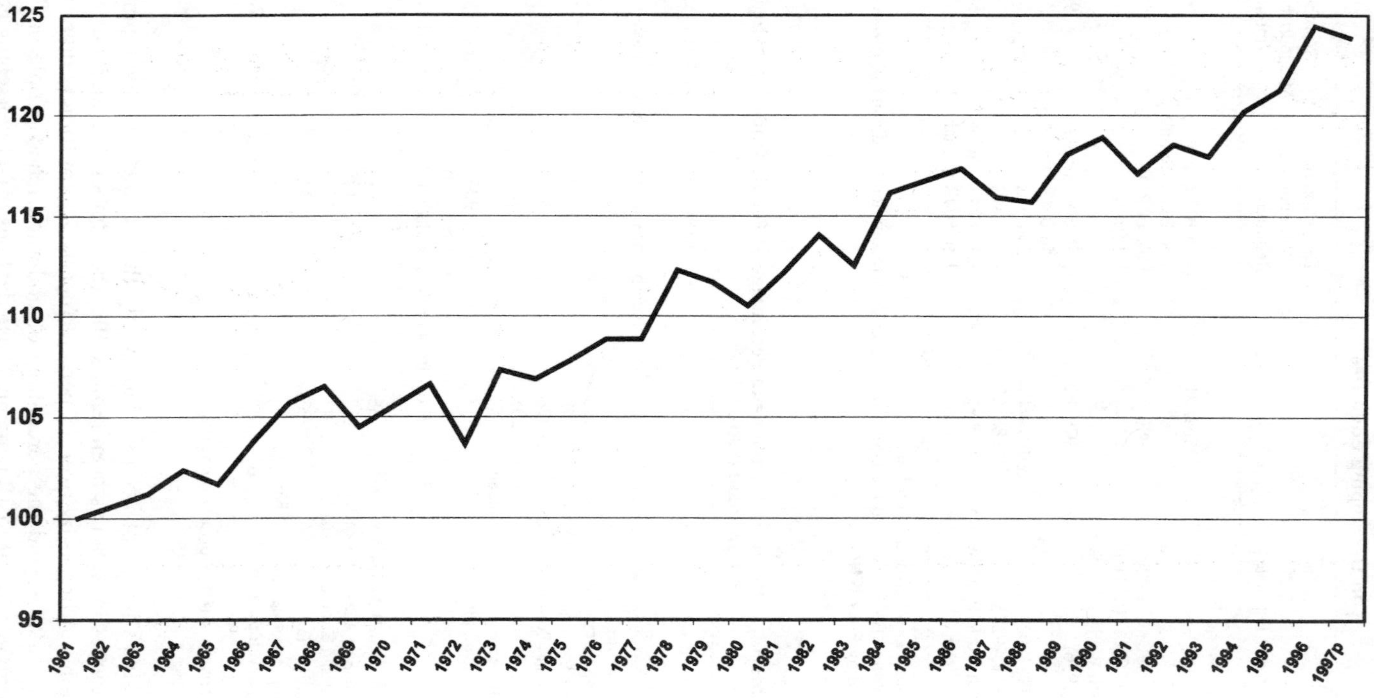

Figure 5.2   Index of Real Food Prices, 1961–1997

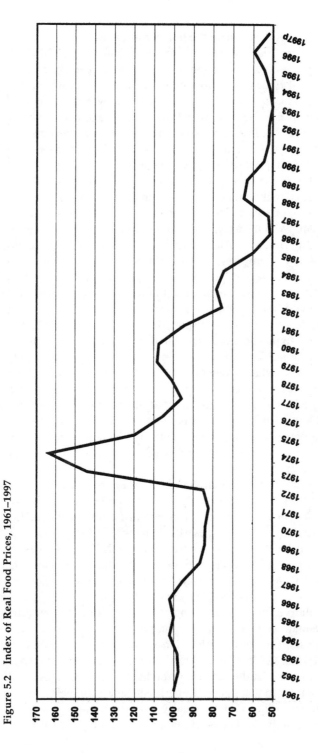

Note: Figures are index of dollar prices deflated by U.S. GDP implicit price deflator.

in sub-Saharan Africa, where the number of undernourished people has increased by over 200 million, and the percentage of population that is undernourished has increased from 38 percent to 43 percent.

Additional evidence of a long-term trend of an improving food situation
is shown in Figures 5.1 and 5.2. These show that worldwide food production
per capita increased steadily from 1961 to 1997, and that world food prices
fell over the period. Figure 5.2 shows that food prices jumped around quite
a bit. They took a huge jump between 1972 and 1974, and then fell sharply.
At their low point (1993) food prices were about half the level of 1961, less
than one-third of the peak price level in 1974. Over the last 10 years, prices
have fluctuated, but with no discernible trend up or down.

Is the progress since the 1960s merely the latest installment of steady
improvement? With the acceleration of technology during the nineteenth and
twentieth centuries, the Western world developed considerable confidence in
the inevitability of progress. We have almost come to the point of expecting
that "everyday in every way we are getting better and better"—that our present state of development is the result of an almost continual improvement
since the days of the caveman. We sometimes imagine life in preagricultural
societies as "nasty, brutish, and short" (to quote Hobbes in *The Leviathan*).

It is easy to presume that our abundant life today is the culmination of
progress on a multitude of fronts, one of which is certainly nutrition. In
Chapter 3, we cited data suggesting that, during the past 100 years, entire
populations have grown taller in Europe, Japan, and India. It comes as
something of a shock then, to find that during the past few decades eth-
nologists, anthropologists, paleopathologists, and agronomists have suggested that perhaps life was not completely bad before the development of
agriculture, which supposedly released us from the brutish life of the
hunter-gatherer (Box 5.1).

One of the first chinks in the armor of the progressivist thesis was a
famous and widely quoted study by Richard Lee (1968:30–48) of the
!Kung Bushman of the Kalahari desert in Southern Africa. Lee found,
when he studied a group of these Bushman of the Dobe area, that, "In all,
the adults of the Dobe camp worked about 2 1/2 days a week. Since the
average working day was about 6 hours long, the fact emerges that !Kung
Bushmen of Dobe, despite their harsh environment, devote from 12 to 19
hours a week to getting food" (p. 37). If 15 hours a week gathering food
is representative, that is only about two hours a day! Such a life leaves
more time than we had previously supposed for the preagricultural societies to spend on activities such as creative arts, crafts, and other activities.

Jack Harlan (1975:10), in a survey of the literature on preagricultural
societies, reports that the pattern of food gathering among Australian abo-
rigines is similar to that of the !Kung Bushman. Both males and females in
Australian aboriginal society usually work for two days and keep every
third day as a holiday. The working adults can supply food for the entire

Box 5.1 Did Settling Down Improve Human Lives?

Mark Cohen

A long-standing debate among prehistorians concerns the impact of early improvements in food-related technology on human health and well being. A traditional view, still popularly held, argues that the development of agriculture, which occurred at various places around the world between 5,000 and 10,000 years ago, generally resulted in the improvement of human health, improvements in the quality and reliability of human food supplies, and the overall lessening of labor demands in the food quest.

Beginning in the 1960s, stimulated by the work of economist Esther Boserup and ethnographer Richard Lee, an alternative view of prehistory was put forward. According to this theory, early farming permitted more mouths to be fed without necessarily increasing leisure—and in fact often increasing the work load. This view also suggested that the adoption of agriculture might have resulted, at least in some areas, in a decline in the nutritional quality of the food supply.

At the same time, according to the new theory, human health began to deteriorate as the intensity of early agriculture increased. Modern epidemiology suggests that many human diseases that pass from person to person in the air or water by touch will be transmitted more readily by larger, sedentary farming communities than by small, mobile bands of hunter gatherers. Diseases vectored by human feces such as hookworm and various kinds of diarrhea should pass more readily; diseases such as bubonic plague transmitted by rats or other animals attracted to human garbage should become more common; and the increasing size of human groups in combination with increasing trade networks would have permitted some epidemic diseases such as measles, mumps, smallpox, and cholera to appear for the first time.

Whether agriculture increased the reliability of human food supplies is also questionable. Human tending may well protect crop plants from failure; and storage of food certainly helped to alleviate hunger in the short run. But domesticated crops growing under human care are often relatively fragile because human beings have selected them and bred them for qualities other than hardiness and because the crops are often being grown outside the ecological niche to which they were originally adapted. Storage requires that a group be sedentary, which limits options in times of crises. Stored food may spoil, and most important, the storage of food made food supplies vulnerable to expropriation by other human groups for the first time.

Hunter gatherers and early farmers alike probably enjoyed relatively balanced diets; but as intensified farming supported larger populations, agriculture became increasingly focused on individual crops such as maize (corn), wheat, or rice. Diets that rely too heavily on any one crop are likely to create dietary deficiency (anemia, pellagra, beriberi, etc.) as is readily seen in the twentieth century, not among "primitives"—hunter gatherers or farmers—but among the poor of modern states.

(continued)

Box 5.1 Continued

The skeletons of prehistoric populations (of which we now have many thousands) appear to support the new view. If we use stature as a measure of well being, as we like to do, it is worth noting that prehistoric hunter gatherers more often than not are taller than the populations that replace them. In fact, the general trend in human stature since prehistory is downward, the modern trend in Western countries being an exception. The skeletons of hunter gatherers commonly display fewer signs of anemia than the farmers that succeeded them (whether this results from better diets or fewer parasitic infections is unclear). Hunter gatherers also commonly show fewer signs of infection than later farmers. Some specific diseases identifiable in the skeleton, such as tuberculosis, appear relatively recently in prehistory among densely populated, settled groups.

From this perspective, the adoption and intensification of agriculture seems to be a series of compromises with growing numbers—increasing numbers of mouths to feed and increasing competition among groups, rather than "progress."

Source: Adapted from Cohen 1984.

group with only about three to four hours of activity per day (Sahlins 1968).

Not only have we evidence that preagricultural societies had plenty of leisure time, we also believe that they ate rather well. Lee (Harlan 1975: 11) reports that !Kung Bushman consume 93 grams of protein per day, most of which comes from meat and nuts. Their food supply is not only abundant most of the time, but reasonably well balanced. We see further evidence that preagricultural societies ate quite well from the records of nutrition they left in their bones. (Bone length is one indicator of nutritional status.) The heights of eastern Mediterranean people at the beginning of agriculture appear to have exceeded the heights of the ancient and modern Greeks (Figure 5.3).

Around the world since the beginnings of agriculture, as populations have grown and exerted increasing pressures on land, people have concentrated their food consumption on those crops that make the most efficient use of the land for converting the sun's energy to food. Jack Harlan (1975:57) again:

> The trend for more and more people to be nourished by fewer and fewer plant and animal food sources has reached the point today where most of the world's population is absolutely dependent on a handful of species. . . . This is a relatively recent phenomenon and was not characteristic of the traditional subsistence agricultures abandoned over the past few centuries. . . .
> Man once enjoyed a highly varied diet. He has used for food several thousand species of plants and several hundred species of animals. . . .

Figure 5.3 Relative Height of Eastern Mediterranean Adult Males Since 9000 BC,
Based on Correlations Between Leg Bones (from Burial Remains)
and Height

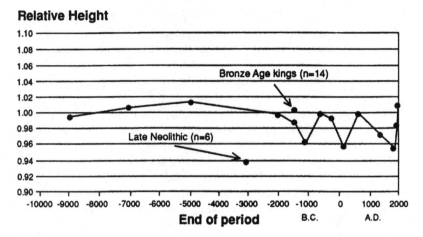

Source: Adapted from Kates et al., 1988:26; data from Angel 1984.

With the beginnings of agriculture there was a tendency to concentrate on the species that were more productive and the most rewarding in terms of labor and capital invested.

If, as the new thinking implies (see Box 5.1), substantial blocks of modern society are less healthy and less well nourished than was preagricultural society, our present-day much-vaunted accomplishments appear tarnished. We should be all the more motivated to improve the level of health and nutrition of modern mankind, at least to the level attained by our preagricultural hunter-gatherer ancestors!

■ THE SEASONALITY OF UNDERNUTRITION

People at risk for undernutrition are not usually at risk all the time; it tends to come in fits and starts. We are all aware of the periodicity of famine—the word connotes a time of extreme food scarcity as contrasted with normal times when food is less scarce. But we are less aware that Third World hunger usually follows the rhythm of the seasons. In the Third World, a strong seasonality is usual in the production, price, and availability of food, as well as in the availability of employment (Sahn 1989). All these factors can influence the nutritional status of a family at risk for undernutrition.

The seasonality of undernutrition is often linked to the agricultural year, which in the tropics is usually heavily dependent on rainfall patterns. In monsoon Asia, for instance, rice is planted at the beginning of the wet monsoon that typically starts in July. For those using the "Japanese method," which involves transplanting seedlings taken from a nursery, a particularly heavy labor demand arises during transplanting (Figure 5.4), which follows planting by a couple of weeks. Harvest begins about four months after planting. With irrigation, farmers can harvest more than one crop per year, but most of the rice starts during the wet monsoon.

Consequently, the price of rice is lowest just after harvest and rises gradually as supplies dwindle. During the growing season, supplies may become short and prices may rise more sharply. The pattern of seasonal variation in the Philippines is shown in Figure 5.5. Compare this with consumption rates in Table 5.4. Consumption is at its lowest in September when the price has been high for three months, and picks up during the following months when the price falls below the annual average.

Because of the relationships between food prices, food availability, and the agricultural year, a hunger season is often timed to the onset of the wet season, when food prices are approaching their peak. Some germs die when they dry out or get cold, and so do some diseases—such as diarrhea—spread more easily during the warm, wet season. With the onset of the wet season, increased communicability and lowered resistance caused by reduced food consumption combine to increase infection rates, exacerbating the effects of reduced consumption (the story is told more eloquently in Box 5.2).

■ WHO IS UNDERNOURISHED?

In which countries is the problem of undernutrition the worst? Table 5.5 shows that the answer to this question depends on the way in which the extent of undernutrition is measured.

If we look at calories available per person as a percentage of average requirements, the worst-off countries are Afghanistan, Chad, and Ethiopia. If we look at mortality rates for children under five as an indicator of undernutrition, we conclude that Niger, Angola, and Sierra Leone are the worst-off. If we look at the percentage of children who are underweight, we identify Bangladesh, India, and Ethiopia.

Note that Asian countries have substantially higher percentages of underweight children than food availability would lead one to expect. Ramalingaswami and colleagues (1996) discuss this problem. They suggest the explanation may be a combination of the following:

- "Girls and women in South Asia are less well regarded and less well cared for than in sub–Saharan Africa." Poor nutrition among pregnant women causes low-birth-weight babies.
- "Differences in standards of hygiene between the two regions

Figure 5.4   Seasonality of Women's Employment, Rural Tamil Nadu, India

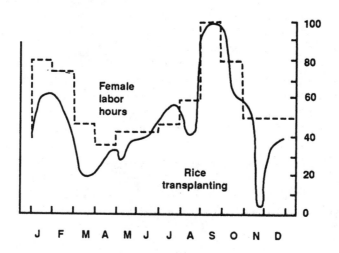

Source: Adapted from Payne 1985:13.

Figure 5.5   Seasonal Price Variation in Rice, Philippines

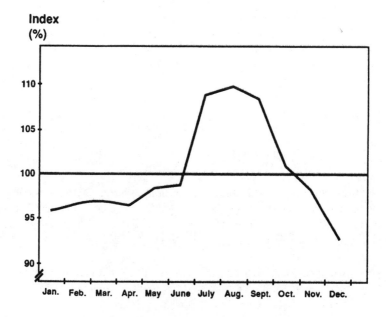

Source: Adapted from Philippines Ministry of Agriculture 1981b.

Table 5.4   Annual Rate of Consumption of Rice and Rice Products, Phiippines, 1980–1981

		Kilos per Capita per Year
1980	March	108.4
	June	110.4
	September	98.2
	December	103.6
1981	March	103.4
	June	115.1

Source: Philippines Ministry of Agriculture 1983.

Box 5.2   The Seasons of Poverty

Robert Chambers, Richard Longhurst, David Bradley, and Richard Feacham

While this is a generalized scenario drawn as a composite from many settings, it illustrates relationships between variables that many settings seem to share. In particular, there is a widespread tendency for adverse factors to operate concurrently during the wet seasons and for these to hit the poor segments of the population harder than the more well-to-do. Typically the scenario develops as follows.

Toward the end of the dry season, water becomes scarce. There is a rise in the labor and energy required to fetch water and to water livestock, and also to gather food and to clear and manure fields. The poorer people begin to suffer more than others. They have less food because they have been able to grow less, because they have fewer livestock, because they may lose a higher proportion of their food reserves in storage, and because they have less money. They may eat less in order to save food for the crucial time of cultivation. Work is scarce and wages are low at this time of year. Some migrate in search of work and food.

The rains bring the start of crisis and of the "hungry season" or "lean period."

For both small farmers and laborers, heavy manual labor for land preparation (often by men), for transplanting (often by women), and for weeding (often from women) comes at this time when food is short. Laborers benefit from being able to get work, but many are in negative energy balance and lose weight. At the same time, food prices are high and transport problems in the rains make it difficult for either central authorities or the open market to relieve local shortages. Anticipating hard work, mothers give their children only a diminished and less regular food supply with their milk. Food preparation becomes more hurried and the diet less varied and nutritious. Less time is spent in cooking, housecleaning, water collection, fuel gathering and childcare, and more of the women's time is spent on agricultural operations.

(continued)

Box 5.2   Continued

Diseases vary in their seasonality, but some of the more serious and debilitating peak during or just after the rains. These usually include malaria and sometimes diarrheal diseases, especially where the wet season is also the hot season. Guinea worm also peaks at this time, as do infections of the skin. The development of protein-energy malnutrition contributes to low immune response. Coinciding with a peak labor demand, when failure to cultivate, transplant, weed, or harvest may critically affect future income and food supplies, infections increase the risks and vulnerability of rural people. This is when the poorer people must work in order to earn enough to tide them over until the next agricultural season. This is also a bad time for mothers and children. Births peak, but body weights of mothers and of babies at birth are both low, and neonatal mortality also peaks. The calorific value of the milk supply of lactating mothers is low. Pregnant and lactating women are weakened by disease and work. Those in the poorer, smaller families are especially vulnerable because of the need to work when work is available.

At harvest time wages are high, but the work is also hard—both the harvesting proper and the post-harvest processing. Furthermore, morbidity is still marked and weakness lingers from the food shortages and sicknesses of the lean season. Weight loss is now at its greatest. Mortality, especially among older adults, peaks in response to the high energy demands and the weakened physical condition.

After harvest, things improve for a time. Food is available, and food intake recovers in both quantity and quality. Body weights rise. Morbidity and mortality decline. There are ceremonies, celebrations, marriages. There is a peak in rates of conception. And then gradually the cycle begins all over again.

Source: Extracted from Chambers et al. 1979.

[South Asia and sub–Saharan Africa] are very pronounced. . . . This all-round poor hygiene increases the burden of illness, and [causes] significantly higher levels of malnutrition among South Asia's children."

- Quality of childcare is higher in sub–Saharan Africa than in South Asia.

Table 5.6 lists 20 countries that appear on the list of "worst 50" countries by all three measures of undernutrition. This list gives us a clearer picture of where undernutrition is most prevalent. Sixteen of the 20 countries are in sub-Saharan Africa. (Other sub-Saharan African countries fail to appear only because data are not available on all three measures.) Three neighboring countries—India, Pakistan, and Bangladesh—are also on the

Table 5.5   **25 Most Seriously Undernourished Countries According to Three Different Measures**

Country	Daily per Capita Calorie Supplies as a % of Requirements	Country	Under-5 Mortality Rate per 1000 Live Births	Country	% of Children Underweight
Afghanistan	72	Niger	320	Bangladesh	65.8
Chad	73	Angola	292	India	63.9
Ethiopia	73	Sierra Leone	284	Ethiopia	47.7
Mozambique	77	Mozambique	277	Mauritania	47.6
Angola	80	Afghanistan	257	Vietnam	45.0
Somalia	81	Guinea-Bissau	231	Pakistan	40.4
Central Afr. Rep.	82	Guinea	223	Indonesia	39.9
Rwanda	82	Malawi	221	Burundi	38.3
Sierra Leone	83	Liberia	217	Sri Lanka	38.1
Burundi	84	Mali	214	Myanmar	38.0
Bolivia	84	Gambia	213	Bhutan	37.9
Zambia	87	Somalia	211	Laos	36.7
Sudan	87	Zambia	203	Niger	36.2
Peru	87	Chad	202	Nigeria	35.7
Malawi	88	Eritrea	200	Haiti	33.9
Bangladesh	88	Ethiopia	200	Guatemala	33.5
Haiti	89	Mauritania	199	Philippines	32.9
Kenya	89	Bhutan	193	Madagascar	32.8
Nigeria	93	Nigeria	191	Mali	31.0
Uganda	93	Zaire	186	Yemen	30.0
Lesotho	93	Uganda	185	Papua N. Guinea	29.9
Ghana	93	Cambodia	177	Tanzania	28.8
Burkina Faso	94	Burundi	176	Sierra Leone	28.7
Zimbabwe	94	Central Afr. Rep.	175	Rwanda	28.6
Niger	95	Burkina Faso	169	Malawi	27.2

Source: Per Capita Calories, UNICEF, http://www.unicef.org/sowc96/swc96t2x.htm
Under-5 Mortality, UNICEF, http://www.unicef.org/sowc96/swc96t1x.htm
Underweight Children, WHO, http://sun1.who.ch/whosis/cgrowth/bulletin.htm

list. (Neighboring Afghanistan is not on the list because data for the country are not available regarding percentage of children underweight.) These countries have large populations: Each of them is larger than the biggest sub-Saharan African country (Nigeria), and together the three have more than 20 percent of the world's population. Outside these areas, the only country to appear on the list is Haiti.

Of course, in raw numbers, countries with large populations have large numbers of undernourished people. Nearly 75 percent of undernourished children in the world live in India, China, Bangladesh, Pakistan, Indonesia, Nigeria, and Vietnam.

Within any given country, malnutrition is likely to be more prevalent in rural areas. The World Bank (1990:238) calculated that, among the 42 countries they classified as low-income in 1988, rural people represented

Table 5.6   Countries That Rank High in All of Three Undernutrition Measures

Country	Ranking by Calories per Capita	Ranking by Infant Mortality	Ranking by Underweight Children
Ethiopia	3	16	3
Sierra Leone	9	3	23
Niger	25	1	13
Burundi	10	23	8
Malawi	15	8	25
Nigeria	19	19	14
Zambia	12	13	29
Bangladesh	16	41	1
Mali	29	10	19
Rwanda	8	32	24
Haiti	17	37	15
Madagascar	26	26	18
Tanzania	27	27	22
Pakistan	40	34	6
Ghana	22	36	26
India	45	39	2
Lesotho	21	28	47
Togo	41	35	30
Senegal	37	42	37
Cameroon	28	46	50

Source: Derived from UNICEF and WHO data.

65 percent of the population. Rural incomes are usually considerably below urban incomes and, because undernutrition is so closely associated with low-income populations, a pretty strong argument can be made that the majority of the world's hungry are rural. Because of this and because so many policies affecting the price and availability of food to both rural and urban consumers impinge on the rural sector of the economy, we make a heavy emphasis in this book on policies affecting the rural sector. The tension that exists between the rural and urban sectors of the Third World is discussed in some detail in Chapter 18. As the world moves into the twenty-first century, Third World economies are expected to become increasingly urban, but even then, rural-oriented policies will remain especially significant among those affecting undernutrition.

Children as a group are by far the most vulnerable to undernutrition, especially at weaning time—that transitional period during which an infant's diet is changed from 100 percent breast milk to 100 percent other foods—a transition that can be abrupt but that, in the Third World, often takes place during an 18-month time span, say, between six months and two years of age. While infants are being moved from breast milk toward other foods, their requirements for a calorie- and protein-dense diet are still very high, and in cultures where the diet is dominated by grains, providing an appropriate diet for weaning children takes a special effort.

Pregnant women and lactating mothers are the next most vulnerable to undernutrition, and evidence is gathering that old women may be next in line. For example, notice again, in Figure 3.3, how the older Indian village women fell further below the NCHS standard than did their older male counterparts.

During times of extreme food shortages or famines the above groups are almost always the most at risk, but at these times a broader segment of the population, including large numbers of able-bodied men, is likely to be affected also.

We hear occasional reports of food deprivation based on gender. Roger Winter (1988), director of the U.S. Committee for Refugees, writes about the Dinka people in Sudan, who have been plagued both by drought and a scorched-earth strategy the Sudanese army used to subdue the Dinka's rebellious tendencies. Winter reports that many refugee groups consist chiefly of physically weakened young men and boys: "Women and children often are left behind, displaced and without access to international assistance or protection. They are dying in shockingly large numbers. In some areas, virtually all children under 3 are dead. Young girls are rare: In a society beset by war, with an economy based on cattle herding, girls are allowed to starve so that resources can be devoted to their brothers."

The Punjab in northwest India has the highest ratio of males to females in India. A study of the area (Das Gupta 1988) reported that the youngest daughters in families with many children are often selectively deprived of both medicine and the more nutritious foods in order that their brothers may be better cared for. Although we looked, we did not find evidence of this practice during our 1981 study of Bagbana village.

When examining the at-risk groups, the emphasis on women and children does not mean that undernutrition never affects adult working men. Although clinical signs of undernutrition are rare in this group, significant numbers appear to suffer an energy depletion that limits work capacities and productivity.

So far we have examined the number of people suffering from undernutrition, as well as the trends, geographic location, and seasonality of hunger, and the people most vulnerable to it. But undernutrition occurs in individuals on a case-by-case basis. If we can identify the characteristics of a family that predispose them to an occurrence of undernutrition, we may, at the same time, uncover clues as to appropriate policies for reducing its prevalence.

Arnold and his colleagues (1981) examined data collected in 1979 by the National Nutrition Council of the Philippines. Their sample contained 722 families from seven provinces. To be included in the sample, a family had to have at least one preschool child. The purpose of the study was to see if family data could be used to predict the presence of an undernourished child. So the preshool child with the lowest level of nutrition of all a family's preschoolers was chosen as the subject. This child, therefore, became the dependent variable, and what Arnold's group tried to predict was the percentage of standard weight-for-age of this child. See Table 5.7 for some of the main findings of the study. Variables with a positive correlation coefficient have a positive influence on percentage of weight-for-age. That is, the higher the value of the variable, the more likely the subject child is to be well-nourished. Some of the relationships are fairly obvious. The more education the father and mother have and the more income the family has, the better nourished the subject child is likely to be.

The importance of weaning age becomes clear when you think about it. The Philippines is a country of rice eaters, and rice is low in both protein and fat. Therefore, the longer a child is breast-fed, the longer is the time it is receiving an appropriately protein-rich, calorie-dense diet.

Variables with a negative correlation coefficient (those at the bottom of Table 5.7) have a negative influence on percentage of weight-for-age. Thus, mothers who bottle-fed their babies almost exclusively were more likely to have undernourished children than those who breast-fed exclusively. Children of mothers who mixed bottle- and breast-feeding tended to be better off than those who were bottle-fed only and worse off than those who were breast-fed only. Children in large families were more likely to be undernourished than children in small families. And within the same family, children born later were more likely to be undernourished than their older siblings. Speculation has it that mothers sometimes give up, if slightly, on the youngest child after they have already borne three or four children (S. Scrimshaw 1978:389; 1984).

Another study has shown that the age of the mother at the time of giving birth may influence nutritional status. Children of mothers who at the time of their children's births were younger than 20 or older than 30 are

Table 5.7   Correlation of Socioeconomic Variables with Percentage of Standard Body Weight-for-Age, Philippine Preschoolers (Under Six Years Old), 1979

Socioeconomic Variable	Correlation Coefficient	Number of Families Sampled
Number of years of formal education of the mother	.27	721
Number of years of formal education of the father	.26	716
Income, farming families	.12	213
Income, nonfarming families	.35	499
Age of weaning if subject child is weaned	.34	545
Type of infant feeding	−.37	718
1 = breast alone, 2 = mixed, 3 = bottle alone		
Total number of household members	−.25	722
Birth order of subject child	−.21	722

Source: Arnold et al. 1981.

Note: All variables were significant at the .01 level except income, which was significant at the .07 level.

more likely to be undernourished than are children born of mothers between 20 and 30 (Rustein 1984).

Sometimes special circumstances exacerbate an already unfortunate situation and increase still further the possibility that a child will be undernourished. In 1980, we had occasion to visit a number of Filipino families, each of which had at least one third-degree undernourished child. In most cases, in addition to the usual problems of low income, low education of the parents, and a number of children in the household, some special situation or stressor existed that might have significantly contributed to child undernutrition; for example, the mother suffered from tuberculosis and was always tired; the mother liked to gamble and left her one-year-old in the care of her four-year-old; the mother had borne twins and thought they carried a curse; the father was living with another woman; or the father was working in the city and came home only every other Sunday.

■ PART 2

CAUSES OF UNDERNUTRITION

The main causes of undernutrition can be traced to economic, demo-graphic, and health variables. Part 2 is devoted to each of these causes of undernutrition, or *nutrition impact vehicles,* as they were called in Chapter 1. The concept of food security demonstrates the interrelatedness of these nutrition impact vehicles, and with this in mind we begin Part 2.

□ 6

The Concept of
Food Security

The world has ample food. The growth of global food production has been faster than the unprecedented population growth of the past forty years. . . . Yet many poor countries and hundreds of millions of poor people do not share in this abundance. They suffer from a lack of food security, caused mainly by a lack of purchasing power.
—Reutlinger et al. 1986:1

In the early 1970s, rising fertilizer prices, spurred by the Organization of Petroleum Exporting Countries (OPEC) oil cartel, and a couple of years of lackluster grain harvests that included a bad crop year in the Soviet Union combined with gradually increasing demand to draw down worldwide grain reserves and send the price of grain skyrocketing. The spike in food prices during the early 1970s is illustrated in Figure 5.2. Worldwide end-of-crop-year stocks of wheat, coarse grains, and rice carried over to 1975 and 1976 were below 140 million metric tons (Gilmore & Huddleston 1983), whereas the carryovers of these grains in the 1980s generally ran some 300 million metric tons or more (FAO 1989:29).

In 1974, the shock of finding that "the global grain bin was nearly empty" (Gilmore & Huddleston 1983:31) channeled food-policy thinking in the direction of the security of national and international grain reserves. The phrase *food security* entered the literature, and food security was discussed as a problem of grain-importing nations (e.g., Chisholm & Tyers 1982).

But, as the worldwide food shortage seemed to evaporate in the 1980s, while the numbers of hungry remained high, the thinking on food security shifted from concern over national food supplies to concern over hungry people. Reutlinger and his colleagues (1986:1) captured this shift toward a concern for people when, in 1986, they defined food security as "access by all people at all times to enough food for an active, healthy life."

By focusing on people, food security thinkers sometimes shift the main emphasis concerning the world hunger problem away from food production and toward the purchasing power of those families at risk for undernutrition. We do not say that food production is no longer considered important in the hunger problem; it is. Food shortages result in high prices for food, which in turn make it difficult for the poor to purchase adequate supplies. A broader recognition now exists of the hunger problem: that food production, income of the poor, and a mix of other variables all influence the incidence of undernutrition.

■ THE FOOD SECURITY EQUATION

Anderson and Roumasset (1985) have developed a series of inequalities for conceptualizing the risk of food insecurity on a national scale. By adapting these inequalities to the household level, we can better understand the concept of food security as well as what delivers the risk of food insecurity to a household.

In its simplest form, the food security equation compares the value of the food production deficit in a household with the income and liquid assets that household has available to purchase food. Almost any household, even that of a landless worker, can raise *some* food at home, if nothing more than a tomato plant near the back door, so we can assume that any household at risk for food insecurity has a food production deficit that must be made up with food purchases. In simplest form, therefore, we can develop the food security equation as follows:

$$\text{Value of food production deficit in a household (HH)} \leq \text{Income and liquid assets available to purchase food}$$

The food production deficit in a household is that food needed, over and above any home production, in order to provide all household members at all times with enough food for an active, healthy life. The value of that deficit is simply the minimum cost of purchasing such a supply of food.

Families make decisions on how to allocate their expenditures among such competing needs as food, housing, clothing, medical care, and entertainment. The right-hand side of the equation says that, for food security, the income and liquid assets (including savings) available in the household's food budget must be at least enough to purchase enough food to cover the food production deficit.

A household becomes more food-secure when the right-hand side of the equation is bigger relative to the left. It becomes less food-secure when the left-hand side of the equation is bigger relative to the right. The risk of food insecurity is the probability that the left-hand side of the equation will be bigger than the right.

We said above that, by focusing on people, food security thinkers tended to shift the emphasis on the world hunger problem away from food production and toward the purchasing power of those families at risk for undernutrition. But the beauty of an equation is that it forces you to look at the balance between variables. In the food security equation, we concern ourselves not only with the right-hand side, the income and liquid assets available in the family's food purchase budget, but equally with the left-hand side, the value of the household's food production deficit. This left-hand side of the equation can be factored into two components, the food purchase requirement and the price of food, for the value of the food production deficit is the product of these two variables. So the equation can be rewritten as follows:

$$\begin{matrix} \text{Food purchase} \\ \text{requirement} \end{matrix} \times \begin{matrix} \text{Price of} \\ \text{food} \end{matrix} \leq \begin{matrix} \text{Income and liquid assets} \\ \text{available to purchase food} \end{matrix}$$

Now we can demonstrate how the price of food affects food security. If the price goes up, the left-hand side gets bigger, and we see a greater risk of food insecurity. If the price goes down, the risk of food insecurity is reduced.

The food purchase requirement in our equation can be shown as the difference between two factors: household food consumption requirement and household food production. The greater the household's food production the less the food purchase requirement; the smaller the household's food consumption requirement the smaller the food purchase requirement. We can rewrite the equation again:

$$\left\{ \begin{matrix} \text{HH food} \\ \text{consumption} \\ \text{requirement} \end{matrix} - \begin{matrix} \text{HH food} \\ \text{production} \end{matrix} \right\} \times \begin{matrix} \text{Price of} \\ \text{food} \end{matrix} \leq \begin{matrix} \text{Income and liquid} \\ \text{assets available} \\ \text{to purchase food} \end{matrix}$$

For any given family, to the extent that we can adopt policies to assure the left-hand side of the above equation is smaller than the right-hand side, we will reduce the risk of food insecurity. Therefore, it makes sense to examine each variable in the equation separately and to discuss what sorts of things influence it.

□ Household Food Consumption Requirement

The household food consumption requirement is affected by the number of people in the household and, as was pointed out earlier, by their age, sex, and working status. (Other things being equal, a family with few children will have an easier time feeding itself than a family with many children— a situation sometimes overlooked.) Because, as we discussed in Chapter 2, good health reduces the need for food, good health reduces the household food consumption requirement. Childbearing increases the food needs of the mother during pregnancy and lactation and thus increases the consumption requirement.

☐ Household Food Production

The poorest people in the world are generally landless, and the relationship between household production and food security is mainly relevant to families with land. Nevertheless, many families have no rights to farmland on which to grow small amounts of food around their houses or to keep a few productive scavenging animals such as chickens, ducks, a pig, a goat, or a cow.

The level of food production in a farming household is influenced by a complex set of variables including the amount and quality of land available and the education of the farm manager and his workers. The quantity and quality of technology and capital available is important; how this technology and capital are used is also important and is usually heavily influenced by a multitude of government incentives and disincentives that can include tariffs, export taxes, price controls, and subsidies of purchased inputs. Agricultural research and education have a powerful influence on quantity produced.

The level of food production of households taken together influences the next variable in the equation—the price of food.

☐ The Price of Food

The price of food is influenced by the quantity produced, as discussed above. But all that is on the supply side. The price of food is also influenced by the demand side: the size of the population as well as the per capita income and the tastes and preferences of consumers. Governments often attempt to influence the price of food with tariffs, export taxes, price controls, and subsidies of purchased inputs.

☐ Income and Liquid Assets Available to Purchase Food

The income and liquid assets position of a household is the result of complex factors, among them the education of its members, its capital position, its land position, its employment opportunities, attitudes toward work, the cost of transportation to and from work, and health.

From all of the above, we see that there are a multitude of influences on each of the variables in the food security equation.

■ IMPORTANCE OF THE FOOD SECURITY EQUATION

In much of the rest of this book we build on the concepts we introduced in the food security equation. Once you understand the food security equation and the influences on the variables within it, you will be well along the road to rational thinking about policies that can reduce the risk of food insecurity.

The food security equation is summarized in Box 6.1 on p. 100.

Box 6.1 The Concept of Food Security

$$
\begin{array}{l}
\text{Value of food production} \\
\text{deficit in a HH}
\end{array}
\quad \le \quad
\begin{array}{l}
\text{Income and liquid} \\
\text{assets available} \\
\text{to purchase food}
\end{array}
$$

$$
\begin{array}{l}
\text{Food purchase} \\
\text{requirement}
\end{array}
\;\times\;
\begin{array}{l}
\text{Price of} \\
\text{food}
\end{array}
\quad \le \quad
\begin{array}{l}
\text{Income and liquid} \\
\text{assets available} \\
\text{to purchase food}
\end{array}
$$

$$
\left\{
\begin{array}{l}
\text{HH food} \\
\text{consumption} \\
\text{requirement}
\end{array}
-
\begin{array}{l}
\text{HH food} \\
\text{production}
\end{array}
\right\}
\times
\begin{array}{l}
\text{Price of} \\
\text{food}
\end{array}
\quad \le \quad
\begin{array}{l}
\text{Income and liquid} \\
\text{assets available} \\
\text{to purchase food}
\end{array}
$$

You are more food-secure as the left-hand side gets smaller relative to the right, or as the right-hand side gets bigger relative to the left. The risk of food insecurity is the probability that the left-hand sides are bigger than the right.

Factors influencing each element in the final equation are listed below:

- HH food consumption requirement
    Number of people in household
    Age, sex, working status of individuals
    Health status of individuals
    Childbearing status (pregnant, lactating)
- HH food production
    A complex set including amount of land, technology, capital, education of farmer
    Government policies (tariffs, price controls, export taxes, input subsidies, research, etc.)
- Price of food
    Quantity produced
    Size of population
    Income of population
    Government policies (tariffs, price controls, export taxes, input subsidies, research, etc.)
- Income and liquid assets available to purchase food
    A complex set including education of members of household, capital position of household, land position, employment opportunities, attitudes toward work, transportation cost to and from work, and health

☐ 7

It Is Not
Food Versus Population

Land, unlike people, cannot be multiplied. . . . Unlike population, land does not breed.

—Heilbroner 1953:82 (paraphrasing Malthus)

■ THOMAS MALTHUS

The debate over food versus people started, you might say, with an argument between the young reverend Thomas Robert Malthus and his father. The elder Malthus was impressed by a recently published book that promised a future world devoid of "disease, anguish, melancholy, or resentment" (Godwin 1793). Young Thomas was not similarly impressed. In fact, he was so skeptical about such a utopian future that he wrote down his objections (Malthus 1803–1826). The father was so struck with Thomas's words that he encouraged his son to publish them (Heilbroner 1953:69–70). First issued anonymously in 1798 as *An Essay on the Principle of Population as It Affects the Future Improvement of Society*, Malthus's "essay" was never short and by its sixth edition, still claiming to be an essay, covered some 600 pages of detailed argument.

The Malthusian thesis postulated that the reproductive capacity of humans must put continual pressure on the "means of subsistence." Human numbers, he said, could increase by "geometric" progression: 2, 4, 8, 16, 32, 64, 128, 256 (we now call this progression *exponential*). Malthus did not see how subsistence could increase any faster than an "arithmetic" progression: 1, 2, 3, 4, 5, 6, 7, 8, 9 (we now call this progression *linear*). Unlike people, land does not breed, and Malthus thought that the potential for human numbers to increase exponentially must therefore put continuous pressure on our food supply.

Malthus enumerated a long list of checks to population growth, including war, "sickly seasons, epidemics, pestilence, and plague." Humans themselves, Malthus thought, would be unable to check their own population growth because the only way he knew how to limit family size was through, as he put it, "moral restraint." (The technology of contraception was next to nonexistent at the time.) And in Malthus's view, given the "passion between the sexes," moral restraint was not strong enough to effectively limit human fertility. Therefore, lurking in the shadows, always ready to impose the ultimate check on population growth, would have to be famine. "Famine stalks in the rear, and with one mighty blow, levels the population with the food of the world" (Heilbroner 1953:83).

There was plausibility to the Malthusian argument. It was, in fact, a precursor to the now widely accepted ecological principle that any population will expand until it fills the ecological niche available to it. What Malthus did not foresee was that there would eventually be other checks to human population growth besides war, pestilence, and famine; that changing attitudes about family size, a kind of "small is beautiful" philosophy, could combine with a new technology in the form of effective and simple contraception to limit population growth. Nor did he foresee the enormous increases in agricultural production that would accompany the application of science to farming.

Important as Malthus's book was for the thesis it espoused, it was more important as a stimulation to thinking among people who read it. Charles Darwin, for instance, reports that he happened to read Malthus "for amusement," yet this reading inspired the theory of natural selection and survival of the fittest that would dominate his *On the Origin of Species* (Bettany 1890; Herbert 1971).

Others were not amused. As one biographer put it, "Malthus was not ignored. For thirty years it rained refutations" (James Bonner, as quoted in Heilbroner 1953:76). In the storm of protest that followed the publication of his essay, Malthus was compared to Satan and denounced as an immoral, revolutionary, hard-hearted, and cruel atheist (Bettany 1890:ix). But the strongest refutation of the seeming inevitability of a perpetual tendency toward famine that Malthus postulated lies in what has happened since he wrote his essay.

Since 1800 the population of the world has, in fact, grown exponentially—dramatically so (Figure 7.1). On the other hand, the growth of world population seems destined to stop eventually through a process demographers call the demographic transition.

■ THE DEMOGRAPHIC TRANSITION

The world appears to be going through a pattern of growth known as the *demographic transition*. Originally described by Frank Notestein (his definition

Figure 7.1 Growth of Human Population

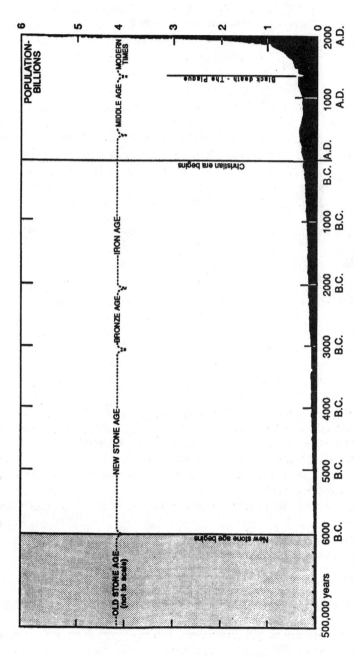

Source: The 0.002 percent estimate, Frejka 1973:15; figure is adapted from Cook 1962:5; other material taken from the Population Reference Bureau.

Note: It took many thousands of years of man's existence on earth for the population to reach a billion, around the year 1830. Up until about 1700 the human population had grown very slowly; the average rate was probably less than 0.002 percent per year. Then the growth rate began to gradually increase. In the early 1970s it rose above 2 percent, over 1,000 times the rate of growth of the ancients. In 1998 the world's population growth rate was down to 1.35 percent. Current projections are that world population growth should approach zero around the year 2100.

is found in Box 7.1), the literature contains a number of ways of defining the term. We adopt and paraphrase from a conceptualization by Carl Haub (1987:19) of the Population Reference Bureau in Washington, D.C.

The theory of demographic transition offers a general model for the gradual evolution of a population's birth and death rates from the preindustrial to the modern pattern, which results in an S-shaped curve of population growth through time. Sweden is illustrative of the transition, which goes through four stages:

Box 7.1   Terms Commonly Used by Demographers

Crude birth rate, or birth rate: The number of births per year per thousand individuals in the population

Crude death rate, or death rate: The number of deaths per year per thousand individuals in the population

Annual growth rate, or growth rate: Crude birth rate minus crude death rate divided by 10, which expresses the rate as a percentage

Doubling time: The number of years it takes the population to double, growing at the present annual growth rate, compounded. (You can figure out how long it will take a population to double, if it grows at a constant annual rate compounded, by dividing the number 70 by the annual, percentage, growth rate.)

Total fertility rate, or fertility rate: The total number of births a female has during her lifetime

Gross reproductive rate (GRR): The number of female children a newborn female will have during her lifetime if current levels of fertility by age of female continue through time

Net reproductive rate (NRR): The expected number of daughters per newborn female, after subjecting those newborn females to a given set of mortality rates. (NRR is lower than GRR because some of the newborn females will die before completing their reproductive years.)

Demographic transition: A pattern of population growth experienced by Western industrialized democracies and involving an S-shaped curve of total population change through time. Frank Notestein (1945) identified three stages in the transition: (1) High growth potential: birth and death rates are high, life expectancy is short, and population growth is slow; (2) transitional growth: birth rates remain high but death rates are falling; population growth rates increase, sometimes to the point that there is said to be a population explosion; (3) incipient decline: the birth rate follows the death rate downward; population continues to grow until birth rate reaches the death rate.

(continued)

Box 7.1 Continued

Population momentum: The tendency for population growth to continue beyond the time that replacement-level fertility has been achieved; that is, even after the net reproduction rate has reached one. The momentum of a population in any given year is measured as a ratio of the ultimate stationary population to the population of that year, given the assumption that fertility remains at replacement level. Using this definition, the *World Development Report 1989* provides population momentum figures for 129 countries and an example of how the calculation is done (World Bank 1989: 214–215).

Population pyramid: A graph of the population distribution according to age and sex. Two basic kinds of pyramids are used: The first type, a numerical pyramid (such as Figure 10.2), plots numbers of people in each age and sex group; the second, a relative pyramid (such as Figure 10.3), plots the percentage distribution of people according to age and sex. The major difference between the two kinds is that the numerical pyramid increases in area as the population grows, while the relative pyramid always maintains a constant area (you can think of it as 100 percent). Thus, the two kinds of pyramids may appear to exhibit different dynamic characteristics.

Age cohort, or cohort: All the people in a population within a given age range. (Each bar in a population pyramid represents a particular age cohort.)

Life expectancy at birth, or life expectancy: The average expected age of death of newborns who follow a given age-specific mortality schedule

Infant mortality rate: The number of babies who die during their first year of life per 1,000 babies born

Dependent children: (Usually) those people who are under 15 years old

Dependent adults: (Usually) those people who are 65 or over

Dependent population: Dependent children and dependent adults

Dependency ratio: The ratio of dependent to working-age adults—those from 15 to 65 (percentage of the population dependent divided by the percentage of working age)

Child dependency ratio: The ratio of the dependent children to working-age adults

1. Pre-industrial stage: Birth rates are high and fertility uncontrolled, with the birth rate exceeding the death rate and generally within the range of 25 to 45 per thousand. Periodic famines, plagues, and wars cause brief periods of population loss. Population grows, but slowly. In the decades before 1805, Sweden was in the last phase of this stage (Figure 7.2).

Figure 7.2   Birth and Death Rates, Sweden, 1751–1984

Rate per 1,000 population

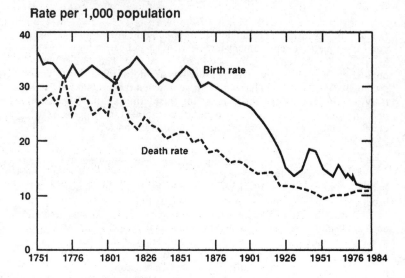

Source: Adapted from Haub 1987:20.

2. Mortality decline before fertility decline: With better public health
   services and more-reliable food and water supplies, death rates fall
   and life expectancy increases. If no accompanying decrease in the
   birth rate occurs, the population growth rate rises and population
   grows rapidly (in Sweden this period covers the 70 years between
   1805 and 1875).
3. Fertility decline: At some point, usually as the country urbanizes and
   industrializes, the birth rate decreases in response to desires to limit family size. Population continues to grow rapidly for a while. But eventually birth rates approach death rates, and population growth slows. The
   growth rate may even fall to zero or below. (The fertility decline in
   Sweden covers the one-hundred-year period between 1875 and 1975.)
4. Modern stage: By this point both the birth rate and death rate are
   low, around 12 per thousand. After the birth rate falls as low as the
   death rate, population size stabilizes if the total fertility rate remains at two children per woman. If the total fertility rate creeps up
   slightly from two, population size increases slowly, although family size remains small.

   In what are today's developed countries, the demographic transition is
essentially finished (look at recent birth [fertility] and death [mortality]
rates in the industrial market economies in the World Development Report

table on health [World Bank 1997:198–199). But the transition is only midway through in the Third World. Compare the demographic transition as shown in Figure 7.2 (with Sweden as representative of the developed world) and Figure 7.3 (with Mexico as representative of the Third World). The death rate decline in Sweden began shortly after 1800 and took approximately 150 years to fall from 30 to 10. The more dramatic death rate decline in Mexico did not begin until about 1915 and took only 40 years to fall to 10 per thousand. Birth rates in Mexico remained above 40 per thousand until the early 1970s, when they began a rapid decline. Consequently, by the early 1970s Mexico's population growth rate was above 3 percent, yielding a doubling time of fewer than 23 years.

The start of the rapid death rate decline in Mexico preceded that of most developing countries, which did not experience rapidly falling death rates until they benefited from the spread of modern medical and hygienic practices after World War II.

Although the Third World is in the fertility decline stage of the demographic transition, its dramatic death rate decline has produced a period of rapid Third World population growth that, according to authoritative projections, will raise world population levels many billions before the numbers stabilize. Figure 7.4 shows, for both the developed world and the world as a whole (whose population numbers are dominated by the population of the Third World), the S-shaped population growth curve expected from the completion of the demographic transition.

Figure 7.3   Birth and Death Rates, Mexico, 1895/99–1980/85

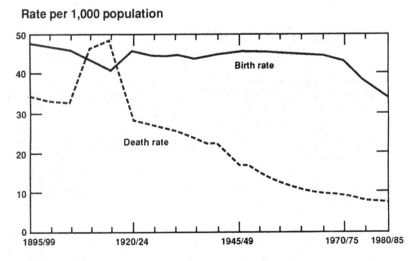

Source: Adapted from Haub 1987:20.

Figure 7.4   Past and Projected World Population, AD 1 to 2150

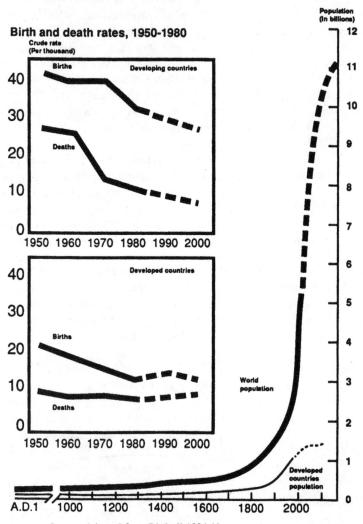

Source: Adapted from Birdsall 1984:11.

Lester Brown and Hal Kane point out a less happy road to population stabilization. Criticizing the optimistic view of demographic transition, they say:

As we approach the end of the twentieth century, a gap has emerged in the [demographic transition] analysis. The theorists did not say what happens when second stage population growth rates of 3 percent per year begin to overwhelm local life-support systems, making it impossible to sustain the economic and social gains that are counted on to reduce births. Unfortunately, trends that lead to ecological deterioration and economic decline are also self-reinforcing: Once populations expand to the point where their demands begin to exceed the sustainable yields of local forests, grasslands, croplands, or aquifers, they begin directly or indirectly to consume the resource base itself. . . .This . . . reduces food production and incomes, triggering a downward spiral in a process we describe as the demographic trap. All countries will complete the demographic transition, reaching population stability with low death and birth rates, or will get caught in the demographic trap, which eventually will also lead to demographic stability—but with high birth rates and high death rates (Brown & Kane 1994:55–56).

Nevertheless, there seems to be evidence that reduced growth rates predicted by the theory of demographic transition are coming to pass. Data from the U.S. Census on the world population show clearly that the rate of growth in population has declined gradually but substantially since the early 1960s. (Note that the rates of growth are still positive—world population continues to grow; but the *rate* of growth is slowing over time.) In addition, the U.S. Census predicts that the rates of growth in population will continue to decline for the next 50 years.

If the world's population growth does, in fact, stop as projected, humans will have succeeded in controlling their own numbers without war, pestilence, and famine—something Malthus did not expect.

■ PROJECTIONS OF FUTURE WORLD POPULATION

As we consider the future prospects for world food supply and demand, we think first of population. How many mouths will there be to feed? The U.S. Census Bureau, basing its statistics on the growth rates shown in Figure 7.5, projects that by the year 2050, world population will be about 9.35 billion, 60 percent higher than the current (1997) population of 5.85 billion (see Table 7.1).

The UN has also made population projections into the future. The UN projections are based on assumptions about how the life expectancy will change in the future, and about how fertility rates will change.

Life expectancy at birth is assumed to increase as average nutrition continues to improve, and as average incomes continue to rise. For males, if a country's life expectancy is less than 60 years, it is assumed that life expectancy will increase at about 0.5 years per year. In other words, if boys born in 1996 have a life expectancy of 54, boys born in 1997 are projected to have a life expectancy of 54.5, and boys born in 2000 are projected to have a life expectancy of 56. After life expectancy in a country reaches 60 years, its rate of increase begins to slow down. The figures for females are similar.

Figure 7.5 Annual Growth Rate of the World Population, Historical and Projected, 1950–2049

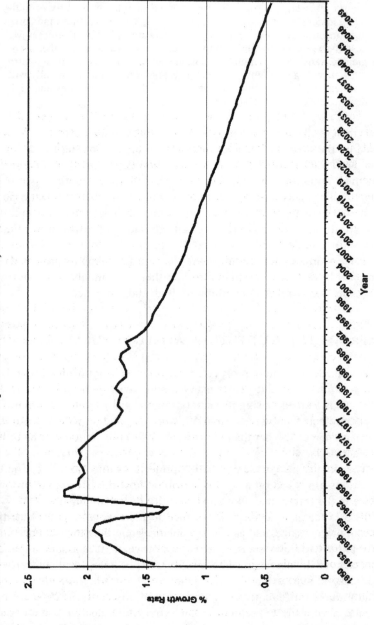

Source: U.S. Census Bureau.

Table 7.1   Population in the Year 2050: Four Projections

Projection	Population Size in 2050 (millions)	Percentage Increase from 1997	Average Annual Rate of Growth (%)
UN low variant	7,900	37	0.568
U.S. Census Bureau	9,350	61	0.889
UN medium variant	9,850	70	0.988
UN high variant	11,900	105	1.349

These assumptions mean that life expectancies are projected to increase substantially in some parts of the world. Babies born in Africa in 2050 are expected to live 20 years longer than babies of their grandparents' generation born in 1990 (FAO technical paper 10 for the World Food Summit). This may sound like quite a dramatic increase. But life expectancy has increased by substantial amounts in other areas: Life expectancy in Saudi Arabia increased from 53.9 years from 1970 to 1975 to 69.7 years from 1990 to 1995; in Indonesia, the increase over the same period was 13.4 years, from 50.3 to 65.2; in South America as a whole, the increase was from 60.7 to 68.5 over the same twenty-year period (World Resources Institute 1997). The UN's assumption is, therefore, within the range of historical experience.

It is more difficult to make reasonable assumptions about future levels of fertility. As a result of this difficulty, the UN presents three possible scenarios, or *variants*. The *medium variant* assumes that fertility declines (from its current level of about three children born to an average woman of childbearing age) until it reaches a *replacement* level of 2.1 children per woman. (This is the number of children each woman would give birth to, on average, to ensure that two children survived to puberty. Even if the fertility rate fell to the replacement level, population would continue to grow because of increases in life expectancy.) In the *high variant*, fertility is assumed to decline until it reaches 2.6 children per woman. In the *low variant*, fertility is assumed to decline until it reaches 1.6.

Again, to put these projections in historical context, let us examine recent experience. For the world as a whole, fertility rates dropped from 4.5 in 1970–1975 to 3.1 in 1990–1995. In Asia, where economic growth has been exceptionally strong in the last 20 years, fertility rates dropped from 5.1 in the early 1970s to 3.0 in the early 1990s. In Europe, fertility was at the replacement rate of 2.1 in the early 1970s; over the next 20 years, the number dropped to 1.6 (World Resources 1997). Thus, the UN's low variant assumption is that fertility worldwide will drop to levels currently observed in Europe.

Based on these assumptions, the UN's three population projections are shown in Table 7.1. The medium variant is quite close to the U.S. Census Bureau's prediction.

As of this writing, in the late 1990s, the specter of AIDS hangs over any discussion of future population. The UN estimates that at the end of 1996 about 22 million adults and three-quarters of a million children were infected with the virus (human immunodeficiency virus or HIV) that causes AIDS. Although the world hopes that medical science can make progress on AIDS treatment, it is still the prognosis that almost all of these 22–23 million people will die from AIDS during the next five to ten years. To put this number in perspective, recall that over 50 million people died in 1995 from all causes. If all HIV-positive people died within five years, that would increase the number of deaths during the period by about 10 percent. One review of the literature concludes:

> At the world level, AIDS is unlikely to suppress population size or growth rates. However, the impact of AIDS may be felt by some individual countries. For example, the U.S. Bureau of the Census predicts that in some countries populations in 2020 will be considerably smaller as a result of the AIDS pandemic—45 percent smaller in Uganda, 35 percent in Rwanda, and 30 percent in Malawi (Lynn Brown 1997).

■ CURRENT TRENDS IN PER CAPITA FOOD PRODUCTION

Not only did Malthus not expect humans to willfully control their own population size, he did not expect our food supply to keep up with a dramatic, exponential growth in our population. The last half of the twentieth century experienced the most rapid growth of population in the entire history of the world, yet during this period of breakneck population growth, food production grew even faster; so per capita food production gradually increased.

The factors contributing to growth in food production will be discussed in Chapter 11. Here we simply note the facts: Food production has continued to grow faster than population. As Figure 7.6 shows, worldwide food production per capita has increased steadily over the past 35 years, growing about 5 percent per decade. Food production per capita in the developed world, where population growth is slow, has grown much more rapidly. In the developing world, food supply grew faster than population from the early 1960s until 1990. Since 1990, food production has continued to grow, but at a slower pace than population, so production per capita has declined.

A World Bank Study (Mundlak, Larson & Crego 1996) concludes that worldwide food supply is growing faster than food demand: "Has supply lagged demand? If that were so, agricultural prices would have risen. They didn't." They find that median price to farmers dropped by 0.61 percent during the 1967–1992 period, and that 71 percent of world production

Figure 7.6   Indexes of Food Output per Capita, Selected Country Groups, 1961–1997

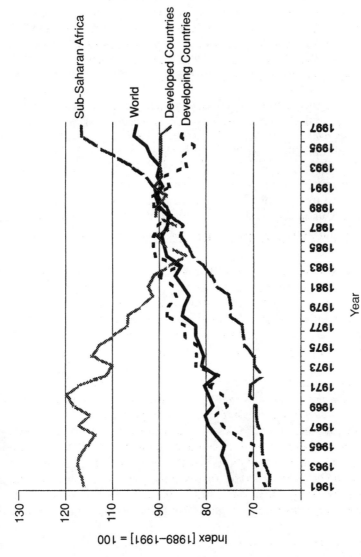

Source: FAO statistics.

from 1967 to 1992 came from countries in which (inflation-adjusted) farm prices fell. This study finds that median growth rate in agricultural production was 2.25 percent per year. (*Median growth rate* means that one-half of the world's food production takes place in countries with agricultural growth rates of less than 2.25 percent.) The study confirms that in most countries, per capita agricultural production grew—food became more plentiful.

FAO data on nutrient availability per capita also shows steady improvement. As Figure 7.7 shows, since 1961, worldwide calories per capita have increased over 20 percent, from 2,235 calories per person per day to 2,712 calories per person per day. Similarly, protein availability has increased about 17 percent to 72.4 grams per person per day. These levels of nutrients are sufficient for an adequate diet for the average person. One interpretation of this states that *if the world's food supply were evenly divided among the people of the world, there would be enough food for everybody.*

So an important question in a discussion of the incidence and permanence of world hunger is how the world's food supplies are allocated among the people of the world. In the next chapter, we look at purchasing power—and its components, income and food prices—as the immediate problem explaining why certain people in the world are unable to afford adequate nutrition.

Figure 7.7 Indexes of Nutrient Availability per Capita, Worldwide, 1960–1995

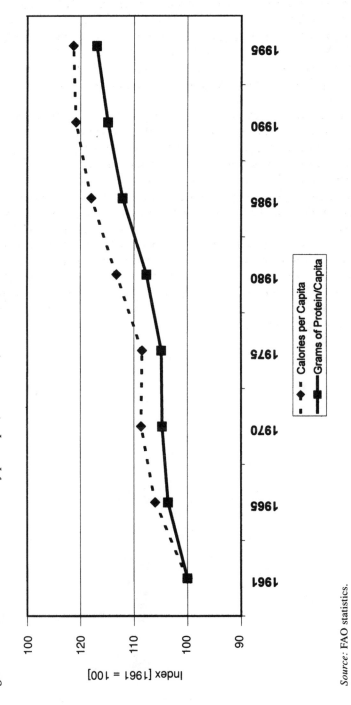

Source: FAO statistics.

□ 8

Purchasing Power:
Income and the Price of Food

Anti-hunger efforts need to focus on the poor, wherever they are: the urban underemployed and unemployed, the rural landless, the rural farmers with inadequate land or other resources. Targeted efforts to alleviate hunger thus need to use poverty as their main criterion, rather than focusing on a particular sector of the economy or region of the country. Similarly, the alleviation of poverty should be the criterion of success.
—Rogers 1988a

■ WHO ARE THE POOR?

There is widespread agreement that a leading cause of undernutrition is low purchasing power or poverty. The World Bank (1996) lists nine countries with per capita income of less than $200 and 52 countries with per capita income of less than $800. It's hard for most of us to imagine how a person could feed herself on a little over $2.00 per day. And people have needs besides food. Merely to survive, a person needs clothing, shelter, cooking fuel, and cooking utensils.

Who are the poorest of the poor? They live in the Third World. They are landless or nearly so. If they do have a bit of land, typically they earn more than half their livelihood working for others. Whether they live packed tightly into city slums or sprinkled across the countryside, they are poorly educated, often illiterate, and commonly superstitious. When employed, they accept the most menial of jobs. Some are subsistence fishermen. Some live in relative isolation in upland farming areas. Often they are squatters, neither owning nor renting the land on which they put up their huts. Their food larder is usually almost empty.

Box 8.1   Could You Survive for a Year on $100 Worth of Food?

Could one adult survive for a year on what it might cost a couple to eat dinner in a good restaurant?

Let us assume a very simple diet, yet one not far from what some of the world's poorest live on: corn grits and cooking oil. Actually no one probably lives on a diet that is this simple. People switch from one food to another as prices change during the year, they pick leaves and munch on them as they walk through the countryside, and they vary their diet on special days like holy days. But the basic diet of the world's poorest comes close to this level of simplicity.

Take the 3,000 calorie recommendation for a moderately active adult male, found in both the FAO and National Academy of Sciences recommendations, and, using the Philippine prices in Table 2.2, do some arithmetic. We will provide 2,400 calories as corn grits and 600 as cooking oil, yielding a diet that is just over 20 percent fat and provides 57 grams of protein daily. A thousand calories of corn grits costs P 1.11, so 2,400 (663 g) would cost 2.66. Multiply this by 365 (days per year) and you have P 970 per year for grits.

The fat makes the diet a lot more palatable (and healthier too, since you need linoleic acid, found in vegetable fat, for survival). The tables of recommended amounts do not include fat because fat adequacy is not normally a problem. However, you do need more fat in the diet than would be supplied by corn grits alone. To get 600 calories as fat you need 67 grams of cooking oil (there are 9 calories per gram of fat), which, at P 2 per 100 grams, will cost P 1.24. Multiplying by 365 gives P 452 per year.

The annual cost of this diet is P 1,424 or about $72. Nobody is going to claim that this is a balanced diet. It is short on iron and vitamins, especially the B vitamins, but it provides more calories than some of the poorest people on earth eat, and its deficiencies are representative of common Third World nutritional deficiencies.

Their households are often fragmented, with one or more members away trying to find work so they can send money home. They may be in debt, to wealthier relatives, to friends, to employers, or to the local moneylenders. The household head is often young, not yet having found good employment, but already burdened with the responsibility of raising children. (For a good essay on the poor of a particular region, see Carner 1984.)

■ THE IMPORTANCE OF ELASTICITY

Purchasing power equals income divided by price. Purchasing power can therefore be increased by increases in income or by decreases in prices. (For a simple illustration of the concept, see Box 8.2.)

Box 8.2   Purchasing Power
Equals Income Divided by Price

Purchasing power can be upgraded by increases in income or by decreases in price. A simple illustration shows how important both income and price are in determining purchasing power. Suppose you spend all your income on purchasing rice; now consider the following three situations.

	Income	Price of Rice per Kilogram	Kilograms Purchased
A	$100	$0.20	500
B	$200	$0.20	1,000
C	$100	$0.10	1,000

Start with situation A. By doubling income from situation A to situation B, you can double the amount purchased. But you can accomplish exactly the same increase in purchasing power by cutting the price of the rice in half, as in going from situation A to situation C.

In the real world, prices and incomes are constantly changing, with corresponding changes in purchasing power. As purchasing power changes, people make changes in their spending patterns. Some of the changes they make involve food purchases that, in turn, influence people's nutritional status. As a result, policymakers concerned with nutrition must be concerned with the income of the poor as well as with the price of the food they eat. And to know the nutritional impact of policies that affect income and prices, they need to know how people change their spending as prices and incomes change.

By making use of consumption surveys taken at different times, we can learn how people's purchasing patterns change in response to changes in prices and income. How much, and in what directions, they change their purchasing in response to certain changes in prices and income is called their *elasticity of demand,* or, for short, their *demand elasticity.* Understanding changes in food consumption that result from changes in prices or income is so important to nutrition policymaking that we devote the rest of this chapter to the concept of elasticity.

■ **TYPES OF ELASTICITY**

In 1973 the Soviets, after a bad harvest, entered the world grain market and for the first time bought substantial quantities of wheat. Around the world, prices responded. In the United States, the prospects of high livestock feed prices sent up the price of beef, and consumers drastically cut back beef consumption. Some even organized boycotts of beef at supermarkets. The change in consumption of beef resulting from this change in price was an expression of the elasticity of demand for beef with respect to price. This type of response is often called *own-price elasticity,* because it is about a change in the consumption of a commodity caused by a change in its own price.

At the same time people were boycotting beef, they were looking around for substitutes, or at least ways to stretch the more limited quantities of beef they were purchasing. Many turned to Italian foods such as spaghetti, ravioli, and pizza, which are usually laced liberally with tomato paste. Tomato paste became scarce and its price shot up. The tomato paste consumption response to the change in the price of beef is called an expression of *cross-price elasticity* because it shows the consumption response to a change in the price of something across the marketplace.

A change in your consumption of, say, orange juice, as a result of a change in your income would be an expression of *income elasticity of demand.* In most cases we expect consumption of a product to increase as income increases, whereas increases in price are expected to decrease consumption. Those few products for which people decrease consumption as their income increases are called *inferior goods.*

Recapitulating the above, we find three kinds of demand elasticity: own-price; cross-price; and income. We will deal mostly with the two most important—own-price elasticity and income elasticity. On occasion we will refer to own-price elasticity simply as price elasticity.

Because the consumption response to a change in the price of a commodity, such as rice, is different from the consumption response to a change in income, we need to examine income and price elasticity of demand separately.

☐ **Income Elasticity of Demand**

How food consumption changes with income. In simplest terms, income elasticity of demand is the percentage change in the consumption of something, such as rice, when a 1 percent change occurs in income. You can easily see that this elasticity will change depending on your income level. If a poverty-stricken Indian villager suffered a 1 percent decrease in income, he might decrease his consumption of rice by half a percent or so. But a wealthy stockbroker who suffered a 1 percent decrease in income might not change her rice consumption at all! (She might spend less on recreational travel, for instance. But this is getting ahead of our story.)

Let us look at some general ways in which food consumption changes as income rises or falls. Table 8.1 provides an illustration, for a Third World country, of how consumption of calories and protein increases as income increases or decreases. (In Table 8.1, expenditure subgroup is used as a proxy for income category.) The table, by the way, provides yet another illustration of the relationship between low income and undernutrition.

In Figure 8.1, more general than Table 8.1, we see differences in food consumption, converted to an equivalent amount of cereal grains, as income changed in a number of countries between 1966 and 1982. The curve is a best-fit trend line for the data. Notice how the rate of increase in consumption falls off as income increases. What is happening is that the proportion of the household budget spent on food decreases as income increases. The first person to write about this was Ernst Engel, and the phenomenon has become known as *Engel's law.*

In Figure 8.2 we can see, in some detail, changes in food consumption patterns associated with changes in income for a low-income region of East Java, Indonesia. Only the families in the top half of the income groupings (the right-hand half of Figure 8.2a) were receiving at least the 1,900 calories cited in Table 8.1 as the minimum appropriate for Indonesians. Figure 8.2b provides a second illustration of Engel's law: As income rises, the percentage of income spent for food declines from 75 for the lowest-income families in the sample population to 60 for the highest-income families. Figure 8.2c shows how the food expenditure mix changes as income increases. As income grows, the East Javanese spend a smaller proportion of their food budget on starchy staples—cassava, rice, maize, and wheat

Table 8.1   Calorie and Protein Intake Estimated from the Fifth National Socioeconomic Survey (Susenas V), All Indonesia, 1976

Expenditure Subgroup (Rupiahs per Capita per Month)	Percentage of Total Population	Calories per Capita per Day	Grams Protein per Capita
Less than 2,000	15.3 }39.1	1,387	22.2
2,000–2,999	23.8	1,870	32.3
3,000–3,999	19.5	2,034	40.2
4,000–4,999	13.6	2,084	47.0
5.000–5,999	8.8	2,288	52.7
6,000–7,999	9.4	2,533	60.9
8,000–9,999	4.2	2,794	69.7
10,000–14,999	3.8	3,066	79.1
Over 15,000	1.6	3,284	93.3
Total	100		
Average		2,064	43.3

Source: Hutabarat 1990, as quoted in Dixon 1982:6.

Note: Dixon (1982:4) reports that minimum nutritional requirements for Indonesia are 1,900 calories and 39.2 grams of protein per day, based on the 1973 FAO/WHO recommendations and the distribution by age and body weight of Indonesians. Groups below that amount can therefore be considered undernourished. Note that, because of wastage in marketing and preparation, the amount available for consumption must be greater than the actual calorie or protein intake. For Indonesia, the minimal daily requirements of food available are 2,100 calories and 45.9 grams of protein. In 1976 the exchange rate for rupiahs were U.S. $1 = Rp 145.

Figure 8.1   Food Consumption and Income, Selected Countries, 1966–1982

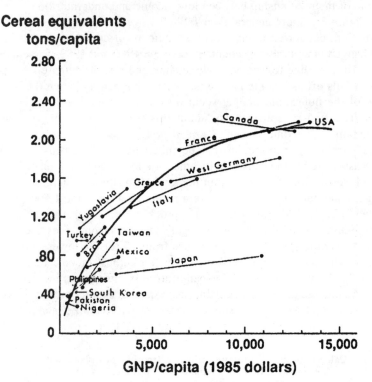

Source: Adapted from Rask 1986.

flour—and a larger proportion on other items, especially animal products. This phenomenon is called *Bennett's law,* which states that the *starchy staple ratio* (the ratio of starchy foods such as cereals and root crops to other foods in the diet) falls as income increases. Figure 8.2d shows how the energy derived from various food sources shifts as income rises. The lowest-income people in the sample derive half their food energy from cassava (see Box 8.3); but as income rises, they quickly substitute other foods, especially rice, for cassava.

Commodities such as cassava, which people consume less of as their incomes rise, are known by the ignominious name of *inferior goods.* In Figure 8.3, we see that, for the world as a whole, diet changes follow Bennett's law. Starchy staple carbohydrates make up about 75 percent of the dietary calories of the lowest-income countries and only 30 percent of the dietary calories of the highest-income countries. For the world as a whole, then, the cereals and root crops are inferior goods. Contrast this income consumption response to the change in consumption of fats and sugars as income increases.

Figure 8.2   Relationships Between Income Level and Nutritional Status, East
Java, 1977–1978

a. Energy (Kcal)

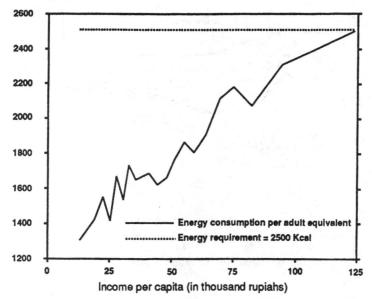

Income per capita (in thousand rupiahs)

b. Food expenditures (percentage of income)

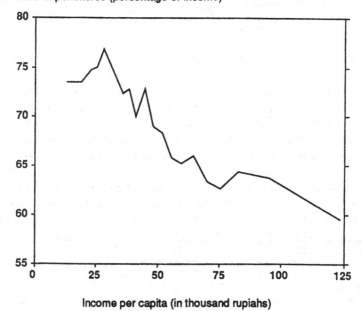

Income per capita (in thousand rupiahs)

(continued)

Figure 8.2   Continued

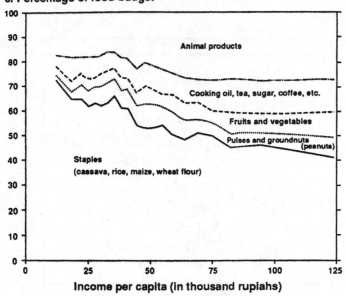

c. Percentage of food budget

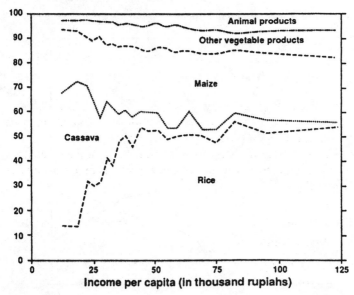

d. Percentage of total energy consumption

Source: Ho 1984.
   Note: Income is shown in thousands of Rupiahs. An income of Rs. 125,000 in 1977/78 was worth something over $200. The study region included Madura and the nearby regency of Sidorajo.

Box 8.3 Cassava

Cassava is a common food source in the tropics, especially among low-income people. It is a member of the spurge family (genus *Manihot*) and, in Africa, is usually called manioc. The fleshy rootstock is high in the starch known to English speakers as tapioca.

One source (Indonesia Oleh Direktorat Gizi Department Kesehatan R. I. 1979:19) gives the major nutritional constituents for 100 grams of dried cassava as: calories, 338; protein, 1.5 g; fat, 0.7 g; and carbohydrate, 81.3 g. There is some feeling among nutritionists that the protein in cassava is largely unavailable. If this is the case, consuming cassava is very close to consuming straight starch.

In the tropics cassava is so easy to grow it has been called "the Lazy Man's Crop." If you want some, just cut a foot or so of stalk from a live plant and stick it in the ground where it can get plenty of sunshine and some rain. Wait six to nine months and dig up the rootstock. The tuberous roots will keep only a week or so out of the ground, but if you are in no hurry do not dig it up; it will usually store for a year or so in the ground. Thus it can be used as insurance against famine during periods of food scarcity.

It is unfortunate that cassava leaves are seldom eaten, for they are high in vitamin A.

To some people, a full-grown cassava plant resembles a miniature papaya tree, while to others it looks more like an overgrown marijuana plant.

The charts shown so far in this chapter certainly do not define the diet for every individual in each of the income categories shown. They do, however, identify clear tendencies toward changes in consumption patterns with changes in income.

Quantifying income elasticities. As we said earlier, income elasticity of demand is the percentage change in the consumption of something, such as rice, when there is a 1 percent change in income.

For very small changes in income—for instance, when the percentage change in income is 1 percent or less—we can express income elasticity of demand algebraically as:

$$E = \frac{\%\text{ change in consumption}}{\%\text{ change in income}} = \frac{\dfrac{QD_2 - QD_1}{QD_1}}{\dfrac{Income_2 - Income_1}{Income_1}}$$

where: E = Elasticity of demand with respect to income

QD_1 = Quantity demanded at old income level (Income 1)

QD_2 = Quantity demanded at new income level (Income 1)

Figure 8.3   Percentage of Calories Derived from Fats, Carbohydrates, and Proteins by Annual GNP per Capita, 1962

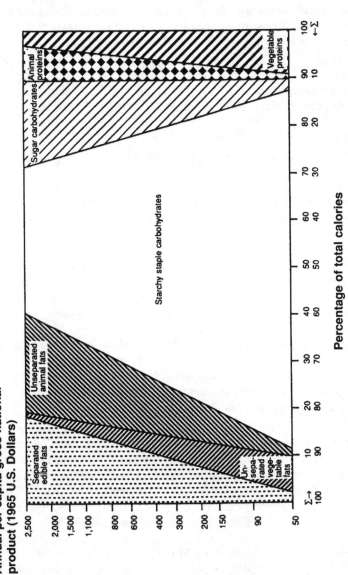

Source: Adapted from Perisse et al. 1969:2.

Note: The regression is based on 85 countries. The GNP data are shown with a ratio scale. Separated edible fats are fats that have been separated from their original source such as butter (made from milk) or peanut oil (made from peanuts). Unseparated fats are fats consumed with their natural carrier such as the butterfat in whole milk (unseparated animal fat) or peanut oil in whole peanuts (unseparated vegetable fat).

In the real world of constantly changing incomes and prices, trying to estimate demand elasticities is a lot more difficult than the above equation suggests. I leave descriptions of how this is done to others (e.g., Deaton & Muellbauer 1980; Huang 1985; Johnson, Hassan & Green 1984). For purposes of this discussion we accept elasticity estimates done by others and concentrate on their meaning and implications for policy planners.

T. J. Ho (1984) calculated income elasticity for the East Javanese consumers whose food consumption patterns were outlined in Figure 8.2. She found the income elasticity of expenditure on food to be 0.58. That is, for this community, a 1 percent increase in income will produce a 0.58 percent increase in spending for food.

For purposes of illustration, let us hypothesize that this community spends half its income on food and, to make the computations simple, let us assume that its income is $100. A 1 percent increase in income raises income to $101. If food spending increases by 0.58 percent, these people will spend 29 cents more on food, for a total of $50.29. The remaining 71 cents of increased income will be spent on nonfood items, bringing the total for that category (housing, clothing, paying off debts, etc.) to $50.71. We can deduce, therefore, that the income elasticity of demand for nonfood items in this community is 1.42.

Had this community increased its spending on food by exactly the same percentage (and in this case exactly the same dollar amount) as its spending on nonfood items, that would indicate that the income elasticity of demand for both food and nonfood items is exactly one (1.0).

In a 1992 paper, Bouis and Haddad review the literature and report a wide range of calorie-income elasticities, from 0.01 in Nicaragua to 1.18 in India. They argue that the wide range is attributable in large part to the different methods different studies use to collect data on calories and the different conceptual measures they have of "income." They conclude that if appropriate measures are used, elasticity estimates fall in the 0.08–0.14 range.

Ho estimates the income elasticity of demand for calories to be 0.28 and for protein to be 0.52. These elasticities condense some of the information in Figure 8.2d. Review this graph and notice again how these people are substituting rice for cassava as their incomes increase. To a lesser extent, they are substituting animal products and other vegetable products for cassava at the same time. Calories from cassava are cheaper than calories from rice, other vegetables, or meat. Therefore, as they increase their spending on food, they buy fewer calories per rupiah and more of other food properties like protein and flavor. That is what the income elasticity figures (low for calories and high for protein) are telling us.

If you find this hard to grasp, here is another way of looking at those elasticity figures for calories versus protein. A 1 percent increase in income yields only a 0.28 percent increase in consumption of calories but a more generous 0.52 percent increase in protein consumption. That is, as income changes, these people change their consumption of protein more (in percentages) than they change their consumption of calories. While you could easily have come to this conclusion without the aid of the elasticity figures, what you get from the elasticity calculations is how much the people of East Java change their consumption of these two nutrients when income changes. That is the beauty—and the importance—of elasticity! It quantifies things.

Of course, people do not go to the market and buy nutrients like calories and protein. They buy food. So let us look at some income elasticity figures for particular commodities and see how these elasticities change with income.

How income elasticity changes as income changes. Table 8.2 shows some income elasticities for three income groups in rural Brazil. Notice that, except for cassava flour, the income elasticity figures are positive. That is, for most foods, consumption increases as income increases. Cassava flour, with a negative income elasticity, is an inferior good.

Notice also that the absolute value (value without regard to sign) of the numbers in this table tends to decrease from low- to high-income consumers. That is, food consumption among low-income consumers is considerably more responsive to changes in income than it is among high-income consumers. This phenomenon is found among all Third World populations.

When the low-income consumer in the Brazilian sample receives a 1 percent increase in income, he tends to increase his rice consumption by about 2 percent. But the high-income consumer tends to change his consumption of rice by less than two-tenths of a percent when his income

Table 8.2   Income Elasticities for Calorie Intake, Selected Foods, by Income Group, Rural Brazil, 1974–1975

	Income Group		
	Lowest 30 Percent	Middle 50 Percent	Highest 20 Percent
Cassava flour	−3.50	−1.59	−.356
Rice	1.99	.172	.173
Milk	2.27	.147	.172
Eggs	1.93	.630	.114
Mean per capita calorie intake	1,963	2,432	2,771

Source: Gray 1982:26.
Note: The 1974–1975 National Household Expenditure Survey (ENDEF) of the Brazilian Geographical and Statistical Institute was used as the data base from which to calculate these income elasticities.

changes by 1 percent. We call the low-income family's consumption response on rice *elastic*. That is, a 1 percent change in income yields a greater than 1 percent change in consumption. On the other hand, we call the high-income family's consumption response on rice *inelastic*. A 1 percent change in its income produces a less than 1 percent change in consumption. If a family changed its consumption of rice by exactly 1 percent when its income changed by 1 percent, we would say it had an income elasticity of demand for rice of one—neither elastic nor inelastic.

Remember that the elasticity figures show percentage change in consumption with a 1 percent change in income. The income elasticity of demand for rice in rural Brazil is about the same as the income elasticity of demand for eggs. But because rice makes up 15 percent of the total calories consumed among this income group, and eggs only one-half of 1 percent, a 1 percent change in income results in a far greater change in actual consumption of rice than of eggs (see Table 8.3). The nutritional significance of an elasticity, therefore, depends not only on the magnitude of the elasticity but on the magnitude of consumption of the goods under consideration.

□ Price Elasticity of Demand

How food consumption changes with price. As we noted in Box 8.2, purchasing power can be increased either by an increase in income or a decrease in price. The consumption response to a decline in the price of a food item can be complex. Let us think about what might happen to consumption among the poorest 30 percent, in terms of income, in Brazil if the price of rice were to fall substantially.

A fall in the price of rice would likely result in the consumption of more rice. But it might well be that not all the increased purchasing power

Table 8.3   Changes in Calorie Consumption Resulting from a 1 Percent Increase in Income, Selected Foods, Lowest 30 Percent of Consumers by Income, Rural Brazil, 1974–1975

	Kilo-Calories	Percentage of Total Kilocalories Consumed	Income Elasticity	Change in Kilocalories Consumed Resulting from a 1 Percent Increase in Income
Cassava flour	440	22.4	–3.50	–15.4
Rice	296	15.1	1.99	5.9
Milk	41	2.1	2.27	.9
Eggs	7	.5	1.93	.1
Other	1,152	59.9		
Total kilocalorie intake	1,963		.46	1,940
Total change in entire diet				9

Source: Calculated from Gray 1982:20, 26.

that results from a fall in the price of rice will be spent on rice. Some of it might be spent on purchasing more of other foods, such as eggs, and some of it might be spent on purchasing nonfood items, such as entertainment.

This percentage change in rice consumption as a result of a 1 percent change in the price of rice is its own-price elasticity. The percentage changes in the consumption of a variety of other things, from eggs to entertainment, resulting from a 1 percent change in the price of rice (a fall in price, in this case) are the cross-price elasticities of demand.

Cross-price elasticities tend to be small. The cross-commodity price impact of a change in the price of rice, for instance, may be spread across a multitude of goods and services. Data on cross-price elasticities are harder to come by and may be less reliable than income and own-price elasticities. Furthermore, much sound analysis of the nutritional impact of policy alternatives can be done with what we know about income and own-price elasticities. Therefore, as mentioned earlier, in this book we will not deal much with cross-price elasticities.

Quantifying own-price elasticities. Remember that price elasticity of demand is the percentage change in consumption of something, like rice, when a 1 percent change occurs in its own price.

For very small changes in price (for instance, when the percentage change in income is 1 percent or less) we can algebraically express elasticity of demand with respect to price as

$$E = \frac{\text{\% change in consumption}}{\text{\% change in price}} = \frac{\dfrac{QD_2 - QD_1}{QD_1}}{\dfrac{Price_2 - Price_1}{Price_1}}$$

where: E = Elasticity of demand with respect to price
QD_1 = Quantity demanded at old price
QD_2 = Quantity demanded at new price

As with income elasticity of demand, estimating these elasticities is a lot more difficult than the above equation suggests. So again we leave descriptions of how this is done to others.

Table 8.4 shows a set of income and price elasticities for major food groups in Indonesia. These figures are for the complete spectrum of incomes, not broken down by income groups. Notice that for Indonesian society as a whole, all the income elasticities are positive and all the price elasticities are negative. This is normal.

Elasticities quantify consumers' behavior in the face of changing purchasing power. If income increases 1 percent, you can expect most consumption responses to be positive. But if price increases 1 percent, you can

Table 8.4   Income and Price Elasticities for Selected Foods, Indonesia

	Income Elasticity	Own-Price Elasticity
Corn and cassava	.3	−.26
Spices	.3	−.25
Rice	.7	−.63
Coconut	1.1	−.88
Tea and coffee	1.1	−.90
Vegetables and fruits	1.2	−.97
Prepared food	1.2	−1.01
Fish	1.3	−1.04
Sugar	1.4	−1.15
Drinks	2.1	−1.71
Livestock and livestock products	2.2	−1.73

Source: Boediono 1978:362.

expect the usual consumption response to be negative. It is so common for price elasticities to be negative that the minus sign is often omitted. We will use the minus sign when quoting specific price elasticities to remind you of the inverse relationship between change in price and change in consumption.

Elasticity figures show you the relative importance consumers attach to the various foods in their diets. Items considered essential or necessary tend to have elasticities below one. Think of it this way: When income falls by 1 percent, consumption of necessities falls by less than 1 percent. Or if the price of a necessity rises by 1 percent, consumption falls by less than 1 percent. From Table 8.4 it appears that, by and large, Indonesians regard corn and cassava, spices, and rice as necessities.

Conversely, items considered luxuries tend to have elasticities above one. If income falls by 1 percent, the consumption of luxuries falls by more than 1 percent as people cut back on luxuries and concentrate what income is left on necessities. If the price of a luxury rises by 1 percent, people are more likely to cut back substantially on consumption of that luxury than if the price of a necessity rises by 1 percent. Table 8.4 shows that Indonesians generally regard livestock and livestock products as luxuries. This is commonly the case in Third World countries.

How price elasticities change as income changes. Per Pinstrup-Andersen and colleagues (1976; Pinstrup-Andersen & Caicedo 1978) were the first to show that one could estimate price (and income) elasticities by income groups as well as by the community as a whole. They divided their Cali, Colombia, sample population into five income groups, and estimated elasticities for each income group as well as for their entire sample. Some of the elasticities calculated in their path-breaking study are shown in Table 8.5.

Notice how responsiveness to change in price generally diminishes as you move from low-income to high-income consumers. From this table it appears that high-income consumers in Cali could not care less about

Table 8.5   Estimated Direct Price Elasticity of Demand by Income Group, Cali, Colombia, 1969–1970

	Low Income			High Income		
	I	II	III	IV	V	Average
Cassava	−.23	−.28	−.25	−.00	−.00	−.19
Potatoes	−.41	−.42	−.31	−.00	−.00	−.26
Rice	−.43	−.40	−.40	−.26	−.18	−.35
Maize	−.63	−.55	−.44	−.00	−.00	−.44
Bread/pastry	−.65	−.56	−.32	−.24	−.00	−.31
Beans	−.82	−.78	−.64	−.45	−.25	−.60
Peas	−1.13	−1.13	−.76	−.59	−.52	−.70
Eggs	−1.34	−1.23	−1.26	−.75	−.35	−.92
Oranges	−1.39	−.96	−.79	−.64	−.29	−.69
Milk	−1.79	−1.62	−1.12	−.64	−.20	−.77
Pork	−1.89	−1.61	−1.12	−.82	−.70	−1.01
Daily calorie intake as percentage of requirement	89	99	117	132	1,718	119

Source: Pinstrup-Andersen et al. 1976:137–138.

small changes in the price of cassava, potatoes, maize, or bread. And even for pork, which the average consumer considers just over the edge into the luxury category, high-income consumers have a demand elasticity with respect to price of less than one (a 1 percent change in the price of pork will generate a less than 1 percent change in pork consumption among these consumers). In contrast, low-income consumers are fairly responsive to changes in food prices. They consider cassava, rice, potatoes, bread, and beans necessities, but they regard animal products and fresh fruit as luxuries.

Since this pioneering study, a number of other studies have been done that relate food price elasticities to income. Alderman provides a useful survey of those studies as of 1986.

■ ELASTICITIES, NUTRITION ECONOMICS, AND PUBLIC POLICY

Armed with their complete set of food elasticity figures by income groups, Pinstrup-Andersen and his team went on to show how price elasticities could be useful in analyzing the differential impact of various agricultural production changes on the nutrition of the poor. Let us look at this subject now.

Reexamine the elasticity formula on page 130. Notice that this elasticity compares two rates of change: rate of change in consumption and rate of change in price. If we know an elasticity and one of the rates of change, we can easily calculate the other rate of change.

We have been looking at price elasticity from the point of view of a 1 percent change in price. In other words, elasticity is the percentage change in consumption when price changes by 1 percent. Once we know the elasticity for a commodity, say cassava, we can look at things the other way around and ask: How much will price change if consumption changes by 1 percent? And if we have a closed economy (no imports or exports) and assume that all cassava offered to the market is consumed (a reasonable assumption), then consumption equals production. So, given the elasticity equation, we can just as easily ask: How much will price change if production changes by 1 percent?

Table 8.5 shows the average price elasticity of demand for cassava to be −0.19. For ease of computation let us call it −0.2. If the elasticity is −0.2 and we set the top half of the elasticity equation to 1—for a 1 percent change in production (which is also consumption)—then the bottom half of the equation must be −5. In other words, with an elasticity of −0.2, an increase of 1 percent in the production of cassava will yield a 5 percent decrease in the price.

Using this type of computation, once you have the elasticity figures by income groups, you can estimate changes in consumption among income groups given various production changes. This is useful to do because governments often successfully promote the production of a particular agricultural commodity or set of commodities, and policymakers may want to know the nutritional consequences of such agricultural policies.

Pinstrup-Andersen and colleagues went through calculations similar to the above for agricultural production in Colombia. For a number of agricultural commodities, they assumed a 10 percent expansion in the quantity supplied to the market and then looked at the resulting amount consumed by the various income groups. The increases in amount consumed are of most interest among the poorest income group, because, as Table 8.5 shows, all the other income groups are either adequately supplied with calories (group II) or oversupplied (groups III, IV, and V). Calories consumed by the groups with incomes higher than group II's are, by and large, wasted.

Notice in Table 8.6 that, although the lowest-income groups have the highest demand elasticity for what they consider the luxuries—peas, eggs, oranges, milk, and pork—they will share in only a small proportion of a 10 percent increase in production of these commodities. This happens because the quantity of these goods they consume is so small that, even though they are relatively responsive to price changes, they do not change their consumption, in absolute terms, as much as do the higher-income groups.

The Colombian government might therefore be well advised to promote production of those commodities in the top half of Tables 8.5 and 8.6. The low-income group, which contains 18 percent of the sample population, would consume a larger proportionate share of the increase in production of these commodities. Notice (Table 8.5) that, by and large, the highest-income consumers simply are not going to bother with changing their consumption

Table 8.6   **Percentage of a 10 Percent Expansion in Quantity Supplied Expected to Be Consumed by Income Group I (the Calorie-Deficient Stratum), Cali, Colombia, 1969–1970**

Commodity and Its Price Elasticity of Demand	Percentage Consumed
Cassava (–.23)	30.4
Potatoes (–.41)	27.5
Rice (–.43)	20.2
Maize (–.63)	27.8
Bread/pastry (–.65)	25.0
Beans (–.82)	19.1
Peas (–1.13)	8.0
Eggs (–1.34)	12.5
Oranges (–1.39)	12.4
Milk (–1.79)	12.0
Pork (–1.89)	11.1

Source: Pinstrup-Andersen et al. 1976:138.

of those commodities in the top half of the table when their prices change. However, a greater than proportionate share of the increases in production of those commodities in the bottom half of the table go to those who already have adequate or more than adequate calories. The Colombian government might equally want to take this into account in allocating resources to agricultural production promotion programs for those commodities.

☐ **Relating Demand Elasticities to Different Incomes and Commodities**

We have examined elasticity data from three Third World countries— Brazil, Indonesia, and Colombia. We have used these data to illustrate some interesting and useful generalizations about the relationships between demand elasticities, income, and commodity type in the Third World. We will now represent these generalizations in geometric diagrams as well as in prose. We introduce the geometric diagrams here because, in the literature, relative demand elasticities are often represented as lines with different slopes.   ·

Income level and income elasticity. As income rises, elasticity of demand for food with respect to income falls (e.g., Table 8.2). That is, low-income people spend a greater proportion of an increase in their income on food than do high-income people. We represent this geometrically with Figure 8.4. In this figure, movement from 1 to 2 represents a 1 percent increase in income. Movement from A to B represents the consumption response of a poor family to the income shift. Movement from E to F represents the (less dramatic) consumption response of a wealthy family to a 1 percent increase in income. The lines labeled C are the locus of points tracing out the consumption responses as income increases. They are like a consumption function. The more steeply sloped line represents the less elastic consumption response (see Box 8.4).

Income level and price elasticity. As income rises, elasticity of demand for food with respect to price falls (e.g., Table 8.5). That is, low-income people are more responsive to a change in the price of food than are high-income people. We represent this geometrically with Figure 8.5. In this figure, movement from 2 to 1 represents a 1 percent decrease in price. Movement from A to B represents the consumption response of a poor family to the price shift. Movement from E to F represents the (less dramatic) consumption response of a wealthy family. The lines labeled D are the locus of points tracing out the consumption responses as price falls.

Figure 8.4   Influence of Income Level on Income Elasticity of Demand for Food

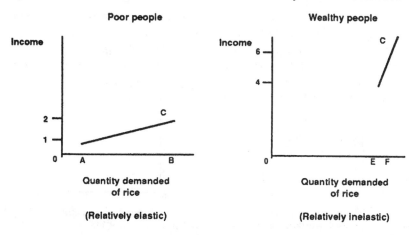

Box 8.4   Talking About Elasticities

Whether positive or negative, whether income or price, an elasticity value

	is called:	
of 1		one, or unity
between zero and 1		inelastic
above 1		elastic
greater than another		more elastic, or relatively elastic
less than another		less elastic, or relatively inelastic

Figure 8.5   Influence of Income Level on Price Elasticity of Demand for Food

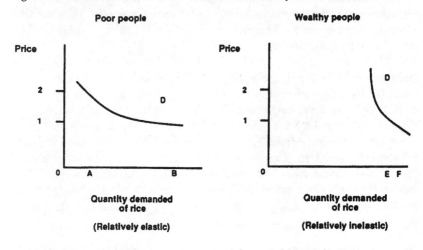

Figure 8.6   Relation Between Commodity Type and Income Elasticity of Demand for Food (Average Consumer)

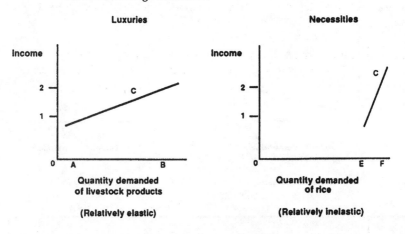

They are demand functions, or demand curves. The more steeply sloped line represents the less elastic demand curve (consumption response).

Commodity type and income elasticity. As income changes, people change their consumption of luxuries by a greater percentage than they change their consumption of necessities. That is, the income elasticity of demand for luxuries is greater than it is for necessities. Third World consumers generally consider rice a necessity, but often regard livestock products as a luxury (e.g., Table 8.4). Alderman (1986:81) cites several examples of studies that found income elasticity of demand for livestock products at above one for low-income Third World consumers. This phenomenon is represented graphically in Figure 8.6, where the consumption response to an increase in income of our Third World consumer is shown to be more elastic for livestock products than for rice.

Commodity type and price elasticity. For a necessity, a 1 percent change in price will elicit a relatively small change in consumption. For a luxury, a 1 percent change in price will elicit a relatively large change in consumption. This is true for consumers across the income spectrum as well as for the average consumer (e.g., Table 8.5). Figure 8.7 is a geometric representation of this phenomenon.

☐ Nutrition Policy Implications

From our discussion of elasticities we can derive two policy recommendations and two policy dilemmas, all of which are of interest to those who would improve Third World nutritional status. The geometric representations of behavior that we just discussed will be helpful in developing these recommendations and in understanding the dilemma.

Increase the income of the poor. Increasing the income of the poor is one of the most fundamental things that can be done to reduce Third World undernutrition. Because poor people have a much greater income elasticity of

Figure 8.7   Relations Between Commodity Type and Price Elasticity of Demand for Food (Average Consumer)

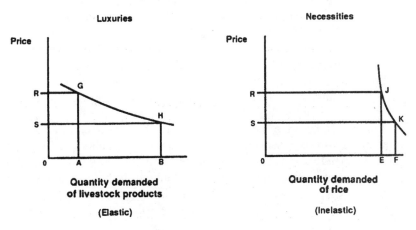

demand for food than do rich people (represented in Figure 8.4), a greater proportion of any increase in their incomes will go to food consumption. Wealthy people are, by and large, overconsuming calories. Increases in income of the wealthy are far less likely to improve nutrition. In fact, because a tendency exists to induce health risks through gaining excess weight and overconsuming fat as income increases, we could make a case that an increase in the income of the wealthy may be detrimental to nutrition.

Promote the production of foods with low elasticities of demand with respect to price. Increasing production of food commodities will lower their price. People at risk for undernutrition benefit most from price declines among those products having low overall elasticities of demand with respect to price. There are two important reasons for this.

First, the foods with low demand elasticities are the foods the poor spend most of their food budget on, the necessities (cassava, potatoes, rice, maize, bread, and beans) shown in the top half of Table 8.5, for instance. Even though poor people have greater demand elasticities for the luxury items, they spend such a small proportion of their food budget on them that reductions in their price are not particularly helpful to the poor's nutrition. Notice in Table 8.3 that rural low-income consumers in Brazil get only 2.1 percent of their calories from milk and 0.5 percent from eggs. Rural high-income consumers in the same sample population consume three and a half times as much milk and four and a half times as many eggs as do their low-income counterparts (Gray 1982:20). Benefits from price decreases resulting from increasing the production of these livestock products, which have relatively high demand elasticities, will go chiefly to the wealthy, who are already well fed—perhaps overfed.

The second reason for increasing the production of foods with low demand elasticities is that increases in the production of these foods will result in greater percentage declines in price than will similar percentage increases in the production of foods with high demand elasticities. This is illustrated in Figure 8.7. Look at the substantial price drop (from R to S) resulting from a small increase in production (from E to F) of the necessity diagrammed in the right-hand side of the figure. Compare that to the very small price drop expected (from R to slightly below R) in the price of the luxury commodity if production increased a small amount from A toward B in the diagram on the left-hand side of the figure.

The substantial price declines associated with increased production of commodities with low demand elasticities are of particular benefit to the poor, who spend most of their food budget on these items. The rich, who spend a smaller proportion of their food budget on these low-elasticity items, will benefit less, proportionally. The increase in purchasing power resulting from a decline in the price of low-elasticity foods enhances the purchasing power of the poor by a greater percentage than it does the purchasing power of the rich.

The farm product promotion dilemma. In a closed economy where the market clears, production and consumption will be equal. In this situation, or in situations close to it, an increase in the production of a commodity with a demand elasticity of less than one will result in a decline in total revenue to the producer. You can reason this through using either the elasticity formula or a demand diagram (for a more detailed discussion of this subject see Miller, Rosenblatt & Hushak 1988).

Imagine a commodity with a demand elasticity of –0.5. Substitute –0.5 for elasticity in the equation on page 130. For the elasticity to be –0.5, the top half of the elasticity formula must be half the value of the bottom half. In other words, the market responds to an increase in production (which equals consumption) in such a way that price changes twice as much as production. If production increases by 1 percent then price will fall by 2 percent. And when price falls by a greater percentage than production increases, total revenue to the farmer decreases.

Now let us look at the same situation as diagrammed on the right-hand side of Figure 8.7. Total revenue is price times quantity produced. The total revenue from the sale of rice in this diagram is the price, OR, times the quantity produced (demanded), OE. This total revenue can be represented graphically as the box, ORJE (length times width equals area). If the price of rice falls from R to S, the new total revenue box is represented by OSKF. Notice that, for a product with an inelastic demand such as rice, the size of the total revenue box decreases when price falls.

Conversely, for products with demand elasticities greater than one, an increase in production will yield an increase in total revenue. Go through the exercise again, only this time assume a price elasticity of demand of –2. The top half of the formula in the price elasticity equation (percentage change in consumption [production]) will have to be twice as big as the bottom half (percentage change in price). Now look at what happens to the size of the total revenue boxes for the luxury product diagrammed in the left-hand side of Figure 8.7. As price falls from R to S, the size of the total revenue box increases!

Now here is the dilemma: When government successfully promotes the production of a farm product with an inelastic price elasticity of demand, such as a grain crop, unless other factors intervene in the market, farmers see their total revenues decrease. Low-income consumers are better nourished, but farmer revenues fall.

When government successfully promotes the production of a farm product with an elastic demand with respect to price (in the Third World, livestock products are sometimes in this category, or often close to it), farm revenue increases, but the majority of the benefits from the lower prices go to the wealthy, who do not really need to consume more food.

Governments want to make everyone happy. But the agricultural policy that does the most to improve nutrition happens to be the policy that is most likely to damage the welfare of farmers.

The prosperity–food price dilemma. A second dilemma exists because food demand increases as income grows. Therefore, governments successful in pursuing policies that create general prosperity will discover that the new prosperity raises food demand, which, in turn, creates higher food prices. In developing countries, where income elasticity is relatively high, the effect is largest. The result is that it is more difficult than it may first appear to improve the purchasing power of the very poor. In practice, of course, greater prosperity always leads to decreases in involuntary undernutrition. The point here is that the effectiveness of promoting prosperity as a means of reducing undernutrition is likely to be mediated by the effects of the programs on food prices. The empirical importance of this is discussed in more detail in Chapter 10. Here we note only the unavoidable links between increased prosperity and upward pressure on food prices.

☐ 9

Undernutrition and the Distribution of Income, Wealth, and Education

"Get off this estate!"
"What for?"
"Because it's mine."
"Where did you get it?"
"From my father."
"Where did he get it?"
"From his father."
"And where did he get it?"
"He fought for it."
"Well, I'll fight you for it!"

—Carl Sandburg 1936:75

■ INCOME DISTRIBUTION AND FOOD CONSUMPTION

☐ Income Elasticity and the Reutlinger Triangles

So far we have presented substantial evidence that, for the world as a whole, low-income people tend to underconsume food while high-income people tend to overconsume it. In an influential monograph published in 1976, Reutlinger and Selowsky attempted to quantify this under- and over-consumption. Figure 9.1 is representative of their work on this subject.

For purposes of developing the data from which Figure 9.1 was drawn, Reutlinger and Selowsky assumed that Third World income elasticity of demand for calories was 0.15. Subsequent estimates based on data from 17 developing countries put the income elasticity of demand for calories at 0.15 or 0.16 (Reutlinger et al. 1986:64) suggesting that this original assumption was reasonable. As noted in the previous chapter, Bouis

Figure 9.1   Calorie Consumption by Income Groups, Latin America, 1965
(with Calorie–Income Elasticity Equal to 0.15)

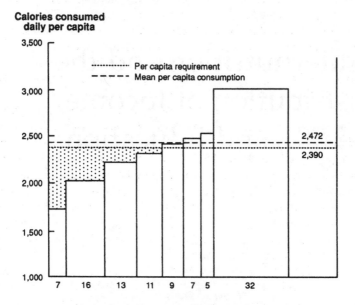

Percentage share of total population by income group,
lowest income on left and highest on right

Source: Adapted from Reutlinger & Selowsky 1976:20.

Note: If an income elasticity of 0.15 seems low to you, remember that income elasticities decline as income rises. The income elasticities we have quoted so far are mostly for very low income. For example, Ho's estimate was 0.58 for the East Javanese sample. The income elasticity estimates shown for calories in Table 8.2 were for rural Brazil, which, by and large, is poorer than urban Brazil, where such elasticity estimates run lower. Remember also that income elasticities for particular foods shown (as in the case of Tables 8.2 and 8.3) tend to run higher than income elasticities for calories as a whole, The median calorie elasticity for low-income families (consuming 1,750–2,000 calories per capita per day) among 19 estimates examined by Alderman (1984:37) was 0.405.

and Haddad conclude, after an extensive review of existing literature, that a number in the range of 0.08–0.14 is a reasonable estimate.

Figure 9.1 plots calorie consumption by income groups in Latin America, given 0.15 as the estimate for overall income elasticity of demand for calories. The dashed horizontal line cutting across the vertical bars represents FAO recommended per capita daily calorie consumption for adult equivalents. The dotted horizontal line close by represents average daily adult equivalent calorie consumption. With a little imagination you can see two stepped triangles in this figure: one (the shaded triangle) represents the total calorie deficit among low-income people, while the other triangle (the boxes above the dotted line) represents overconsumption among the rich. We refer to these as the *Reutlinger triangles*.

Figure 9.1 is a visualization of the nutritional impact of differential purchasing power among Third World income groups. As the rich and the poor both bid for food in the marketplace, the poor simply do not have as much clout as the rich. The rich bid food away from the poor.

As per capita income increases, people, especially the rich, eat more livestock and livestock products. Over the past century the worldwide demand for livestock and livestock products has increased to the point that the world livestock herd, which in the 1800s was largely a scavenging herd (cows ate grass; chickens, pigs, and ducks ate table scraps), is now eating substantial amounts of grain. In 1983 and 1984 about one-third of the world's grain production was fed to livestock (Reutlinger et al. 1986:24). As the rich consume meat, milk, eggs, and other livestock products, they are, to some extent, bidding grain away from the poor. To recapitulate: Income distribution is important in nutrition for two reasons: (1) the greater the distance between the rich and the poor, the greater is the capacity and the tendency of the rich to bid food away from the poor; and (2) the greater the concentration of income in the hands of a wealthy few, the greater is their tendency (because of their high incomes) to purchase and consume livestock products. The more the wealthy consume livestock products, the more dependent the livestock herd becomes on grain as it switches from scavenging and eating grass. The more the price of grain is bid up to satisfy the wealthy's demand for animal products, the harder it is for the poor to buy the grain they need for minimal nutrition.

☐ The Redistribution-Incentive Paradox

Programs that transfer purchasing power from the rich to the poor will reduce the size of both of the Reutlinger triangles, thus improving nutrition (the upward-sloping line that is the hypotenuse of the right triangles will become more horizontal). By eliminating all differences in income, the Reutlinger triangles could also be eliminated, and food would, presumably, be fairly evenly distributed across the population.

Two major and vastly different countries—China and the Soviet Union—have experimented with programs that greatly reduced differences in income. As they succeeded, they reduced differences in food consumption, but at the same time they experienced difficulties with food production.

Before their respective socialist revolutions, both countries enjoyed healthy agricultural economies. In 1917, the year of the Russian Revolution, the world's leading agricultural geographers (Finch & Baker 1917: 13) wrote that "the Russian Empire leads the world in both acreage and production of wheat. . . . Nearly one-fifth of the average harvest is exported."

China's socialist revolution was completed after World War II. Before that war, China accounted for 93 percent of the world's soybean exports (Economist Intelligence Unit 1959:33).

Both Russia and China went from being major food exporters before their socialist revolutions to major food importers afterwards. And during the 1980s both countries tried to reintroduce market-oriented incentives, in part to bolster their flagging agricultural productivity.

There appear to be nutritional gains from reducing the size of the Reutlinger triangles through redistributing income, yet income redistribution, carried to extremes, appears to introduce incentive problems that could conceivably lead to low levels of food consumption for all. It seems, then, if your goal is to improve nutrition for all, there is not much point in debating the relative merits of laissez-faire, free-enterprise capitalism (which can produce large Reutlinger triangles) versus extreme socialism (which appears to lead to problems in agricultural productivity), for both of these extremes may lead to widespread hunger problems. In reducing undernutrition, then, the appropriate debate with reference to income redistribution should center on how much and by what methods to do it. That is, to what extent should the rich be taxed, and how should the money going into the tax till be spent?

In much of the last part of this book we will consider the question of policies that affect nutrition, which heavily involve the issue of how to allocate the money going into the tax till. We concentrate here on income distribution and redistribution. We will look at methods of measuring income distribution, some factors influencing income distribution (such as education, fertility control, and the adoption of new technology), and finally at the relationship between these factors and the pace of economic development.

■ COMPARING AVERAGE INCOMES IN DIFFERENT COUNTRIES

In an international economy, prices are influenced by consumption in all countries. The affordability of food for poor people in one country is influenced by the consumption patterns of affluent people in other countries. As we look at the distribution of income in the world, we note that average per capita incomes are very different from one country to another (see Tables 9.1 and 9.2). To pick the most dramatic example, in 1995, per capita income in Mozambique was $80 per year, while per capita income in Switzerland was $40,630. The average person in Switzerland earned over 500 times the amount earned by the average person in Mozambique (World Bank 1997).

Table 9.1   Income and Population Distribution, Selected Countries

	1995 GNP ($ million)	Percentage of World Total GNP	1995 Population (millions)	Percentage of World Total Population
United States	7,098,951	25.6	263.1	4.6
Japan	4,963,443	17.9	125.2	2.2
Germany	2,252,216	8.1	81.9	1.4
France	1,450,919	5.2	58.1	1.0
United Kingdom	1,094,567	4.0	58.5	1.0
Italy	1,088,020	3.9	57.2	1.0
China	744,149	2.7	1,200.2	21.2
Brazil	579,568	2.1	159.2	2.8
Canada	573,764	2.1	29.6	0.5
Spain	532,322	1.9	39.2	0.7
Korea, Rep.	435,055	1.6	44.9	0.8
Netherlands	371,040	1.3	15.5	0.3
Australia	337,971	1.2	18.1	0.3
Russian Federation	331,957	1.2	148.2	2.6
India	315,982	1.1	929.4	16.4
Subtotal	22,169,925	80.1	3,228.2	56.9
World total	27,684,197	100.0	5,673.0	100.0

Source: World Bank.

Note: These are the 15 countries that have the largest GNP of all countries. The eight countries with the highest per capita income would be a different list and would show a greater intensity of income concentration.

Table 9.2   1995 GNP per Capita for Selected Countries, Using Exchange Rate Comparison and Purchasing Power Parity Comparison

Exchange Rate Comparison		Purchasing Power Parity Comparison	
Country	GNP per Capita ($)	Country	GNP per Capita ($)
Mozambique	80	Ethiopia	450
Ethiopia	100	Rwanda	540
Tanzania	120	Mali	550
Rwanda	180	Tanzania	640
Mali	250	Mozambique	810
India	340	India	1,400
China	620	China	2,920
Brazil	3,640	Brazil	5,400
United States	26,980	Germany	20,070
Germany	27,510	Japan	22,110
Japan	39,640	Switzerland	25,860
Switzerland	40,630	United States	26,980

Source: World Bank, World Development Report, 1997.

Incomes, as the term is used here, refers to the gross national product (GNP) or the closely related concept gross domestic product (GDP), which measure the total value of goods and services produced in the economy. The richest 10 countries in the world have less than 10 percent of the world's population but produce over 60 percent of the world's goods. The poorest 56 countries support more than 50 percent of the world's population but produce less than 5 percent of the world's goods.

☐ **Global Redistribution:
Do Incomes Grow Faster in Poor Countries?**

How can such enormous differences exist between countries? One obvious answer to this question is that much more investment in productive capital occurs in rich countries; people in those countries are more productive because they have more and better capital, better equipment in their workplaces, better roads and communications, and better education. Many economists believe that as time passes, income per capita in poor countries will catch up with income in rich countries; in other words, incomes per capita will *converge*. Investors will discover that investing in poor countries with low levels of capital has a higher payoff than investing in rich countries where there are high levels of capital; this investment will increase the capital stock in poor countries and therefore increase production per person in those countries.

In Table 9.3, we see mixed evidence about whether this *convergence theory* is correct. Income per capita is growing faster in low-income countries (3.8 percent per year) than in middle-income (–0.7 percent) or upper-income (1.9 percent) countries. But the high growth in the low-income-country category reflects strong growth in India (3.2 percent annual growth) and China (8.3 percent)—two countries that between them have over 2 billion people or two-thirds of the population of low-income countries. When those two countries are removed, per capita incomes are dropping by 1.4 percent per year in low-income countries.

However, this bad news reflects in part the large negative growth rates observed in parts of the former Soviet bloc; during the 1985–1995 period, these economies underwent severe problems adjusting to a new economic system. This is reflected in low- and middle-income countries in Europe and Central Asia, where per capita income dropped an average of 3.5 percent per year. If we eliminate both groups of countries—China and India with their high positive growth rates and the former Soviet bloc countries with their high negative growth rates—we find that middle- and low-income countries had an annual rate of growth in per capita income of –0.38 percent. This is still far less than the positive growth rates of 1.9 percent per year in the high-income countries.

☐ **An Alternative Way of Comparing Incomes in
Different Countries: Purchasing Power Parity**

Some economists have expressed doubt about whether the usual method of comparing GNP per capita in different countries gives an accurate view of

Table 9.3   **GNP per Capita and Average Annual Growth Rates, for Country Groups**

Country Group	Population (millions)	1995 GNP per Capita ($)	Average Annual Rate of Growth in GNP per Capita 1985–95
Low-income economies	3,179.9	430	3.8
Excluding China and India	1,050.3	290	−1.4
Middle-income economies	1,590.9	2,390	−0.7
Upper-middle-income	438.3	4,260	0.2
Lower-middle-income	1,152.6	1,670	−1.3
Low- and middle-income	4,770.8	1,090	0.4
High-income economies	902.2	24,930	1.9
Low- and middle-income countries in:			
South Asia	1,243.0	350	2.9
East Asia and Pacific	1,706.4	800	7.2
Europe and Central Asia	487.6	2,220	−3.5
Sub-Saharan Africa	583.3	490	−1.1
Middle East and N. Africa	272.4	1,780	−0.3
Latin America and Caribbean	477.9	3,320	0.3
World	5,673.0	4,880	0.8

Source: World Bank, World Development Report, 1997.

the quality of life in those countries. The usual method—as reflected in the numbers in the previous section—translates the value of goods and services in a country from the local currency to U.S. dollars by using the market exchange rate. In effect, this measure translates local currency into dollars by considering how many units of the local currency it would take to buy a dollar on the foreign exchange market.

An alternative method translates local currency into a dollar equivalent by comparing the purchasing power of the local currency to the purchasing power of the dollar. In effect, this measure translates how much it would cost in the local currency spent in the local market to buy the same quantity of goods that could be purchased in the United States with one dollar. Using this conversion method, the richest country (the United States, by this measure, rather than Switzerland) has a per capita income 50 times larger than the per capita income of the poorest country (Ethiopia, by this measure, rather than Mozambique). (See Table 9.2.) Compare this factor of 50 to what we reported above—that the average income in the richest country was 500 times that of the poorest country—based on exchange rate comparisons of GNP per capita.

This *purchasing power parity* (PPP) measure of GNP per capita provides a little more support for the convergence theory, which indicates that poor countries are catching up with richer countries. By the PPP measure (and including only those countries for which complete data are available), the 61 lowest-income countries had per capita incomes equal to 6.7 percent of the level in the United States in 1987; by 1995 that had risen to 8.3 percent. Even leaving out China and India, we see the numbers for the remaining low-income countries rise from 8.0 percent to 8.4 percent. In other words, incomes in the poorest countries are catching up with income in the United States, although very slowly. Middle-income countries did not do any catching up during the 1987–1995 period. For 35 middle-income countries (with PPP GNP per capita of between $4,000 and $14,000 in 1995), incomes stood at 25.6 percent of those of the United States in 1987, but that number fell to 23.3 percent in 1995. Twenty-three upper-income countries made a little progress compared to the United States, moving from 82.6 percent of the U.S. level in 1987 to 83.8 percent in 1995.

■ MEASURING INCOME DISTRIBUTION WITHIN A COUNTRY

☐ Pareto's Law

For a typical town, when you rank family or individual incomes from low to high and graph them, the result is suggestive of a J. The J-shape is especially pronounced if you graph just the richest people in the town (Figure 9.2).

In the late 1800s the Italian mathematician-economist-sociologist Vilfredo Pareto examined income distribution among the rich and moderately rich in a number of countries and found the J-shaped distribution pattern among them to be remarkably consistent. Furthermore, he was able to fit this pattern to a mathematical formulation that soon became known as *Pareto's law.* Pareto's law had its problems, and, as it turned out, one of the main benefits of Pareto's work on income distribution was to stimulate

Figure 9.2   Stylized Representation of Income Distribution Among the Rich in a Typical Community

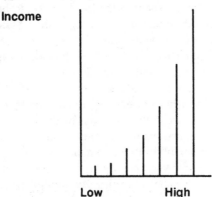

Note: Each vertical bar represents the total income of one individual or family. A line traced across the top of the bars resembles a "J."

others to think about alternative methods of measuring it. (For a concise discussion of Pareto's work on distribution see Steindl 1987.)

☐ The Lorenz Curve

In 1905, the U.S. statistician Max Lorenz proposed a method of comparing distributions of income and wealth through a cumulative income or wealth curve, the *Lorenz curve,* an example of which is shown as the dashed line in Figure 9.3. The vertical axis, OC, represents percentage of total income for the group under analysis. The horizontal axis, OE, represents the percentage of individuals (or families) in the group.

To conceptualize how a Lorenz curve is constructed, imagine a group of 100 individuals, each with a different income. Bake a cake that represents the total income of the group. Cut the entire cake into blocks, each block being a length proportional to one individual's income, and distribute the cake accordingly. Now arrange all the individuals in a line according to cake size, with the person having the shortest piece of cake first and the person with the longest piece last. Starting with the person with the shortest piece of cake, have the line pass by a point at which each individual stacks her piece of cake on top of the previous piece until all the pieces are placed in a column. Then the column will represent all the income of the group.

Figure 9.3   A Lorenz Curve

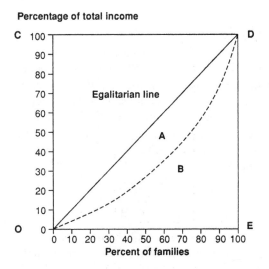

Source: Adapted from Kakwani 1987:244.

As every tenth person places cake on the column, measure the height of the column at that time and calculate what percentage of total income is represented so far. On the Lorenz diagram, plot the percentage of total income accounted for so far against the percentage of population accounted for at that time until every person has walked by. Connect the points with a smooth line and you have a Lorenz curve (Cowell 1977:23).

The straight diagonal line, OD, in Figure 9.3 is called the *egalitarian line*. If everyone in the group under analysis had exactly the same income, the Lorenz curve would correspond to the egalitarian line. If all the income accrued to one individual, the Lorenz curve would be the right angle represented by OED in Figure 9.3. The more the Lorenz curve bends away from the egalitarian line, the greater the inequality of income.

Figure 9.4a shows a Lorenz curve for the distribution of land owned in a Bagbana village, India, during 1968 and 1981. More than 30 percent of the families in this village own no land, which is why both Lorenz curves in Figure 9.4 track the zero line of land owned for more than a third of the way across the horizontal axis. Notice that inequality in land distribution in this village increased during the 13 years from 1968 to 1981.

Figure 9.4b shows the Lorenz curve for farm income in this same village over the same period; more people have farm income than own land (many are landless farm workers). During the 13 years under consideration the inequality of farm income decreased. A possible explanation is discussed later in this chapter in the section on the distributional impact of the green revolution.

In Table 9.4 some raw data from the Philippines is presented, from which several Lorenz curves could be constructed. To fix the concept in your mind you might try constructing a Lorenz curve for Philippine families for 1983.

☐ The Gini Coefficient

The search for a better method of measuring income and wealth distribution did not end with Lorenz. In 1912 the Italian economist Corrado Gini proposed yet another measure of inequality, the Gini ratio, often called the *Gini coefficient* (Dagum 1987). Gini used the Lorenz curve as the basis of his ratio. He simply compared the area of the triangle OED (see Figure 9.3) with the area of the lens-shaped piece taken out of that triangle by the Lorenz curve. Labeling the lens-shaped part A and the remainder of the triangle B, the Gini ratio is:

$$\frac{A}{A+B}$$

If one individual in the group has all the income, the Gini ratio becomes one. If the size of A approaches zero, the Gini ratio approaches zero. The range of the Gini is thus from zero to one. At the bottom of Table 9.4 are Gini ratios for the income distribution data shown in that table.

Figure 9.4 **Lorenz Curves for Farm Land and Farm Income, Bagbana Village, India, 1968 and 1981**

a. Cumulative land

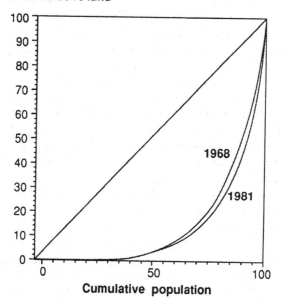

b. Cumulative farm income

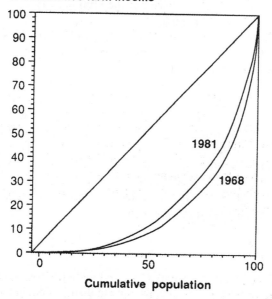

Source: Field surveys by Phillips Foster and his assistants. Lorenz curves by Paul Fishstein.

Table 9.4   Distribution of Total Family Income by Decile and Gini Coefficient,
              Philippines, 1978–1983

Ranking of Families	Percentage					
	1978	1979	1980	1981	1982	1983
First tenth	0.9	0.8	0.8	0.8	1.0	1.0
Second tenth	2.1	2.0	1.9	1.9	2.0	1.9
Third tenth	3.2	3.1	2.9	2.8	3.2	3.2
Fourth tenth	4.1	4.1	3.9	3.8	3.6	3.7
Fifth tenth	5.3	5.4	5.3	5.1	5.0	5.0
Sixth tenth	6.7	6.7	7.0	6.7	6.4	6.5
Seventh tenth	8.6	8.6	8.9	8.6	8.1	8.3
Eighth tenth	11.4	11.3	11.9	11.6	11.2	11.3
Ninth tenth	16.3	16.0	15.4	16.7	16.1	16.1
Last tenth	41.1	42.0	42.0	42.0	43.4	43.0
Gini coefficient	0.521	0.525	0.527	0.534	0.535	0.533

Source: Philippines National Economic Development Authority 1983:157.

Although popular, the Gini coefficient is open to criticism (Paglin 1974). It shows nothing about the location of the concentration of income inequality among high- versus low-income groups. The shape of the Lorenz curve could conceivably change (with the poor better off and the middle-class worse off, for instance) without any change in the Gini. Furthermore, neither the Lorenz curve nor the Gini take account of expected variation in income as people age.

Imagine a group consisting of working adults with ages distributed evenly from 20 to 50 years and with everyone in his twenties paid the same, everyone in her thirties paid the same, but more than those in their twenties, and everyone in his forties paid the same, but more than those in their thirties. Calculate the Gini. (Calculating the Gini is not easy unless you use a computer program. For an explanation on how it is done see Cowell 1977.) It would be greater than zero, although you might feel the income distribution was equitable.

Now imagine another group with the same income by age, but in which young and old ages predominate, with few in the middle group. The Gini would be higher than before, indicating greater inequality, but you might not think the ratio fairly contrasted the two groups.

☐ Relative Income Share

Lorenz curves and Gini ratios make for useful comparisons and appear frequently in the literature of income and wealth distribution, but they are hard for the layman to understand and time-consuming to explain to politicians. Increasingly, the easy-to-understand *relative income share* is being used to describe income inequalities. With relative income share, you array the incomes in the population from lowest to highest and divide the population into equal-sized groups, just as you did on the Lorenz curve. Then you calculate the percentage of the total income in each group. And that is it; you have relative income share.

Given time series data, as in Table 9.4, you can track what is happening to any one income category that you may be interested in, such as the poorest, who are the most susceptible to undernutrition.

Relative income share is equally convenient for making comparisons among countries. A good source of such comparisons can be found in the World Bank's annual World Development Report table on income distribution (e.g., World Bank 1996:196–197).

□ Income Distributions in Different Countries and Changes Over Time

Information on income distributions within different countries has been compiled from various sources by Deininger and Squire (1997). Some of this is presented in Table 9.5. The countries represented in the table account for over 70 percent of the world's population and over 80 percent of the total world income. We can see from the table that there is quite a wide variation in the degrees of income equality. Of the countries reported in the table, the most equal distribution, as reflected by the lowest Gini coefficient, is in Spain (Gini = 25.91); the most unequal distribution is in Brazil (Gini = 59.60). The poorest 20 percent of the population controls 8 percent of the income in Spain, but only 2.5 percent in Brazil. The richest 20 percent of the population controls 35 percent of the income in Spain, but 65 percent of the income in Brazil.

Over the last 30 years, there appears to be a trend toward greater inequality of income in many countries. Table 9.6 illustrates changes in the Gini coefficient over time for a sample of countries. The increase in inequality has been especially pronounced in formerly socialist (Soviet bloc) countries since the end of the Cold War and the breakup of the Soviet Union. For example, the Gini coefficient in Poland went from 25.5 in 1991 to 33 in 1993; in Bulgaria the increase was from 24 in 1991 to 34 in 1993. In addition, the increase for China probably represents reforms in the general economic system. However, the increases in inequality were not limited to countries that were replacing a socialist system with a more market-oriented economy. In both the United States and the United Kingdom, inequality increased gradually but substantially over a period going back to the late 1960s. From 1968 to 1991, the Gini coefficients increased from 33 to 38 in the United States, and from 24 to 32 in the United Kingdom. This trend does not appear in every country. For example, Japan and India show little change. Italy showed a substantial increase in equality, with the Gini coefficient dropping from about 40 in the mid-1970s to about 32 in the early 1990s.

Table 9.5 Income Distribution in Selected Countries

Country	Year	Gini	Quintile 1	Quintile 2	Quintile 3	Quintile 4	GDP as % World Total	Population as % of World Total
United States	1991	37.94	0.0450	0.1520	0.3180	0.5590	25.64261	4.6381
Japan	1982	34.80	0.0590	0.1770	0.3487	0.5818	17.9288	2.207178
Germany (pre-unified)	1984	32.20	0.0659	0.1938	0.3735	0.6112	8.135386	1.443136
France	1984	34.91	0.0658	0.1901	0.3575	0.5803	5.240966	1.023446
United Kingdom	1991	32.40	0.0764	0.2025	0.3621	0.5916	3.953761	1.031784
Italy	1991	32.19	0.0841	0.2158	0.3929	0.6257	3.930112	1.008357
China	1992	37.80	0.0602	0.1672	0.3253	0.5835	2.687994	21.15711
Brazil	1989	59.60	0.0248	0.0740	0.1655	0.3482	2.093498	2.806667
Canada	1991	27.65	0.0768	0.2136	0.4032	0.6516	2.072534	0.521876
Spain	1989	25.91	0.0839	0.2271	0.4139	0.6472	1.922839	0.690976
Korea, Rep.	1988	33.64	0.0739	0.1968	0.3595	0.5776	1.571491	0.790606
Netherlands	1991	29.38	0.0692	0.2107	0.3997	0.6364	1.340259	0.272519
Australia	1989	37.32	0.0560	0.1631	0.3388	0.6012	1.220808	0.318245
Russia (USSR)	1993	30.53	0.0743	0.2007	0.3788	0.6223	1.199084	2.61229
India	1992	32.02	0.0880	0.2130	0.3750	0.5890	1.141379	16.38215
Mexico	1992	50.31	0.0413	0.1192	0.2445	0.4466	1.101274	1.61874
Indonesia	1993	31.69	0.0868	0.2095	0.3724	0.5930	0.684186	3.406968
Pakistan	1991	31.15	0.0840	0.2127	0.3814	0.6030	0.21585	2.289885
Bangladesh	1992	28.27	0.0935	0.2286	0.4010	0.6209	0.103829	2.111197
Nigeria	1993	37.47	0.0399	0.1292	0.2729	0.5070	0.104504	1.961452
Vietnam	1992	35.71	0.0780	0.1920	0.3460	0.5700	0.063697	1.295172
Philippines	1988	45.73	0.0520	0.1430	0.2760	0.4750	0.260166	1.20915

Source: Deininger & Squire 1997.

Note: The numbers listed under each quintile are the percentage of national income earned by that quintile and all poorer quintiles combined. Thus, for the U.S., the poorest 20% of the population earns 4.5% of the national income, the poorest 40% of the population earns 15.2% of the national income, the poorest 60% earns 31.8%, and so on.

Table 9.6   Changes in Gini Coefficients Over Time for Selected Countries

	U.S.	U.K.	Taiwan	Japan	Italy	India	China
1968	33.50	24.10	28.90	34.90		31.86	
1969	33.64	24.90		35.70		31.47	
1970	34.06	25.10	29.42	35.50		30.38	
1971	34.30	25.70		36.90			
1972	34.46	26.00	29.02	33.40		31.85	
1973	34.42	25.10	33.60	32.50		29.17	
1974	34.16	24.20	28.09	33.60	41.00		
1975	34.42	23.30	31.20	34.40	39.00		
1976	34.42	23.20	28.40	33.90	35.00		
1977	34.98	22.90	28.00	33.70	36.30	32.14	
1978	35.02	23.10	28.43	32.90	35.98		
1979	35.06	24.40	27.70	33.90	37.19		
1980	35.20	24.90	27.96	33.40	34.29		
1981	35.62	25.40	28.15	34.30	33.12		
1982	36.48	25.20	28.51	34.80	32.02		
1983	36.70	25.70	28.45		32.87	31.49	27.20
1984	36.90	25.80	28.81		33.15		25.70
1985	37.26	27.10	29.20	35.90			31.40
1986	37.56	27.80	29.29		33.58	32.22	33.30
1987	37.56	29.30	29.65		35.58	31.82	34.30
1988	37.76	30.80	30.02			31.15	34.90
1989	38.16	31.20	30.41	37.60	32.74	30.46	36.00
1990	37.80	32.30	30.11	35.00		29.69	34.60
1991	37.94	32.40	30.49		32.19	32.53	36.20

Source: Deininger & Squire 1996.

■ FACTORS INFLUENCING INCOME DISTRIBUTION

Because unequal distribution of income contributes to Third World undernutrition, we need to examine the causes of unequal income distribution so that we can, later, consider policies that might reduce undernutrition through changes in income distribution. The causes are many and complex and not fully understood.

□ Traditional Thinking: Heredity and Environment

Traditional thinking on the causes of differences in income concentrated on heredity and environment; we can develop a list of the leading schools of thought on this subject. Condensing each school in a purposely over-simplified sentence provides an efficient way of leafing through the diversity of opinions. Each school of thought (the list here is excerpted from Chu 1982:18–19) purports to offer at least a partial clue as to that basic income distribution question: Why is A's income greater than B's?

"Because A is smarter," says the *ability school.*

Box 9.1
World Distribution of Income: Who is Rich?

Who is rich? Would you say that all people in the top half of the income distribution are rich? Or do you have to be in the top quarter, or the top 10 percent, or the top 5 percent? Or would you say that only the richest 1 percent of the population are "the rich"? This is a subjective judgment, and well-intentioned, well-informed people can come to different conclusions. Once you have decided how you would define "rich," use the table below to gain an idea of how much money a rich person earns.

Using data such as that in Tables 9.1, 9.2, and 9.5, we constructed an estimated world distribution of income. For each country, we calculate the average income in each quantile, and then we assumed that everybody in that quantile earns the average income. Using this simplification, we calculated how many people earn less than $1,000 per year, how many earn less than $2,000, etc.

In the center column below, we show the world distribution of income translated into U.S. dollar terms using exchange rates. (As described in the text of this chapter, this is the usual way to compare incomes in different countries.) In constructing the world distribution of income, we used data on 92 countries accounting for 87.5 percent of the world's population and 93 percent of the world's income.

In the right-hand column, we show the world distribution of income using the *purchasing power parity* (PPP) concept to translate income into U.S. dollar terms. As described in the text, this method of comparing incomes in different countries attempts to adjust for different costs of living, so that a person making $5,000 in one country has approximately the same standard of living as a person making $5,000 in another country. In this calculation, we dropped four countries (Gabon, Moldova, Slovenia, and Vietnam) for which PPP measures of income were not available. The remaining countries account for 86 percent of the world's population and 96 percent of the (PPP adjusted) income. (Therefore, to an even greater extent than in the exchange rate income distribution, the countries omitted are relatively poor countries.)

To put these numbers in perspective, consider the following: A college student might imagine finding a job that pays about $17,000 per year. That level of income would make you richer than 90 percent of the world's population. The average income in the U.S. ($26,980 per person) is higher than the incomes of 90–95% of the world's population. The "poverty line" in the United States is currently about $16,000 for a family of four, or $4,000 per family member. This level of income is higher than 80 percent of the world's population; the "standard of living" of this poverty-line family is better than the standard of living of 60 percent of the world's population.

So: Are you one of "the rich"?

(continued)

Box 9.1   Continued

Distribution of World Income in 1995

The poorest ___ percent of people	earn less than ___ dollars (using the exchange rate comparison of income)	earn less than ___ dollars (using the comparison of income)
10	185	834
20	268	1,131
30	330	1,488
40	489	1,747
50	699	2,545
60	894	3,758
70	1,465	5,338
80	4,224	7,015
90	16,780	17,598
95	32,268	25,611
98	51,654	39,205
99	58,287	56,857

"Because A chose to work harder and/or chose to take more risks, and he was rewarded for this behavior," says the *individual choice school.*

"Because A went to a high-quality, expensive college and got a good education, and she is being rewarded for the educational investment in her," says the *human capital school.*

"Because A came from a well-to-do, supportive family. As a result, he was raised better, learned the habits and attitudes necessary for success, and thus can get and hold a better job," says the *family background school.*

"Because A works in the primary labor market, characterized by large firms and/or labor unions, while B works in the secondary labor market, characterized by small firms and without the protection of labor unions," says the *segmented labor market school.*

"Because A inherited a large fortune from his parents," says the *wealth inheritance school.*

"Because A is a white male and B is a black female," says the *discrimination school.*

"Because A is in her prime years of earnings and B is either substantially younger or older," says the *life cycle school.*

"Because A is lucky," says the *stochastic school.*

Each of these schools of thought could be the subject of considerable discussion as to causes and interrelationships with the other schools. Take the first one, for instance, the ability school. Ability is constrained by both heredity and environment. But we have learned much in this century about how the developmental potential of an individual can be influenced by a

Figure 9.5   Relationship Between Family Size, Birth Order, and Intelligence in 19-Year-Old Dutch Men Tested Between 1963 and 1966, by Occupational Background

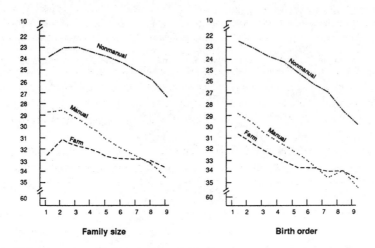

Source: Adapted from Belmont & Marollo 1973:1,100.
Note: The Raven Progressive Matrices test was used to measure intelligence. This test is characterized as one that attempts to be culturally unbiased and has the unusual property that the lower the score, the higher the intelligence rating. N = 137,823 for nonmanual, 184,334 for manual, and 45,196 for farm.

mother's behavior during pregnancy. Poor eating habits, smoking, drug abuse, alcohol abuse, and other activity during a woman's pregnancy can limit the potential of her offspring. Is this part of the family background school?

Intelligence tests conducted on over 386,000 Dutch men as they were inducted into the military were correlated with their family size and birth order (whether they were born first, second, etc.). Belmont and Marolla (1973) found a high level of statistical significance when they correlated intelligence with family size and birth order. With the exception that an only child tended to be less intelligent than children in a family with two or three children total, there was a remarkable tendency for intelligence to decrease as family size and/or birth order increased (Figure 9.5).

In a study in the United States, Blake (1989) found that family size is a major influence on verbal and educational attainment, both of which tend to decrease as family size increases. Do parents, to some extent, determine family size? And if so, is family size a variable that issues from the individual choice school?

We have been examining some of the traditional ways of thinking about the causes of inequality of income distribution, schools of thought based largely on heredity and environment or their interaction. Recent research has caused us to study the impact of other variables, such as technology adoption, education, and fertility control, on income distribution.

☐ **Technology Adoption**

The Kuznets curve. In his 1954 presidential address to the American Economic Association, Harvard economist Simon Kuznets (1955) hypothesized that during the early phases of development Third World countries might experience increasing income inequalities before "leveling forces become strong enough to first stabilize and then reduce income inequalities." His idea that the path of income inequality through time in the Third World would trace the shape of an inverted U became known as the *Kuznets curve.* Subsequent studies have lent support to Kuznets's hypothesis (Adelman & Morris 1973; Ahluwalia 1976b; Chenery, Robinson & Syrquin 1986).

Using cross-sectional data of a sample of 60 countries, including 40 Third World countries, 14 developed countries, and 6 socialist countries, Ahluwalia estimated relative income shares as per capita income changed. The result of one of his multiple regressions, which estimates percentage income share for the lowest 40 percent of the population from income variables, is shown in Figure 9.6. In this diagram the income share of the lowest 40 percent of the population declines from around 17 percent at around $150 per capita to about 12 percent at around $400 per capita, and then is back up to around 17 percent when income increases to $3,000. The U shape in Figure 9.6 is not inverted because the diagram tracks a measure of income equality instead of inequality, as in the original statement of the Kuznets curve.

It seems reasonable to postulate that the poor may benefit less from development than the rich. As development takes place, those in the more advanced sector of the economy are likely to be the first to take advantage of it. Therefore, they reap the first gains. After all, when the new productive techniques come along they often require new knowledge and substantial amounts of capital. The railroads and canals and electric companies, which were originally privately owned, are a case in point. It was difficult for the poor even to imagine "making a killing" in these areas.

Modernization could conceivably make the poor worse off. As Ahluwalia (1976b:330–331) puts it: "An aggressively expanding technologically advanced, modern sector, competing against the traditional sector for markets and resources (and benefiting in this competition from an entrenched position in the institutional and political context) may well generate both a relative and absolute decline in incomes of the poor." He concludes from his research, however, that though the initial stages of development are likely to make the poor worse off relative to the rich, these same initial stages are not necessarily inclined to making the poor worse off in absolute terms.

The distributional impact of the green revolution. Given this background, it was logical for people to be afraid that the green revolution

Figure 9.6   **Estimated Relationship Between Income Share and per Capita GNP,
60 Countries, Various Years Prior to 1975**

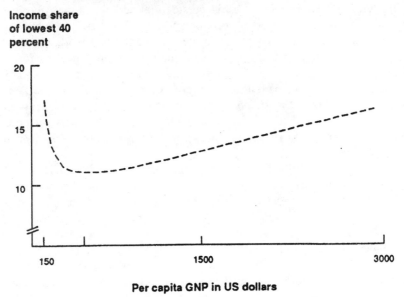

Source: Adapted from Ahluwalia 1976a:133.

might increase inequality of income; indeed, it might make the poor absolutely worse off, in regions where it was adopted (for a brief discussion
on the green revolution see Chapter 11). After all, it has been common for
new agricultural technologies to be adopted earlier by the leading farmers
in a region, who are often those with the biggest or best farms, the best education, and the greatest willingness to take a risk by trying something
new. Furthermore, a tendency exists for public services to be more available to the big farmers than to the small, for technology to carry with it a
labor-saving bias that reduces labor's share of the product, and for technological innovations to be more appropriate to some geographical areas
than to others. Would not wealthy landlords use the benefits from green revolution technology as a stepping-stone to increasing the size of their holdings at the expense of small farmers, thus increasing income inequality?

Some of the above fears turn out to have been justified; most not.
Early adopters did tend to be the bigger, better farmers, but this has not
prevented smaller farmers, who are often slower to change, from adopting
green revolution technology.

Still, the benefits of the green revolution have accrued more to farmers in regions where water, especially irrigation water, is plentiful. Growers of lowland rice (rice that spends much of its early growing days with
its stalks standing in a few inches of water) benefit more than growers of
upland rice. Wheat and rice farmers, who predominate in tropical regions

with 40 inches or more of annual rainfall, benefit more than sorghum and millet farmers, who farm the semiarid tropics where rainfall is usually less than 40 inches per year.

The high-yielding fine grains (wheat and rice) grown with adequate water are far more responsive to fertilizer than are even the best varieties of the coarse grains (sorghum and millet) grown in the dry regions where irrigation water is scarce to nonexistent. The fertilizer subsidies that Third World governments frequently provide to their farmers therefore benefit the fine-grain producers more than the coarse-grain farmers. Thus, the benefits of the green revolution have concentrated mainly in the wetter tropics and especially on the flatter lands where irrigation and water management are easier. This phenomenon may well have increased income inequality between regions.

Nevertheless, within regions "the benefits from adopting modern varieties have been remarkably evenly distributed among farmers differing in size of holding and tenure status": This is the conclusion of a major study commissioned to examine the impact of the international agricultural research centers (Anderson et al. 1985:4).

In a detailed study of the economy of a northern Indian village where modern varieties had been widely adopted, Bliss and Stern (1982:291) found no strong association between size of holding and the intensity of use of inputs associated with the adoption of green revolution technology; in fact, "the adoption of various newer varieties and intensive practices seemed to be particularly associated with the younger educated farmers."

How is it that the benefits could be so evenly distributed among farms of different sizes and farmers of different tenure status? For one thing, the capital requirements of the green revolution are minimal. Unlike hybrid corn, which has done so much to increase corn yields in the United States and Europe, the green revolution fine-grain seeds breed true (i.e., produce offspring almost identical to the parent plant). Hybrid seed corn must be produced annually under technically demanding conditions on specialized farms and sold to farmers each year. A farmer who planted the grain from his hybrid corn crop as seed would be most disappointed in the yield results. Green revolution rice and wheat, although the result of complicated crosses, are not true hybrids. You can plant a little one year, take the resulting grain as seed for next year's crop, and rapidly and cheaply multiply your seed stock. Thus, a handful of green revolution seed is all you need to begin farming—and it usually does not cost any more than traditional seed.

On the one hand, green revolution varieties do require capital in the form of commercial fertilizer. On the other hand, fertilizer, like seed, is almost infinitely divisible, and a farmer need purchase only as much as he needs for his particular plot. Unlike capital investment in a tractor, the capital investment in the green revolution is not "lumpy"—that is, it does not come only in large, indivisible clumps.

A second reason for the evenly distributed benefits is that the green revolution technology is not labor saving. To the contrary, it turns out to be labor using (Hossain 1988b:12; Ranade & Herdt 1978:103; Pinstrup-Andersen & Hazell 1985:11). Much of the Third World grain crop is harvested and threshed by hand, and the increased crop yield requires more labor for harvest. More important, though, the fertilizer applied to the crop turns out to stimulate the growth of weeds as well as grain. Farmers are finding it profitable to remove these weeds, and, in the Third World, weeding a field is labor-intensive (weeds are pulled by hand or chopped with a blade, for example).

Because the poor spend a greater proportion of their income on food than do the rich, the benefits from price drops associated with increased production following the adoption of green revolution technology favor the poor over the rich. Because of the very low overall elasticity of demand for cereals, consumers benefit substantially from the price drop caused by increased production, but farmers as a whole experience a decline in total revenue (see the last part of Chapter 8 for a review of why this happens).

In a study of the social returns to rice research, Evenson and Flores (1978:255) found that in the Philippines, during the period from 1972 to 1975, the annual loss to producers from the adoption of the high-yielding rice varieties was $61 million, while the annual gain to consumers was $142 million, yielding a net annual gain to society of $81 million. Similarly, working with Colombian data, Scobie and Posada (1984) concluded that, during 1970–1974, Colombian rice producers lost $796 million, while consumers benefited by over $1,349 million, for a net gain to society of $553 million. Furthermore, they concluded that "while the lower 50 percent of Colombian households received about 15 percent of household income, they captured nearly 70 percent of the net benefits of the [rice] research program" (p. 383).

The cereal production increases that, because of demand elasticities of well below one, result in the loss of revenue for commercial rice growers may, at the same time, result in an increase in total revenue to the semisubsistence farmer. A semisubsistence farmer is defined as one who purchases less than 50 percent of his food supply in the marketplace. (Almost no one is a subsistence farmer, purchasing no food supplies, not even spices, in the marketplace.)

Consider a semisubsistence farmer who consumes, say, 90 percent of his rice crop. He has a small amount left over for sale in the market. He sees his neighbors on larger farms, who sell most of what they grow, practicing green revolution technology, and copies them, purchasing some seed and fertilizer and irrigating his crop as usual. His yield increases by the same percentage as that of the larger farmers, but, if he consumes the same amount of rice as he used to, the size of the surplus that he has left to sell grows by a much greater percentage than the percentage growth in his total production. Thus, even in the face of sharply declining rice prices, he may experience a gain in total revenue whereas his more commercially oriented neighbors are experiencing losses.

☐ **Education and Fertility Control**

Ahluwalia's study, which estimated a type of Kuznets curve of income distribution (shown in Figure 9.6), also produced evidence of how some variables besides per capita income affect income distribution. Table 9.7 shows the results of two of his multiple regressions on 60 countries, mentioned earlier in this chapter. In these regressions, the variables in the left-hand column are hypothesized to have an impact on the relative income shares.

The numbers in the middle column (equation one) show how the variables in the left-hand column influence percentage income share among the top 20 percent of the population. The numbers in the right-hand column (equation two) show how the variables in the left-hand column influence percentage income share among the bottom 40 percent of the population.

The variables on GNP per capita and GDP growth rate are included to account for the Kuznets curve. The variable at the bottom of the table,

Table 9.7   Cross-Country Regressions Explaining Income Shares

	Dependent Variable: Percentage Income Shares			
	Top 20 Percent		Lowest 40 Percent	
Explanatory Variables	Direction of Influence of Variable	Equation One	Direction of Influence of Variable	Equation Two
Constant	−	9.07	+	77.93
		(0.27)[a]		(4.11)
Log per capita GNP	+	50.35	−	47.28
		(2.13)		(3.50)
(Log per capita GNP)	−	8.16	+	7.65
		(1.98)		(3.35)
Growth rate of GDP	−	0.11	+	0.11
		(0.32)		(0.55)
Literacy rate	−	0.09	+	0.06
		(2.21)		(2.56)
Secondary school enrollment	−	0.14	+	0.02
		(2.48)		(0.74)
Growth rate of population	+	3.59	−	1.19
		(4.29)		(2.56)
Share of agriculture in GDP	−	0.25	+	0.04
		(2.23)		(0.65)
Share of urban population	−	0.10	+	0.06
		(1.68)		(1.79)
Dummy for socialist countries	−	9.41	+	8.57
		(3.27)		(5.35)
R^2		.76		.69
F		22.31		6.21
SEE		4.6		2.6

Source: Ahluwalia 1976a:131.

Note: Note that on each explanatory variable the signs switch between the top 20 percent and the bottom 40 percent of the population.

a. Values in parentheses are T ratios. For this sample, a T value of 1.68 indicates significance at the 10 percent level for a two-tailed test.

dummy for socialist countries, is included to account for the fact that, by and large, socialist countries have a more equal income distribution than nonsocialist countries. The remaining variables in the equation are included to see how they influence relative income share when the influence of the Kuznets curve and socialism are accounted for.

The signs on the numbers are of particular interest to us in examining the regression because they tell us the direction of influence that the related variable has on percentage income share when the other variables are at their average value. (Because the units of measurement of each of the variables influence the size of the regression coefficients—the numbers not in parentheses—and because we do not have these units of measurement, the size of the numbers is not of particular interest to us here. The size of the numbers in parentheses is important because they are the results of a test of significance—the bigger the number, the more likely its variable is to be of significant influence.)

First look at signs for the dummy for socialist countries. In equation one, the sign for this variable is negative, meaning that socialism tends to lower the percentage income share of the top 20 percent of the population. In equation two, the sign is positive. That is, socialism tends to raise the relative income share of the lowest 40 percent of the population.

Now examine the signs for the other variables. Increasing the literacy rate, the rate of secondary school enrollment, the share of agriculture in the GDP, and the share of urban population appears to increase the relative income share of the poor and to reduce the relative income share of the rich.

The share of agriculture in the GDP variable is not significant for the poor (T = 0.65), so we will not consider this variable important. As the percentage of the urban population increases, relative income share of the poor increases. This seems reasonable, because urban people generally enjoy higher incomes than rural people, and as rural people move to the city in search of better jobs the total income distribution may become more equal. However, because of problems of crowding, pollution, crime, and so on associated with growth in Third World cities, it is hard to argue for urbanization as a means to reduce income inequality.

Literacy rate and secondary school enrollment are good indices of overall education among the poor in Third World countries. The wealthy see to it that their children get an education somehow or other; the illiterates and those without even a secondary education are usually the poor. Increasing the rate of literacy and secondary education makes the poor potentially more productive and gives them better access to employment and better-paying jobs, thus reducing income inequality.

The influence of population growth rate on relative income share is harder to understand. It is the only one of the variables considered here for which increasing its value makes the poor worse off relative to the rich. The reasons for this are complex enough that we discuss them in their own chapter.

■ THE IMPACT OF DISTRIBUTION ON THE PACE OF DEVELOPMENT

In an attempt to find how the structure of economies changes with economic development, Hollis Chenery (1971) ran a multiple regression on "about 100" countries, using 1950–1965 World Bank data. From this regression he computed values for the savings rate, school enrollment ratio (percentage of those in school versus those expected to be in school), adult literacy rate, and birth rate per thousand population at different levels of per capita income. The results give a picture of how the magnitude of these variables changes as per capita income changes (Table 9.8).

In Table 9.8 we can see that, normally, increases in the savings rate, school enrollment ratio, and adult literacy rate are associated with increases in per capita income. On the other hand, increases in the birth rate are associated with a decrease in per capita income. The educational and fertility variables in this regression are affecting per capita income in a manner similar to the way they impacted income distribution in the regression shown in Table 9.7.

Could it be that by emphasizing the development of human capital through education and health programs designed to increase literacy and reduce fertility, countries could at the same time accelerate their development and reduce income inequalities? A study in the late 1970s answered this with a tentative yes. Ahluwalia, Carter, and Chenery (1979) examined 12 countries for which they had data on growth and income shares for a 10-year period. They found that the countries most successful in reducing income inequality were also the countries with the highest rates of growth in per capita incomes.

Recently a more comprehensive study by the World Bank (Deininger & Squire 1997) failed to make a strong correlation between growth and income inequality. Of the 88 countries whose per capita GDP grew for a decade, income inequality improved slightly in about half the cases and worsened slightly in the other half. However, the study found that the distribution of *wealth* (as measured by land ownership) does strongly affect growth. Countries having great inequality of wealth grow more slowly than countries with less inequality. For example, 15 developing countries have a Gini coefficient (for land distribution) higher than 70. Of these 15 countries only two showed growth rates higher than 2.5 percent per year during the period 1960–1992.

■ THE REDISTRIBUTION/INCENTIVE PARADOX RECONSIDERED

In Chapter 8 we argued that one of the leading causes of Third World undernutrition is lack of purchasing power among the poor, a combination of low income and the high price of the goods and services they buy. In

Table 9.8   **Normal Variations in Economic Structure with Level of Development**

	Level of GNP per Capita (in 1989 U.S. Dollars)[a]								
	200	400	800	1,200	1,600	2,400	3,200	4,000	8,000
Gross national savings, as % of GNP	9.4	12.0	14.8	16.4	17.6	19.3	20.5	21.5	24.6
School enrollment ratio	17.5	36.2	52.6	61.2	66.9	74.2	78.9	82.3	91.4
Adult literacy rate	15.3	36.5	55.2	65.0	71.5	80.0	85.4	89.4	93.0
Birth rate per thousand	46.6	41.8	36.6	33.8	31.1	28.2	25.3	22.4	17.1

Source: Chenery 1971:19.
Note: All values are computed from multiple regression for a sample of about 100 countries 1950–1965. Underlying data from the IBRD (World Bank), *World Tables*, December 1968.
a. The GNP data were originally in 1964 dollars and have been converted to 1989 dollars using the consumer price index (CPI).

this chapter we argue that inequality of income in and of itself is a cause of Third World undernutrition, producing, as it does, Reutlinger triangles of overconsumption and underconsumption of food.

Income inequality has, at times, been dramatically reduced through draconian measures severely applied throughout the country. For example, land reform with little or no compensation to the landlords, perhaps even their deaths being part of the deal; and banishment of intellectuals to prison camps or forced farm labor, sometimes their eyeglasses being smashed to help "keep them in their place." The collectivization experiments carried out as a result of the revolutions in Russia in 1917, China after World War II, or, more recently, Cambodia (at the hands of the Khmer Rouge) are testimony to the extreme measures that peoples will take in an attempt to reduce income inequality and improve the lot of the masses.

Although these bloody revolutions succeeded in reducing income inequality, and probably simultaneously in reducing the Reutlinger triangles, the resulting erosion of productivity incentives has left these countries struggling to keep up with their neighbors, especially in agricultural output.

This chapter has focused on ways to improve Third World nutrition by reducing the size of the Reutlinger triangles; we find the optimal way of attempting this may be through sponsoring programs that heavily emphasize health, fertility control, and education for all, thus simultaneously upgrading the productivity of the masses, reducing income inequality, and accelerating the pace of economic development.

□ 10

Demographic Factors Influencing Demand for Food

Chapter 7 presented some projections about the size of the world's population—it could grow by over 50 percent during the next 50 years. Does this mean that if food supply grows by 50 percent we will have enough extra food to feed those extra mouths? To answer that question we must first examine the factors that influence food consumption per person. In Chapters 8 and 9, we discussed how demand for food increases as income increases, and we examined some trends in per capita income levels and the distribution of income. In this chapter, we ask the question: What factors influence the amount of food consumed per capita?

■ POPULATION CHARACTERISTICS AND DEMAND FOR FOOD

Before turning to the issue of income and its impact on per capita food consumption, we shall first consider how average demand for food changes as a result of other characteristics of the population. We saw in Chapter 2 that nutrient requirements depend on age, sex, pregnancy and breast-feeding status, and physical activity level.

□ Age Structure

The age composition of a population (*age structure*) is one of the most important features of that population. It is a reflection of the underlying demographic conditions of the preceding decades and at the same time is an important determinant of future demographic patterns.

Population pyramids. The most convenient way to visualize the age structure of a population is through a graph of population distribution according to age and sex, called a *population pyramid*. Conventionally, population pyramids represent age cohorts by five- or 10-year intervals, and place males on the left of a vertical line and females on the right, with the youngest cohort at the bottom. The graphic representation of the age cohorts can be either the actual numbers or the percentage distribution. Figure 10.1 shows a numerical population pyramid for the industrialized nations versus the Third World in the year 1985, with projections to 2025. The horizontal lines across both sets of pyramids mark the dividing lines that are commonly, but arbitrarily, placed to separate the dependent age categories (in this case, below 15 years or above 65 years) from the working-age population. Such numerical population pyramids do a nice job of making visible the differences in actual population size, Third World versus developed world, and they can also show demographic features such as the higher survival rate of older women (notice the difference between the numbers of men and women in the oldest cohort for the 2025 projection for the developed world). But to make comparisons from one country to another, or from one time period to another within a country, pyramids showing percentage distribution (relative pyramids) are usually more helpful.

Figure 10.2 shows relative pyramids for two developed countries (the United States and West Germany) and one Third World country (Mo-

Figure 10.1 Population Pyramids for Less and More Developed Countries, 1985 and Projections to 2025

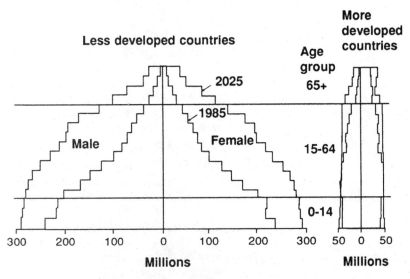

Source: Adapted from Merrick et al. 1986:19.

Figure 10.2   Age Structure in Morocco, United States, and West Germany, 1985

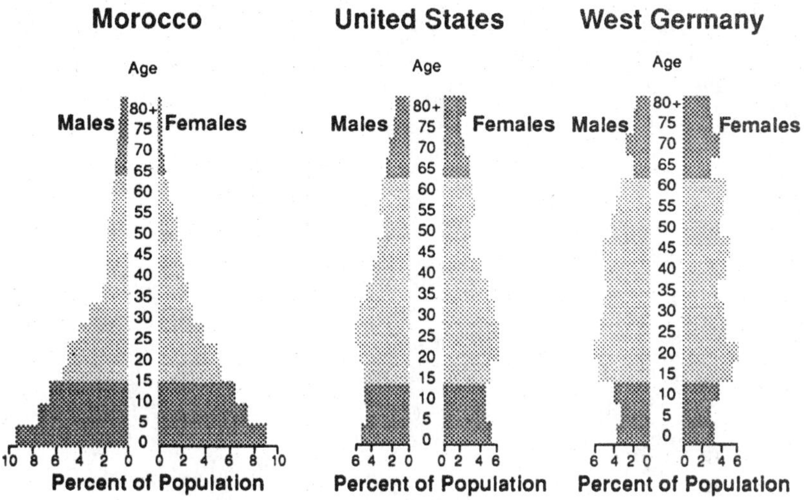

Source: Adapted from Haub 1987:21.

rocco). The total area in each pyramid is exactly the same and represents 100 percent of the population of each country. The relative size of the youngest age cohort (zero to five) is reflective of the magnitude of the birth rate in the previous five years in each country. In 1972, the birth rate in Morocco was 45 per thousand; in the United States it was 16, and in West Germany, 10.

Demographic patterns in the recent past can often be read directly from current population pyramids. For instance, during World War II and immediately afterwards, birth rates in Germany decline. In 1985, the year of the pyramid shown in Figure 10.2, people born between 1945 and 1950 were between 35 and 40 years old. They are shown in the cohort 35. Notice the narrowness of Germany's pyramid during that year. By contrast, the United States experienced a 15-year baby boom starting immediately after World War II, which shows as a bulge in the 1985 pyramid extending from cohorts 25 through 35.

Age structure is of interest to demographers because, as we have noted above, it provides clues about past and future demographic patterns. It is important to policymakers because of its impact on two things we will discuss next: (1) momentum in population growth; and (2) dependency ratios.

Momentum in population growth.   Over a long period, a population would just reproduce itself if individual couples produced exactly the right number of children to replace themselves, allowing for some children to die before they arrived at childbearing age. In most populations this number comes to just over two children (e.g., about 2.1) per couple (or per woman). In this discussion, we assume that 2.1 children, on the average, will handle replacement. If a population has remained constant for a couple of generations and then its fertility rate rises higher than 2.1, it will grow. (We are assuming no net immigration or emigration and no improvements in health care that raise average life expectancy.) If, on the other hand, its fertility rate falls below 2.1, it will shrink. For that reason, a fertility rate of 2.1 is considered the replacement level (Merrick et al. 1986:6).

You might expect that when the fertility rate of a rapidly growing population falls to 2.1, births and deaths would be in balance, and population growth would stop. This is not the case, at least not immediately. The reason is demographic momentum. A population that has had high fertility in the years before reaching replacement-level fertility will have a much younger age structure than a population with low fertility before crossing the replacement threshold. Consider the three countries in Figure 10.2. West Germany has a fertility rate of 1.4. It has already stopped growing, with a population growth rate of minus 0.2 percent. Notice that a substantial proportion of its population is over 35. The United States has a fertility rate of 1.9 and rate of natural increase of 0.7 percent. (Immigration is now causing the United States to grow faster than that.) It also has a more youthful population than West Germany. But an enormous proportion of the population of Morocco, which in 1982 had a fertility rate of 6.9, is below 35 years of age. Morocco's rate of natural increase was 3.2 in 1982. It fell to about 2.6 in 1989. Now suppose that Morocco's fertility rate should suddenly fall to 2.1. Would its population growth stop immediately? No, because of the large numbers of young people in the childbearing years relative to the older years. Would it stop soon? No, because of the large number of people below 15 who will be moving into the childbearing years.

As noted above, the rate of natural increase of population in the United States is 0.7 percent even though its fertility rate is 1.9, just below replacement level. This is caused by momentum. To reinforce your understanding of momentum in population growth, study Figure 10.3. On a worldwide basis, population momentum means that "even if there were a sudden reduction of fertility to the level strictly needed to replace the population, the world population would still increase by more than 2 billion" by the year 2050 (FAO, WFS Background Paper no. 4).

Dependency ratios. When the age structure of a population is known, the dependency ratios can be easily calculated. The dependency ratio is usually defined as the ratio of dependents to working-age adults. As mentioned before, working-age adults are generally identified as those from 15 to 65. But dependents are commonly split into groups by age, and two

Figure 10.3   A Demonstration of Momentum in Population Growth

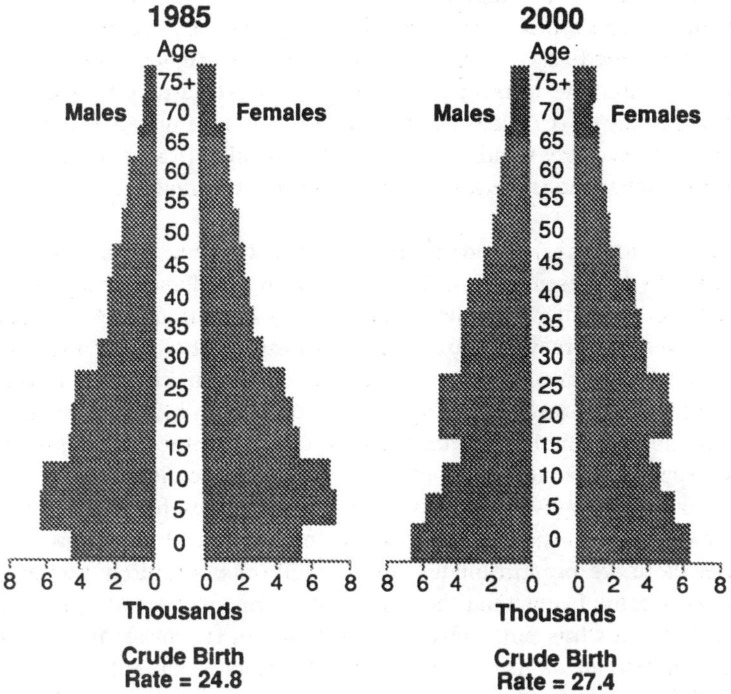

1985
Age
75+
70
65
60
55
50
45
40
35
30
25
20
15
10
5
0

Males   Females

8 6 4 2 0   0 2 4 6 8
Thousands

**Crude Birth
Rate = 24.8**

2000
Age
75+
70
65
60
55
50
45
40
35
30
25
20
15
10
5
0

Males   Females

8 6 4 2 0   0 2 4 6 8
Thousands

**Crude Birth
Rate = 27.4**

Source: Adapted from Haub 1987:14.
Note: The pyramids here demonstrate the effect of age structure on population change. In 1985 this population had a noticeable bulge in the age groups 5–9 and 10–14, the result of a recent baby boom. In this population about half of all the childbearing takes place in the twenties. When the bulge groups reach their twenties, the number of births will rise disproportionately. In this example the total fertility rate is held constant at 3.1, as is mortality. In 1985 the crude birth rate was 24.8 per 1,000 but by the year 2000 it will have increased to 27.4, as a result of the bulge groups reaching childbearing years. The growth rate will have increased from 1.65 in 1985 to 1.84 in the year 2000.

more ratios are then defined: The adult dependency ratio is the percentage of the population 65 and over divided by the percentage of the population between 15 and 65; the child dependency ratio is the percentage of the population below 15 divided by the percentage of the population between 15 and 65.

In a rapidly growing population the burden of dependent children per adult is far greater than in a slowly growing population or one with zero population growth. Compare again the population pyramids in Figure 10.2, this time with regard to the child dependency ratio. In West Germany, which in 1985 had essentially zero population growth, 15 percent of the population was below 15 years of age, and 70 percent was in the age group 15 through 64. The child dependency ratio was thus 0.21; that is, 0.21 children per working adult. Another way of looking at these data is to say that some 4.7 adults were available, on the average, to raise and educate each child.

In Morocco, whose population was growing at just over 3 percent at the time the pyramid was drawn, 42 percent of the people were children and 54 percent were in the working-age group (15–64). That produces a child dependency ratio of 0.77. In Morocco, then, there were only 1.3 adults available, on the average, to raise and educate each child. (Raw data for calculating dependency ratios were furnished by the Population Reference Bureau.)

The age structure of population in the future. What kind of age structure will we see in the future? The theory of demographic transition described in Chapter 7 predicts that as living conditions improve, life expectancy will increase, followed by declining fertility rates. This implies that in the future there will be a smaller percentage of children and a larger percentage of adults. Projections from the Food and Agriculture Organization shown in Table 10.1 are consistent with this theoretical prediction. Life expectancy is increasing—so there will be more older people; fertility rates are declining—so there will be fewer babies for each woman of childbearing age. And future population pyramids will be narrower.

If there are proportionately more adults than children, the need for food will grow faster than the population. The simple example in Table 10.2 illustrates this point. Although population increases by 50 percent, calorie requirements increase by 54 percent because the future population is 66 percent adult rather than the present 60 percent. This effect can also be seen in comparisons of current energy requirements in different geographical areas. Because of the high proportion of children in Africa's population compared to the United States and Canada, average calorie requirements in Africa are 2,150 calories compared to 2,400 in North

Table 10.1 Future Life Expectancy, Fertility Rates, and Population Growth: Africa, Asia, and the World (based on UN medium-variant projection)

	Africa			Asia			World		
Period	Population Growth Rate	Life Expectancy at Birth	Fertility Rates	Population Growth Rate	Life Expectancy at Birth	Fertility Rates	Population Growth Rate	Life Expectancy at Birth	Fertility Rates
1990–95	2.81	53.0	5.80	1.64	64.5	3.03	1.57	64.4	3.10
2000–05	2.56	55.8	4.91	1.38	67.9	2.73	1.37	67.1	2.84
2010–15	2.37	60.5	4.09	1.15	70.8	2.44	1.20	69.9	2.60
2020–25	2.08	63.4	3.37	0.89	73.2	2.19	1.00	72.5	2.38
2030–35	1.62	69.4	2.63	0.68	75.0	2.12	0.78	74.6	2.22
2040–45	1.19	72.3	2.10	0.49	76.7	2.10	0.57	76.4	2.10
2045–50	1.14	73.4	2.10	0.40	77.4	2.10	0.51	77.1	2.10

Source: Adapted from FAO, WFS Background Paper No. 1.

America (FAO, WFS Background Paper No. 4). The projections of the impact of changing age structure on per capita calorie requirements are shown in Table 10.3. In Africa, where the age structure is projected to change the most, per capita calorie requirements are expected to increase by 7 percent (to 2,300 calories per person per day) over the next 50 years. In Asia and Latin America, the increase is 2 percent. In the developed world no change is projected (except for a slight decline in requirements in Europe, attributable to an increase in percentage of elderly people in the population).

□ **Other Demographic Characteristics and Food Requirements**

Average per capita food requirements in a population also depend on other characteristics of the people. In this section, we discuss likely impacts on per capita food requirements over the next 50 years from three factors: (1) the number of pregnant women in the population; (2) the average amount of physical activity in the population; (3) the average height of people.

Table 10.2   An Example Demonstrating How Changing Age Structure of a Population Can Affect Food Requirements

	Present	Future
Number of children (requiring 1,800 calories per capita per day)	4 million	5 million
Number of adults (requiring 2,700 calories per capita per day)	6 million	10 million
Total population	10 million	15 million
Total calorie requirements	23,400 million	36,000 million
Calories per capita per day	2,340	2,400

Table 10.3   Estimated Effects of Demographic Factors in Average Calorie Requirement per Capita per Day (percentage increase or decrease from 1995)

	Africa	Asia	Europe	Latin America and the Caribbean	North America	Oceania
Age structure	+7	+2	−1	+2	no change	no change
Change in percentage of pregnant women	no change	−1	no change	no change	no change	no change
Change in level of physical activity	−3	−4	−1	−2	−1	−1
Change in average height	+2	+2	no change	+2	no change	+1

Source: FAO, WFS Background Paper No. 4.

Pregnancy. Pregnant and breast-feeding women require higher caloric intake. Two opposing trends exist here. As the base of the population pyramid contracts, we see an increase in the ratio of women of childbearing age to total population. On the other hand, the drop in fertility rates means that each woman of childbearing age is becoming pregnant fewer times during her lifetime. As Table 10.3 shows, the FAO estimates no net effect on average per capita food requirements, except for a 1 percent decline in Asia.

Physical activity. Anyone who has ever exercised in an attempt to control her weight knows that physical activity burns calories. On a worldwide scale, what is likely to affect average per capita calorie requirements is not "average visits to the gym," but the average physical activity of adults on the job. Farming (especially in developing countries) requires more physical activity than many city jobs. Therefore, as urban populations grow faster than rural populations in the future, we should expect to see a decline in the average activity level. As Table 10.3 shows, the FAO projects that this change will cause a reduction in per capita food requirements of from 1 to 4 percent.

Height. Good nutrition during infancy and childhood can cause a person to become a taller adult. But taller adults need more calories to maintain their bodily functions. The FAO projections are based on an underlying assumption that food supplies will continue to grow faster than food demand, thus the incidence of undernutrition will decline, and there will be less stunting. Table 10.3 shows that this is expected to add 2 percent to energy requirements in developing countries, and to have no substantial effect in the developing world.

■ PER CAPITA INCOME AND DEMAND FOR FOOD

Compared to the changes in population characteristics described above, growth of per capita income is likely to have a much bigger effect on food demand. Average food demand per person will increase in the future as per capita incomes increase. In other words, the average person will eat more in the future because average income will be higher, and people will purchase more food.

To estimate how large the growth in demand for food per capita will be, we need answers to two questions:

How much will average income per capita grow?
How much will income growth affect food demand?

☐ Growth in Income per Capita

To answer the first question, we can look at economists' predictions about future growth in income per capita, and at historical experience with growth. The World Bank projects growth (during the decade of the 1990s) of 2.9 percent per year in low- and middle-income countries, and growth of 2.1 percent per year in high-income countries. Historical experience shows that during the 1980s, per capita income grew at a 2.4 percent annual rate in high-income countries and at a 1.2 percent rate in low-income countries.

As we saw in Chapter 9, growth in per capita incomes is not the same for all countries. Some countries (notably in Asia) have seen rapid growth, and others (notably in sub-Saharan Africa) have seen negative growth, or declines in per capita incomes. (Note the growth in per capita income described above is "real" income, or income after adjusting for inflation.) If income per capita grows at a rate of between 1 and 3 percent per year, at the end of 50 years, average income will be higher by between 64 percent and 438 percent, as shown in Table 10.4.

☐ Impact of Income Growth on Food Demand

As a person's income increases, that person's demand for food increases. As described in Chapter 8, economists measure the size of that impact by a measure called *income elasticity of demand for food*. Estimates show that the income elasticity for food is between 0.1 and 0.3. This means that a 1 percent increase in a person's income will increase the quantity of food demanded by the person by from 0.1 to 0.3 percent. If we apply this to the growth in income projected in Table 10.4, we obtain growth in per capita food demand of between 6.4 percent (if income grows by 64 percent and income elasticity is 0.1) and 101 percent (if income grows by 338 percent and income elasticity is 0.3).

The most likely scenario remains at the low end of this range of projections for two reasons. First, although average growth of per capita incomes in the 2–3 percent range have been observed for a decade, it may be difficult to sustain this level of growth for 50 years. Second, economists recognize that income elasticities decline as income increases. Therefore,

Table 10.4   The Power of Compound Growth

If income per capita grows at an annual rate of:	Then income after 50 years will be higher by a factor of:
1%	1.64 (about one-and-a-half times current income)
2%	2.69 (over twice current income)
3%	4.38 (over four times current income)

as average incomes increase in the future, the applicable income elasticities may be lower than those currently observed.

Is it reasonable to expect that per capita food demand will grow by 5–20 percent over the next 50 years? Growth of this magnitude would mean that (assuming constant prices) the worldwide average intake of calories per capita might grow from the current 2,720 per day to a level between 2,856 (equivalent to the current average diet of Algeria) and 3,264 calories per day (approximately equivalent to the current average diet of Mexico). For an additional comparison, between the early 1970s and the early 1990s, worldwide consumption of calories per person grew about 11 percent.

☐ **Growth in Population and Growth in Food
per Capita—A Multiplicative Effect**

Notice that growth in per capita food consumption magnifies the impact of growing population. Imagine a country in which 1,000 people consume 2,500 calories per day—total food consumption in the country is 2.5 million calories per day. Now suppose the population grows to 2,000, and per capita calories grows to 3,000; now total food consumption in the country is 6 million calories per day. The population has grown by 100 percent (from 1,000 to 2,000), but food consumption has grown by 140 percent (from 2.5 to 6 million). Not only are there more mouths to feed, but each mouth is eating more. The practical effect of this is illustrated in Table 10.5. If population grows by 50 percent over the next 50 years, and if per capita food demand grows by between 5 and 20 percent, total food demand will grow by between 57.5 and 80 percent.

■ **DIETARY DIVERSIFICATION
AND DEMAND FOR FOOD**

As average incomes go up, people do not simply eat more food; they eat different kinds of food. In particular, they eat more meat and animal products, and they consume fewer calories from cereals. To illustrate this, consider the diets of various countries and country groups shown in Table 10.6.

In the mid-1990s, average calories consumed per day worldwide were about 2,700, with about 400 (15 percent) coming from animal products and about 2,300 from plant sources. According to FAO estimates, it took about 4,800 *plant-derived calories* to produce these 2,700 calories. Thus, it took about 2,500 plant-derived calories to produce the 400 calories from animal products—a ratio about about 6:1. (See Box 10.1 for the FAO's estimates of the number of plant-derived calories needed to produce a human-consumed calorie from various animal products.)

Table 10.5 Growth in per Capita Food Consumption Magnifies the Effect of Population Growth

If population grows by 50% over the next 45 years, and if per capita food demand grows by ___%	then total food demand will grow by ___%
5	57.5
10	65
15	72.5
20	80

Table 10.6 Calories (per Capita per Day) from Cereals and Animal Products in Various Countries and Country Groups, 1995

	Nigeria	India	China	Brazil	U.S.	All Developing Countries	All Developed Countries
Income/capita ($)	260	340	620	3,640	26,980	4,771	24,930
Calories from animal products	79	170	506	543	989	315	861
Calories from cereals	1,057	1,483	1,578	889	847	1,435	1,018
Total calories	2,508	2,388	2,741	2,834	3,603	2,570	3,192

Source: FAOSTAT Statistical Database, 1998.

Box 10.1 Plant-Derived Calories Needed to Produce a Calorie from Animal Products

FAO estimates that it takes:

- 11 plant-derived calories to produce 1 calorie of beef
- 11 plant-derived calories to produce 1 calorie of mutton
- 4 plant-derived calories to produce 1 calorie of pork
- 4 plant-derived calories to produce 1 calorie of poultry
- 8 plant-derived calories to produce 1 calorie of milk
- 4 plant-derived calories to produce 1 calorie of egg

Source: FAO, WFS Background Paper No. 4.

In 1995, people in developing countries consumed about 12.5 percent of their 2,570 calories as animal products. Suppose this percentage rises to 15 percent (approximately the world average today) by the year 2050. Even if caloric intake remained constant at 2,570, this shift to animal products would mean that each person would need 8.7 percent more plant-derived calories. The calculation is as follows: The current diet is 315 calories from animal sources, and 2,255 from plant sources; if 6.25 plant-derived calories are needed to produce one animal product calorie, this means the current diet requires 4,224 plant-derived calories; if calories from animal products rise to 15 percent of 2,570 (385 calories), the future diet would require 4,591 plant-derived calories. This is an 8.7 percent increase in plant-derived calories. To put it somewhat differently: If diets in developing countries were slightly more diversified (15 percent animal products instead of the current 12.5 percent)—even with no increase in calories per capita—the effect on food demand would be the same as an 8.7 percent increase in population.

Consider a different scenario—suppose that by the year 2050, people in developing countries have incorporated meat into their diets to such an extent that their diets resemble diets in developed countries today. In this case, the future developing country diet would be 27 percent animal product calories (693 out of 2,570). Converting this to plant-derived calories, and adding the 1,877 calories consumed directly from plant sources, yields about 6,200 plant-derived calories—a 47 percent increase from the present diet.

■ TOTAL IMPACT OF DEMOGRAPHIC CHANGES ON FOOD DEMAND: ALTERNATIVE SCENARIOS

The same multiplicative effect described above between population growth and growth in consumption per capita applies more generally to all the effects described in this chapter. To review, using examples:

- If population grows by 50 percent, and population characteristics cause food demand to grow by 5 percent per capita, total demand grows by more than 50 percent—demand will be $(1 + .50) \times (1 + .05) = 1.575$, or 57.5 percent above current levels.
- If population grows by 50 percent, and if changes in population characteristics give food demand a 5 percent boost, and if (in addition) income increases demand per capita by 15 percent, total demand grows by 81 percent. (The computation is $[1 + .50] \times [1 + .05] \times [1 + .15] - 1$].)
- If diversification of diets has an additional impact on effective (or plant-equivalent) demand of 10 percent, the total growth in demand is 99 percent.

In these examples, the numbers were chosen to be "in the reasonable range." They are by no means intended as an exact projection.

We can learn two important lessons from the last paragraph. First, notice the impact of taking changes in demographic characteristics into account.

Box 10.2 Can We Solve the World Food Problem by Giving Up Bacon and Eggs?

Arthur Dommen

Some people argue that it is immoral for people in the high-income industrial nations to eat a diet rich in livestock products as long as there are people starving in parts of Africa, Asia, and Latin America who could consume directly the cereals and pulses that are now being fed to cattle, pigs, and chickens. Since approximately a third of the world's grain supply goes to feed livestock, the argument has a certain plausibility to it.

It is certainly true that food energy is lost in putting grain through livestock to convert it to livestock products. For instance, it takes around 2 pounds of grain to produce a pound of chicken, 4 pounds of grain to produce a pound of pork, and 8 pounds of feed (in this case, much of it grass and other materials not usable by man as food) to produce a pound of beef.

The question is, if the rich cut bacon, eggs, steak, butter, and cheese, for example, from their dinner table, to what extent would the grain and pulses currently going to produce these products find their way to the food-short people of the developing countries? To be more specific, how would the food get into the hands of the world's hungry? Who would buy it? Who would store it? Who would ship it? Who would distribute it? How much would it cost? Would the resources spent on this direct feeding activity go further toward solving the hunger problem if spent on alternative activities?

But the story is more complicated than this. Some of the products finding their way into the Western livestock feed market these days are produced by farmers in developing countries—soybeans from Brazil and cassava chips from Thailand, to mention just two. These products enjoy large and expanding markets in Europe and Japan, which do not have enough acreage available to satisfy the feed demand from the livestock sectors of their own countries. These exports of livestock feed add to income in the developing countries.

Even with the enormous grain consumption of the world's livestock herd, there is enough grain-producing capacity left over to feed the world's hungry—if they had the purchasing power to buy the grain they need. Furthermore, the grain-consuming livestock sector acts as an insurance policy against the "seven lean years" or whatever other period of bad harvests we might experience. The commercial livestock sector acts as a huge cushion for human grain consumers. Commercial livestock producers absorb large quantities of grain when supplies are cheap and abundant and reduce livestock feeding when grain supplies are expensive and scarce because of drought or other causes.

The causes of Third World undernutrition are complex. Simple approaches such as giving up bacon and eggs for breakfast may make you feel better about the world food situation, but there are probably more effective actions you can take toward solving the problem.

Arthur Dommen is an agricultural economist specializing in Third World food issues.

Population grows by 50 percent (in the example); but total food demand grows by 99 percent—nearly double the growth in population. Even though none of the demographic effects is large in and of itself—5 percent growth in demand per capita because of population characteristics, 15 percent growth because of income growth, 10 percent growth because of diet diversification—the cumulative effect is large. Second, notice the frequent use of the word "if" in the above example. In making projections about the future, this word has to be used a lot. It is useful to construct alternative scenarios to see how much variation results. Table 10.7 shows a number of scenarios about possible growth in demand for food.

In constructing scenarios, we must be internally consistent. We should not assume that incomes per capita will be stagnant and that a large amount of dietary diversification will take place simultaneously; dietary diversification is a result of growth in incomes. The scenario laid out in the example above—and much of the discussion in this chapter—is based on a fundamentally optimistic outlook. Prosperity is assumed to increase; food supplies are assumed to keep pace with demand. As a result, life expectancy increases and fertility declines; the age structure of the population changes toward fewer children and more adults; average per capita income increases, and with it demand for food; increased prosperity also encourages increased consumption of meat relative to plant sources of calories. The scenario is optimistic—but it is also consistent.

The requirement of internal consistency carries with it a certain element of self-correction of projections. For example, if we adopt more pessimistic assumptions—prosperity declines and food supply fails to keep pace with demand—we see several implications. First, population may grow more rapidly than anticipated—the decline in fertility rates is dependent (according to the theory of demographic transition) on the increase in life expectancy attributable to prosperity. However, the change in age

Table 10.7   **Various Scenarios About Growth in Demand for Food to the Year 2050, Expressed as Percentage Increases**

Scenario	Effect of Population Growth	Effect of Population Characteristics	Effect of Increasing Income	Effect of Dietary Diversification	Total Impact
A	50	5	15	10	99
B	65	5	15	10	119
C	90	5	15	10	152
D	40	5	15	10	86
E	65	0	15	10	109
F	65	0	5	10	91
G	65	0	20	10	118
H	80	0	5	5	98
I	40	0	20	20	101

structure or in average height of the population will not be as large as projected above (and may move food demand in the opposite direction). Similarly, lower growth in incomes will result in a smaller increase in calories per capita and less dietary diversification. Thus, although population growth is larger (under this pessimistic scenario), other factors are less important. Scenario H demonstrates this: Income growth is lower, therefore growth in calories per capita and dietary diversification are smaller, but population growth is larger; the result is that demand approximately doubles—the same as we see in scenario A. Scenario I demonstrates a more optimistic scenario: Income growth and dietary diversification are greater, but population growth is slower; the result is that demand approximately doubles. This demonstrates the *self-correcting* mechanism at work.

11

Agricultural Land, Water, and Yields

The last few chapters helped us analyze the questions: How much food is enough? How many people will need to be fed? How much food will the average person eat? How does the average level and the distribution of income in the world influence the answers to these questions? Next, we turn to the supply side. Will there be enough food? How can we increase the supply of food to make food more affordable? Prices of food are not etched in stone and handed down from on high. They are determined in the market day-by-day and week-by-week through the interplay of supply-and-demand forces. When the supply of food increases, prices drop, food becomes more affordable, and hunger decreases. In this chapter we examine the factors that determine food supply.

■ THE BASIC EQUATION OF FOOD SUPPLY

The typical way to analyze the food supply is to focus on crops and split up output according to the following simple equation:

$$\text{Total output} = \text{Output/Acre} \times \text{Acres}$$

Typically, *output per acre* is referred to by the term *yield*. Of course, one might think that this equation ignores food from animal products. But, as described in Chapter 10, animal food-products require animal feed, and animal feed comes from crops. And only 16 percent of calories worldwide come from meat products. About 50 percent comes from cereal crops (rice, wheat, maize, etc.). Therefore we will discuss food production from the perspective of crop production.

The equation obviously splits into two factors: land area and yield. (FAO estimates that 69 percent of the increase in plant production between 1970 and 1990 was due to improved yields and 31 percent to increases in cultivated areas.) In our discussion in this chapter, we will examine three principal influences on current and future agricultural output:

- Quantity of available agricultural land and water
- Intensity of input use on the land
- Technological change

■ AVAILABLE LAND

Of course, one way to increase food production is to increase the amount of land devoted to agricultural production. Data in Table 11.1 show that agricultural land has increased slowly but steadily. Worldwide, total land in agriculture increased 2.5 percent during the 1960s, 2.5 percent during the 1970s, 3.1 percent during the 1980s, and 0.3 percent during the first half of the 1990s.

But can this rate of increase continue into the future? The FAO reports that compared to current use of 760 million hectares, there are 2.57 billion hectares of "rainfed land with crop potential" in developing countries excluding China. At first blush, this would appear to be very good news. But much of this potential land (67 percent) is hilly, or has poor soil or drainage. As Table 11.2 shows, the potential for increased production on good quality land is considerably more limited. Nevertheless, there does appear to be potential to bring new land under cultivation; the area of this potential agricultural land is perhaps 30 percent of current area. The potential differs significantly from region to region. In South Asia and the Near East and North Africa, little potential exists for expansion. Brazil and

Table 11.1   Worldwide Agricultural Land Use, 1961–1994, in Thousands of Hectares

	Agricultural Land Use	Arable Land	Permanent Pasture
1961	4,486,786	1,266,139	3,141,388
1965	4,533,592	1,279,747	3,171,358
1970	4,597,899	1,302,294	3,208,432
1975	4,662,167	1,313,227	3,257,858
1980	4,710,115	1,331,998	3,282,680
1985	4,775,131	1,347,871	3,330,509
1990	4,860,536	1,356,743	3,397,493
1994	4,872,738	1,353,267	3,398,741

Source: FAOSTAT Statistics Database 1998.

Table 11.2. Land Use and Availability in Developing Countries (in millions of hectares and excluding China), 1996

	Good Soil/Terrain	Poor Soil or Terrain	Total
Currently used for crops	547	213	760
Land with crop potential	848	1,722	2,570
Use as % of potential	64%	12%	30%

Source: Derived from FAO, World Food Summit, Background Paper No. 1, 1997.

Congo-Brazzaville (and surrounding African countries) have large tracts of land that could be brought under agricultural production.

The last paragraph implies that it is possible to increase the amount of land under cultivation significantly, perhaps by 30 percent or more. However, this calculation requires the additional assumption that no land currently under cultivation is lost to agriculture. Three reasons raise concerns that land currently used for agricultural production might not be usable for agriculture in the future. First, as population grows and urban areas expand, some farmland is paved over. The impact of suburban sprawl is obvious in parts of the United States. However, worldwide urban areas and other human settlements take up only 3 percent of the land mass. Therefore, even significant urbanization will have a small quantitative effect on agriculture worldwide. Second, as we will discuss in more detail in the next chapter, global warming may result in expansion of ocean areas and flooding of coastal areas. Third—and of most concern to experts— land currently in production may be *degraded* through soil loss or contamination to such a degree that it can no longer be used to grow crops. This aspect will be discussed in more detail in the next chapter.

Conversely, undoubtedly some potential does exist for increasing production without increasing yields *or* acres. Most significant here is likely to be expansion of double or triple cropping—where a single plot of land is planted with two or three crops sequentially during a year. Double cropping becomes more feasible if agronomists develop crop varieties that require a shorter growing season. Other new technologies may increase the importance of non-land-based food production—most immediately fisheries and aquaculture, but potentially including hydroponics, food from the sea, and food from space.

Taking all these factors into account, some experts are notably more pessimistic than is the FAO regarding the future potential for adding or maintaining land for food production. Kendall and Pimentel cite a lack of arable land as "one of the most urgent problems facing humanity . . . [and also] perhaps the most neglected" (Kendall & Pimentel 1994). In another study, Pimentel calculates that nearly one-third of the world's cropland (1.5 billion hectares) has been abandoned during the past 40 years because erosion has made it unproductive (Pimentel et al. 1995). Gary Gardner of

WorldWatch Institute also concludes that little room exists for large-scale expansion of cropland: "Replacing lost land is likely to be more difficult than many officials think. . . . Optimistic officials often overestimate the potential for expansion by including marginal land, where cultivation may not be sustainable. Indeed, the world's major grain producers have all overexpanded into marginal land in recent years, damaging large areas of land in the process. Many are now pulling back to the land that can be cultivated with a resulting loss of grain production" (Gardner 1996).

■ THE IMPORTANCE OF WATER

Of course, finding new agricultural land is useless unless we also have sufficient water for agricultural production. As Table 11.3 shows, agriculture uses enormous amounts of water, especially in the developing world. Table 11.4 shows the amount of irrigated land has grown steadily over time. Irrigation is especially important in growing rice; indeed, irrigated land produces 80 percent of the food in Bangladesh, 70 percent of the food in China, and over 50 percent in India and Indonesia (FAO Fact Sheet on Water and Food Security 1996). Worldwide, irrigated land provides about 40 percent of total food. Yields on irrigated land range from 30 to 200 percent higher than on nonirrigated land. Irrigation raises corn yields from 1.7 to 3.9 (metric tons per hectare) in Latin America, from 1.2 to 3.1 in Africa, and raises wheat yields from 1.8 to 4.1 in Latin America and from 1.4 to 2.4 in North Africa/Near East; vegetable yields rise from 5.1 to 14.2 in East Asia.

Will it be possible to continue increasing irrigation? The FAO is quite optimistic on this question: "Half or even two-thirds of future gains in crop production are expected to come from irrigated land" (FAO WFS Fact

Table 11.3   Water Use by Continent, 1995

Continent	Africa	Asia	Former USSR	Europe	North & Central Amer.	Oceania	South America	World
% water used in agriculture	88	86	65	33	49	34	59	69
% water used for domestic	7	6	7	13	9	64	19	8
% water used in industry	5	8	28	54	42	2	23	23
Total use cubic km per year	144	1,531	358	359	697	23	133	3,240
Total runoff cubic km per year	4,570	14,410	348	3,210	8,200	2,040	11,760	44,538

Source: FAO, World Food Summit, Background Paper No. 7, 1997.

Table 11.4. Irrigated Land

Year	Arable Land (thousands of hectares)	Irrigated Land (thousands of hectares)	% of Arable Land that is Irrigated
1961	1,266,139	138,813	11
1965	1,279,747	149,740	12
1970	1,302,294	167,331	13
1975	1,313,227	187,559	14
1980	1,331,998	209,233	16
1985	1,347,871	223,304	17
1990	1,356,743	242,185	18
1994	1,353,267	254,027	19

Source: FAOSTAT Statistical Database 1998.

Sheet on Water and Food Security 1996). A World Bank/UNDP study estimated that an additional 110 million hectares of land could be brought under irrigation, producing enough more grain to feed 1.5 to 2 billion people (World Bank/UNDP 1990). Tables 11.3 and 11.4 allow us to calculate that total water use in agriculture was about 2,200 cubic kilometers, amounting to 0.0088 cubic kilometers of water per 1,000 hectares of irrigated land. If 110 million hectares of newly irrigated land were irrigated at this rate, the total additional water requirement would be 968 cubic kilometers, about 30 percent of current water usage.

However, other experts are more pessimistic about future water availability. Sandra Postel concludes that agriculture cannot increase water use much beyond current levels without causing substantial environmental problems. She argues that the approximately 44,500 cubic kilometers of water reported in Table 11.3 as total runoff greatly overstates available water. First, she argues, about 20 percent of that is geographically so remote that it is not available for human use. Of the remaining 32,900 cubic kilometers, about 75 percent occurs during floods, and therefore is not available for irrigation during dry periods. The actual quantity of usable water is then around 12,500 cubic kilometers. "The problem is that water use tripled between 1950 and 1990 as world population soared by some 2.7 billion. . . . Worldwide demand for water cannot triple again without causing severe shortages for crop irrigation, industrial use, basic household needs, and critical life-supporting ecosystems" (Postel 1997). She notes that water shortages are already appearing as depletion of groundwater. She cites evidence that water tables are dropping a meter or more each year in northern China and falling 20 centimeters a year in India's Punjab.

Others belittle this talk of water shortages as "doomsaying." Julian Simon of the University of Maryland is one of the most outspoken optimists about future resource availability. He bases his optimism on a confidence in human ingenuity:

Usable water is like other resources, however, in being a product of human labor and ingenuity. People "create" usable water, and there are large opportunities to discover and utilize new sources. Some additional sources are well-known and already in partial use: transport by ship from one country to another, deeper wells, cleaning dirty water, towing icebergs to places where water is needed, and desalination. . . . [In addition] huge new supplies of groundwater have been found in the Red Sea Province of eastern Sudan, Florida, and elsewhere (Simon 1996:chapter 6).

The FAO makes some small-scale, practical recommendations of ways in which water can be used more efficiently, such as water harvesting (collecting runoff and saving it for periods of need) and drip irrigation (delivering irrigation water directly to the roots of plants). In addition, agricultural scientists have developed crop varieties that require less water to thrive and have developed chemicals that promote water retention in soil.

As we will see in the following chapter, water use in agriculture is a major source of environmental concerns related to agricultural production. Increased irrigation carries the threat of increased soil erosion, increased chemical runoff and resulting water pollution, and increased threat of global warming from paddy-rice production.

■ YIELDS AND INPUT USE: PURCHASED INPUTS

The discussion of water availability and use is a dramatic example of how yields can be increased by adding more inputs to the land. The term *inputs* as economists use it refers to factors or goods that contribute to production. Water, labor, chemicals, and machinery are all examples of inputs. As a general rule, when we increase the intensity of input use on a plot of land, we increase the output of that plot.

The growth in worldwide use of agricultural machinery and fertilizers is shown in Table 11.5. Use of agricultural machinery has approximately doubled since the early 1960s. Fertilizer use has more than quadrupled since 1961. The question for these inputs is not whether we *can* continue to increase their use—we can always build more tractors or produce more fertilizer—but whether we *should* increase their use.

For fertilizers, the question is a relatively simple one. Too much fertilizer can actually result in reduced output; even if the yield does increase, the value of the increased production must be enough to cover the increased cost of the fertilizer. Despite the dramatic growth of fertilizer use, the potential for additional use exists in many parts of the developing world, especially in sub-Saharan Africa. Table 11.6 shows growth in fertilizer use per hectare in selected developing countries compared to a more developed country in the same region. Several facts are worth noting.

Average fertilizer application rates are significantly higher in Asia than elsewhere in the world (reflecting high rates of fertilizer use in rice

Table 11.5 Worldwide Use of Agricultural Machinery and Fertilizer, 1961–1995

	Agricultural Tractors	Harvesters and Threshers	Total Fertilizer Consumption (MT)
1961	11,318,240	2,230,968	31,182,240
1965	13,404,160	2,375,414	47,002,900
1970	16,102,100	2,614,277	69,307,500
1975	18,758,240	3,024,066	91,399,110
1980	21,943,570	3,548,891	116,719,600
1985	24,746,280	3,997,885	128,613,200
1990	26,551,380	4,054,829	138,043,400
1995	26,196,870	4,163,052	130,865,300

Source: FAOSTAT Statistical Database 1998.

production). Fertilizer use in China is now nearly as high (on a per hectare basis) as in Japan. But in other parts of Asia, average rates are still substantially below the levels in China and Japan. Fertilizer use in many parts of Africa is extremely low. The comparison of Congo-Brazzaville (formerly Zaire) to South Africa provides a stark contrast, with use in South Africa 30 times higher than in Congo-Brazzaville. In a paper for the International Food Policy Research Institute (IFPRI), Bumb and Baanante (1996) estimate that fertilizer use will continue to increase, but the rates of increase will slow substantially. The highest growth rate is expected in sub-Saharan Africa (see Table 11.7).

Fertilizer use may be at less than the economic optimal rate in the poorest countries because farmers are unable to borrow money and are unable to save enough money to buy as much fertilizer as they would like. In addition, states the FAO, "In sub-Saharan Africa, where fertilizer use is still very low, consumption is hampered by high distribution costs, the lack of markets for output, lack of a domestic fertilizer industry and poor yield response, and the high risk of using fertilizer in traditional agricultural settings" (FAO WFS Background Paper No. 10).

Of course, the same arguments may apply to machinery—poor farmers with limited access to credit may not be able to buy as much machinery as they would like. But we should be cautious in assuming that machinery can be as efficiently used in the developing world as it is in the United States and other "rich" countries. Agricultural production in the United States tends to be done on large-scale farms using a lot of machinery and relatively little labor. Because the United States is a rich country and a large agricultural exporter, this kind of capital-intensive farming is often regarded as the "modern" and "efficient" method to which all farmers in all countries should aspire. This type of farming *is* efficient in the United States because of its prevailing relative prices of inputs. With labor being relatively scarce, labor wages are high; capital markets are well developed, therefore farm credit is widely available at relatively low interest rates; and gasoline and equipment prices are relatively low.

Table 11.6 Fertilizer Use in Selected Countries in Asia and Africa, 1961–1995

	Japan		China		India		Indonesia	
	MT of Fertilizer Consumed	Rates of Fertilizer Use (kg/ha)	MT of Fertilizer Consumed	Rates of Fertilizer Use (kg/ha)	MT of Fertilizer Consumed	Rates of Fertilizer Use (kg/ha)	MT of Fertilizer Consumed	Rates of Fertilizer Use (kg/ha)
1961	1,584,170	285.44	728,000	7.04	338,300	2.17	135,990	7.56
1965	1,851,500	346.85	2,604,000	25.42	784,600	4.96	94,498	5.25
1970	1,954,600	398.09	4,407,000	44.04	2,256,600	14.05	240,193	13.34
1975	1,801,300	403.88	6,851,600	70.04	3,493,800	21.32	489,100	27.17
1980	1,816,000	422.92	15,334,700	158.08	5,532,600	33.58	1,173,025	65.17
1985	2,034,000	483.25	16,851,600	178.51	8,504,300	51.35	1,971,800	101.12
1990	1,839,000	446.25	27,027,410	289.72	12,584,000	75.87	2,387,000	117.86
1995	1,641,600	413.50	35,527,200	386.26	13,876,100	83.54	2,512,431	146.67

	South Africa		Nigeria		Congo-Brazzaville	
	MT of Fertilizer Consumed	Rates of Fertilizer Use (kg/ha)	MT of Fertilizer Consumed	Rates of Fertilizer Use (kg/ha)	MT of Fertilizer Consumed	Rates of Fertilizer Use (kg/ha)
1961	214,921	17.91	1,394	0.05	270	0.04
1965	364,100	29.84	3,649	0.14	1,400	0.21
1970	557,700	45.08	6,894	0.25	4,700	0.69
1975	772,712	61.47	54,300	1.97	10,713	1.55
1980	1,064,338	85.56	173,900	6.24	7,900	1.12
1985	878,715	71.12	292,000	10.25	6,800	0.94
1990	791,549	58.76	400,340	13.55	6,200	0.86
1995	747,800	49.90	200,000	6.59	12,000	1.65

Source: FAOSTAT Statistical Database 1998.

Table 11.7   Past and Projected-Future Fertilizer Use: Levels and Growth Rates

	Fertilizer Use			Annual Growth	
	1959/60	1989/90	2020 (projected)	1960–90	1990–2020
	(million nutrient tons)			(percent)	
Developed countries	24.7	81.3	86.4	4.0	0.2
Developing countries	2.7	62.3	121.6	10.5	2.2
East Asia	1.2	31.4	55.7	10.9	1.9
South Asia	0.4	14.8	33.8	12.0	2.8
West Asia/North Africa	0.3	6.7	11.7	10.4	1.9
Latin America	0.7	8.2	16.2	8.2	2.3
Sub-Saharan Africa	0.1	1.2	4.2	8.3	3.3
World total	27.4	143.6	208.0	5.5	1.2

Source: Bumb and Baanante 1996.

Note that farm laborers in the United States earn over $6 per hour and gasoline costs $1.20 per gallon. Thirty days of labor costs the same as 1,200 gallons of gas. In some developing countries, 30 days of rural labor costs the same as 30 gallons of gas. Now consider a simple example in which a farmer trying to decide whether to adopt a method of production that uses machinery more intensively—weeding between crop rows with a tractor, for example, rather than by hiring people with hoes. The method will allow the farmer to use less hired labor (suppose it would save 30 days of hired labor per year), but will require the farmer to use more gasoline (suppose it would require 500 more gallons of gasoline each year). For a farmer in the United States, adopting the new method is sensible and efficient. The farmer saves enough money (in reduced labor costs) to buy 1,200 gallons of gas, but he needs to buy only 500 gallons. For a farmer in a developing country such as that described above, adopting the new method not only makes no sense, it is downright inefficient. That farmer only saves enough money (in reduced labor costs) to buy 30 gallons of gas, but he needs to buy 500 gallons.

Of course, "machinery" does not *have* to be the giant large-scale tractors and equipment we find in the United States. In developing countries, farmers are more likely to use smaller-scale farm machinery, or machinery that relies more on human or animal power.

■ POPULATION, LABOR, AND AGRICULTURAL PRODUCTIVITY

In Chapter 7, we saw that under any reasonable assumptions, population will grow substantially over the next 50 years. As population grows, more people become available to work in agricultural production. Of course, future population growth will possibly occur only in the cities. In fact, Mundlak, Larson & Crego found that agricultural labor dropped in 40 percent of countries worldwide from 1967 to 1992. However, it appears likely that population growth will lead to increases in average labor per hectare in many parts of the developing world. Table 11.8 shows trends in agricultural labor forces. In Africa, Asia, the developing world, and the world as a whole, the number of agricultural workers per unit of agricultural land has increased steadily. (Not shown in the table, workers per hectare are decreasing in the developed world and in Latin America. In North America there are about .008 workers per hectare—the average farm worker tends over 300 acres. Compare that to Asia—3 acres per worker—or Africa—15 acres per worker.)

Adding labor to each hectare of land will increase yield as long as productive work exists for the additional workers. Economists describe this situation as one where there is a *positive marginal productivity*. One can imagine a situation in which existing workers are already doing all that is possible, and where adding another worker to a plot of land causes a decline in production as the workers begin to get in each other's way (*negative marginal productivity of labor*).

In those areas that are already under cultivation, what is the marginal productivity of labor in agriculture? That is, by how much would the addition or subtraction of one worker change farm production? In the years before World War II, a considerable literature developed that assumed such a large pool of unemployed and underemployed labor languished in Third World agriculture that substantial amounts could be withdrawn for the industrial labor force with no diminution in agricultural production; in other words, that the marginal product of labor in agriculture was zero (Lewis 1954; Fei & Ranis 1964).

Gary Becker (1975) called that thesis into question with a powerful argument that people attach at least some value to their leisure time. If this is the case, then they will not work their fields up to the point that another minute spent farming yields no product at all. They would rather spend those few minutes at leisure.

Still, we see considerable evidence that the marginal product of labor in agriculture is below the wage rate. A number of studies have shown that yields on small holdings in India, so small that all labor is supplied by the farm family, are significantly higher than yields on large farms where a substantial proportion of the labor force is hired (Berry & Cline 1979). Studies in other locations have arrived at similar results (see Figure 11.1).

Farmers who hire labor are unwilling to hire so much that the product for the last hour worked by the laborer is less than the cost of hiring him for that hour. But when labor is all from the family, for those last few hours worked family members may be willing to work for something less than the going wage, because the family will benefit from those last few

Table 11.8 Agricultural Workforce and Workers per Hectare of Agricultural Land, Selected Regions, 1980–1994

	Africa		Asia		Developing Countries		World	
	Economically Active Agricultural Population (thousands)	Workers per Hectare of Agricultural Land (thousands)	Economically Active Agricultural Population (thousands)	Workers per Hectare of Agricultural Land (thousands)	Economically Active Agricultural Population (thousands)	Workers per Hectare of Agricultural Land (thousands)	Economically Active Agricultural Population (thousands)	Workers per Hectare of Agricultural Land (thousands)
1980	139,903	0.13	816,838	0.71	994,791	0.35	1,069,294	0.23
1985	152,858	0.14	883,776	0.74	1,076,204	0.37	1,143,335	0.24
1990	167,125	0.15	959,776	0.76	1,166,836	0.39	1,229,171	0.25
1994	179,949	0.17	1,011,015	0.80	1,222,273	0.41	1,280,066	0.26

Source: FAOSTAT Statistical Database 1998.

Figure 11.1   Farm Size and Production per Unit of Land in Less Developed Nations

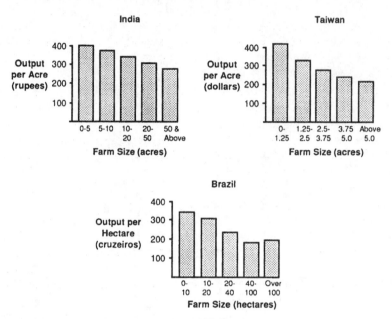

Source: Adapted from Stevens and Jabara 1988:68.

hours and because they may have no higher-valued use for their time (Mazumdar 1965, 1975; Sen 1964, 1966).

All this argues that the marginal productivity of labor in agriculture is low, and comparisons of wages in agriculture versus nonagricultural activities in the Third World support this thesis. The ILO (International Labor Organization 1987) lists the daily wage rate for agricultural activities in the Philippines in 1985 as P 23.74 per day (just over one U.S. dollar), but the daily rate for nonagricultural activities is P 56.48 per day, or 2.4 times the agricultural rate. The ILO lists the daily rate for farm labor in India at about half a dollar and shows the manufacturing wage to be over five times that amount.

Unemployment rates for the Third World are hard to come by. The ILO (1988:4) estimated that there were some 100 million workers unemployed and 500 million underemployed worldwide. Presumably, the majority of these people live in the Third World. The ILO gives the unemployment rate for the Philippines in 1985 as 6.1, and that for Uruguay in 1986 as 11.4. It gives no estimate for India. (The ILO defines unemployment as all people above a specific age who are without work, available for work, and seeking work.)

Underemployment figures are even harder to come by. Underemployment refers to people who are employed part-time or in jobs of lower productivity than their skill levels would allow if appropriate jobs were available. Most of those who hawk cigarettes one by one on a Third World urban street corner could earn more if they could find a better job. The World Bank (1984:88) estimates that underemployment in the Third World ranges "from 20 percent in Latin America to about 40 percent in Africa."

The unemployed, and probably also the underemployed, in the Third World are mostly young males. The ILO 1984 figures for Uruguay show 4.4 times as many unemployed people in the age bracket 14–24 as in the bracket 45–54. For India in 1984, the ILO's figures show 73 times as many unemployed men in the 20- to 29-year-old age bracket as in the 40- to 49-year-old group.

Given the high rates of Third World unemployment, especially among young men, together with the relatively low wage rates in Third World agriculture relative to work outside of agriculture, it is difficult to make a case for enough of a labor shortage in agriculture to make the typical farm family better off with many, rather than few, children. If farm productivity is the main consideration, it appears that the typical Third World farm family would be better off spending more on fertilizer for high-yielding seeds and less on raising extra children.

But we are not yet finished with the arguments about population growth as a stimulant to productivity. A number of thinkers have argued that population growth in and of itself is a stimulant to productivity. One of the writers in this school (Clark 1973) capsulized one of its chief arguments in the title of his article "More People, More Dynamism." That is, society is better off with a large population than with a small "as a result of there being more knowledge creators" in a large population (Simon 1986:169).

Critics of this argument note that in today's high-tech world large numbers of people create little assurance of a high level of knowlege creation. If they did, then India and China, with over a third of the world's population between them, should account for a greater share of the world's technological development than do Germany, France, Great Britain, the United States, and Japan, which collectively account for only 10 percent of the world's population. In the Third World, many Einsteins may be undiscovered for want of a proper education.

Ester Boserup, in her book *Population and Technological Change* (1981:5), argues that population growth creates a kind of crisis situation that stimulates the invention of new technology: "Shrinking supplies of land and other natural resources would provide motivation to invent better means of utilizing scarce resources or to discover substitutes for them." Note that in this "necessity is the mother of invention" argument, it is population growth that drives the creation of technology, and not the creation of technology that expands the capacity of the economy to support more people.

Boserup argues that farming is most intense in the densely settled regions of the world (not that people have tended to gather in those regions of the world where soils are most productive). She argues that, because periods of technological innovation and expanding productivity have usually been accompanied by increases in population, growth of population must have caused the increase in technology and production. Critics of this thesis argue that it is just the other way around, that it is the technological innovation and expanding productivity that have, in fact, made possible the associated increase in population.

Because productivity is related to income, and income is so closely related to food consumption, those who argue that population growth of itself is a stimulant to productivity imply that population growth would help alleviate the world hunger problem, or at the least impose no threat to a solution. This school of thought has to contend with a series of arguments that claim population growth has a detrimental impact on the nutrition of the poor.

■ YIELDS AND TECHNOLOGY

The previous three sections show that yields per hectare can be increased by using productive inputs (water, labor, purchased inputs) more intensively on each hectare of land. Next, we turn to an alternative way of producing higher yields—improved technology. A technological improvement allows us to gain more output from the same quantity of inputs (or the same output using fewer of the inputs).

The *Green Revolution* (described in Box 11.1) grew from an international effort to develop new, higher-yielding seed varieties. Table 11.9 shows the growth in yields for the three main cereal crops—wheat, maize (or corn), and rice. The table illustrates the dramatic yield-growth of all three crops in every geographical area.

How much of the yield increases are attributable to increases in inputs described above, and how much to new technology? This question is hard to answer because of the nature of the new seed varieties. As described in Box 11.1, the new varieties achieved their higher yields in part by being more responsive to fertilizer; in addition, the new varieties were often more sensitive to drought, and thus have been frequently grown on irrigated land. Therefore, the higher observed yields are the result of a complex interaction between technological improvement and additional levels of inputs.

Several researchers have attempted to unravel this complexity. The Consultative Group on International Agricultural Research (CGIAR 1997) reports "22 percent of the developing world's [wheat] production increase

Box 11.1   What Is the Green Revolution?

Dana Dalrymple

In October 1944, about a year before the close of World War II, the Rockefeller Foundation brought to Mexico a young plant scientist to join a team of agriculturalists that had recently stared work to assist in the agricultural development of that country. In a few months, the new man, Norman Borlaug (who was later to be awarded a Nobel Prize for his work in Mexico), was put in charge of the wheat program. He and his team set out to develop new varieties of wheat that would do better than the local varieties. Disease resistance (e.g., resistance to the fungus causing the disease rust) was particularly important at first. In the mid-1950s increased emphasis was given to increasing yields and within a few years varieties had been developed which could produce much more than the traditional ones.

Encouraged by this success, in the 1960s Rockefeller Foundation joined with the Ford Foundation to establish two permanent research stations for the development of high-yielding cereals, the International Rice Research Institute (IRRI) in the Philippines and the International Maize and Wheat Improvement Center (CIMMYT) in Mexico. The success of these centers in developing high-yielding varieties led to such enthusiasm for the idea of international agricultural research centers that by the late 1980s thirteen centers, treating various aspects of improving Third World agriculture, had been set up worldwide, and sponsorship had spread to a consortium of donors worldwide including both foundations and government agencies.

The high-yielding varieties of wheat and rice have spread more widely, more quickly, than any other technological innovation in the history of agriculture in the developing countries. First introduced in the mid-1960s, they

Figure a   Estimated Proportion of Area Planted to High-Yielding Varieties of Wheat and Rice, South and Southeast Asian Nations, 1965/66–1982/83

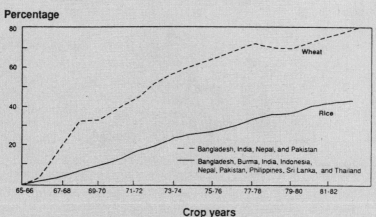

Source: Adapted from Dalrymple 1985.

(continues)

Box 11.1   Continued

occupied about half of these countries' total wheat and rice area by 1982–1983 (Dalrymple 1985). Figure a shows the remarkable growth in adoption of high-yielding varieties in South and Southeast Asia.

Struck by the remarkable speed with which high-yielding varieties of wheat and rice were being developed for the Third World and by their potential to alleviate world hunger, William S. Gaud, who was then administrator of the U.S. Agency for International Development, referred, in a 1968 speech, to the phenomenon of their development and spread as "the green revolution" (Dalrymple 1979:724).

Actually, the green revolution's wheat and rice varieties, also known as high-yielding varieties (HYVs) or modern varieties (MVs), do not do much better than the traditional varieties (they can even do worse) unless they have appropriate amounts of water and fertilizer. In fact, it is largely tolerance of and response to substantial amounts of fertilizer that makes them so successful.

Figure b Lodging and Nonlodging Rice Plants

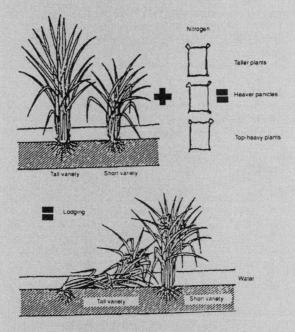

• Plant height increases with nitrogen application and lodging becomes a problem.
• Many leaves on the lodged plants decay since they are soaked in water and do not receive sufficient light.
• Short, stiff stem prevents lodging.
Note: Nonlodging plants are tolerant of fertilizer.
Source: Adapted from Vergara 1979:158.

(continues)

Box 11.1 Continued

The traditional varieties of wheat and rice were not tolerant of significant amounts of fertilizer. When Third World farmers attempted to increase rice or wheat yields by adding fertilizer—especially nitrogen fertilizer—to their fields, their plants would grow so tall that they would fall over. The technical term for this is lodging. What the plant scientists at the international institutes did was to locate plant varieties with genes for shortness and breed these genes into plants that had other characteristics desirable for the Third World. The new plants, called semidwarfs, borrowed dwarfism genes from Japan (for wheat) and China (for rice). When used with fertilizer, they grew taller than without the fertilizer, but not excessively so. Thus they were much more resistant to lodging (Figure b).

Plant scientists did not stop merely with the development of nonlodging plants. They bred into their new varieties a host of other characteristics such as disease resistance.

One of the more intriguing changes in plant design that they accomplished involved rearranging the location of the seed cluster on the plant.

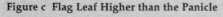

Figure c Flag Leaf Higher than the Panicle

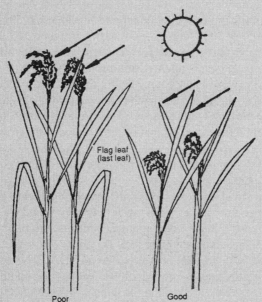

Flag leaf
(last leaf)

Poor   Good

• There is less shading of the upper leaves if the panicle does not extend far above the flag leaf.

Note: Green revolution plant scientists designed a rice plant where the topmost leaves were not shaded by the seed cluster.

Source: Adapted from Vergara 1979:161.

(continues)

Box 11.1   Continued

Traditional rice plants sent their cluster of seeds (the panicle) high into the air. The seeds themselves store energy, but they do not make it. Photosynthesis is concentrated in the leaves. It did not make sense for the seed cluster to shade the highest leaves on the plant, so the scientists bred rice plants whose topmost leaf, the flag leaf, extended well above the panicle, thus taking maximum advantage of the available sunshine (Figure c).

The green revolution, then, is a whole complex of innovations, such as those described above, that combine to make up new plant varieties. The modern plant varieties, when used with a package of appropriate inputs such as fertilizer and water and good management, are dramatically raising crop yields in the Third World.

For more about the green revolution, see Brown 1970; U.S. Department of State 1986a, b; Stackman, Bradfield & Mangelsdorf 1967.

resulting from higher yields is attributed to the gradual spreading of modern or high yielding varieties." A study of Syrian wheat found the increase in wheat yields (which more than quadrupled from the 1950s to the early 1990s) was due to several factors: New varieties accounted for about 35 percent of the increase; better management and increased fertilizer use accounted for 23 percent each; and irrigation accounted for 19 percent of the increase (CGIAR 1995). Peter Oram (1995), in an IFPRI paper, writes: "It is estimated that about 50 percent of the gains in farm yields have resulted from plant breeding and the balance from the application of other improved practices." These suggest that of the average yield growth of 2 percent per year from 1968 to 1997, new technology accounts for between 0.5 and 1 percent per year, and input growth accounts for the remaining 1 to 1.5 percent per year.

The technological improvements shift out the aggregate supply curve for food and cause food prices to be lower than they would otherwise have been. CGIAR reports that in developing countries, prices for crops targeted by CGIAR have dropped more than the prices for non-CGIAR crops. The United States Department of Agriculture (USDA 1991) estimates that research into improvements in agricultural production methods has reduced the average yearly food bill in the United States by $400 per person.

Can crop yields continue to grow? And if so, at what rate? The answers to these questions go a long way to determining whether the future food supply will keep pace with demand. Above, we reviewed the different opinions about the prospects for adding irrigation, fertilizer, and labor to agricultural production. Even the most optimistic projections see input usage growing more slowly than in the past. But what about technology?

Table 11.9 Yields of Wheat, Rice, and Maize, for Various Geographical Areas, 1961 and 1997, in Hectograms per Hectare

	Wheat			Rice			Maize		
	1961	1997	% change	1961	1997	% change	1961	1997	% change
Africa	7,154	17,439	144	14,823	21,837	47	10,408	15,942	53
South Asia	8,447	25,192	198	15,802	28,814	82	10,437	15,826	52
East and S.E. Asia	6,781	8,901	31	17,482	33,761	93	10,344	22,755	120
Latin America	11,905	23,977	101	18,004	32,937	83	12,132	25,051	106
Near East	9,119	19,136	110	29,505	58,136	97	17,510	48,352	176
Transition economies	10,794	20,651	91	21,188	26,399	25	20,877	40,751	95
Western Europe	19,655	52,760	168	53,401	61,100	14	25,436	88,316	247
Oceania	11,569	17,273	49	42,529	86,765	104	21,533	67,517	214
United States	16,070	26,725	66	38,227	66,091	73	39,184	79,740	104
World	10,902	26,846	146	18,669	38,252	105	19,418	40,854	110

Source: FAOSTAT Statistical Database 1998.

Figure 11.2 Average Growth Rates in Cereal Yields, 1961–1997

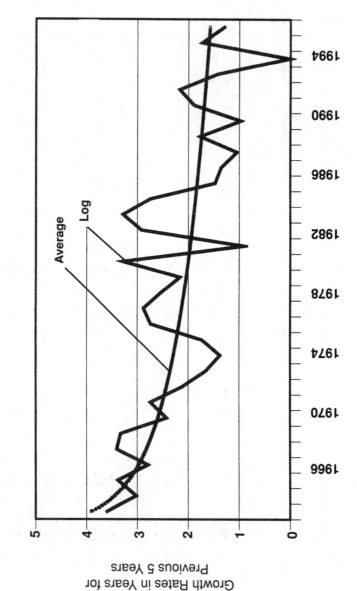

Figure 11.3   Worldwide Cereal Yield, 1961–1997

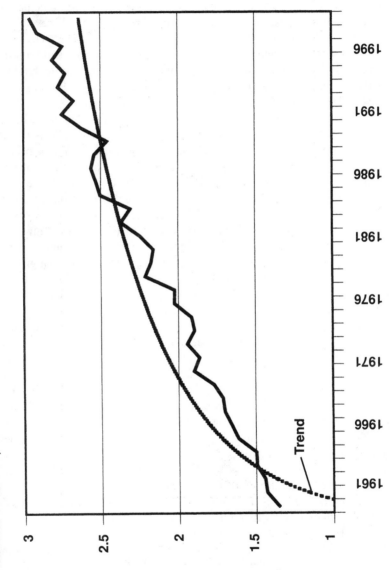

Can technological advances pick up the slack caused by slower growth in input use? We find optimists and pessimists on this question.

The pessimists point out that growth in yields has been slowing (see Figures 11.2 and 11.3). Imagine (say the pessimists) that crop yields are growing according to an S-shaped curve; we have gone through a period of rapidly rising yields, but we are now reaching the top, where yields become flat: "Countries that have doubled or tripled the productivity of their cropland since mid-century are the rule, not the exception. But with many of the world's farmers already using advanced yield-raising technologies, further gains in land productivity will not come easily" (Brown & Kane 1994:132).

Some pessimism about yields is based on a belief that scientists cannot discover new ways to increase yields. "Rising grain yield per hectare . . . must eventually give way to physical constraints. . . . Yields may now be pushing against various physiological limits such as nutrient absorption capacity or photosynthetic efficiency" (Brown & Kane 1994: 138). Thomas Sinclair, a horticulturist at the University of Florida, Gainesville, explained to *Science* magazine: "To grow corn, . . . you have to have leaves, stalks, and roots, so there's got to be mass committed to what you don't harvest. . . . At the beginning of this century, . . . many crops had harvest indexes on the order of 0.25 of their weight in grain, and now many crops are approaching 0.5. . . . Maybe you could go up to 0.6 or 0.65, but beyond that you can't have a viable plant" (quoted in Mann 1997:1,042).

Another source of pessimism about yields is concern about whether they are "environmentally sustainable." According to this school of thought the current high yields have been obtained by putting extreme pressure on the natural environment. The environment can stand this pressure for only a short time; yields then naturally begin to decline. The interaction between agricultural production and the environment will be explored in more detail in the next chapter.

Perhaps in response to these legitimate concerns about environmental impact of agricultural production, the emphasis of international agricultural research has shifted (during the 1990s) from increasing yields to reducing environmental impact. But this may help explain why yields in experiment stations (the laboratories of crop production) have leveled. A related explanation is that international crop research has been underfunded (Pardey & Alston 1995). Alexandratos (1995) argues that the slowdown in yield growth is less a result of technological feasibility and more a result of low farm-level prices (see Box 11.2). Finally, worldwide average crop yields have been brought down during the 1990s by a large drop in yields in the former Soviet Union, probably a temporary phenomenon. If you accept any of these explanations about the slowdown in yield growth, you may be more optimistic about future growth in yields.

Box 11.2 Why the Supply Curve Slopes Upward

There is a physical and a cost basis for the relationship between price and the amount that a farmer will try to produce. Let us start with the underlying physical relationship, using as our example the relationship between the amount of seed planted in one field (say a hectare of land) and a crop yield. The raw date we assume are given in Table a and plotted in Figure a. The top curve in Figure a represents the total yield from varying amounts of fertilizer (total physical product or production function). The bottom curve represents the yield added by each successive increment of 10 units of seed (marginal physical product).

Table a Hypothetical Yield Response to Varying Amounts of Seed

Seed	Yield	Marginal Physical Product
0	0	39
10	39	13
20	52	9
30	61	5
40	66	0
50	66	−2
60	64	

Figure a Hypothetical Total Physical Product and Marginal Physical Product from Use of Seed on a Fixed Quantity of Land

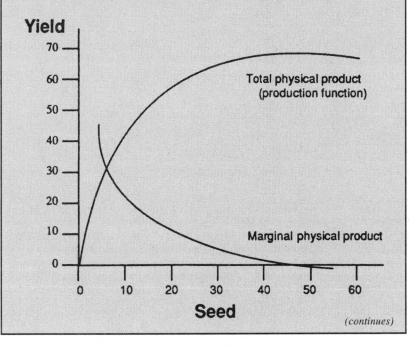

(continues)

Box 11.2 Continued

What we have in Figure a is a graphic representation of the fact that, as we increase the amount of an input used, holding other inputs constant, we experience diminishing returns to successive inputs (thus the downward-sloping marginal physical product curve—which is often called diminishing marginal returns). The functional relationships we are talking about here are based on observations that have been made in the real world.

Now let us combine the variable inputs commonly used to increase production on our hypothetical one hectare of land. As we increase production we not only add more seed, but more fertilizer, more labor, and maybe other inputs such as irrigation water and pesticides. These things cost money. As we increase production, we could, at various amounts produced, add up the costs of the things we are using to increase production and plot these sums to get a cost curve.

The cost curve would say very much the same thing that Figure a says, except that it would measure costs, instead of seed, along the horizontal input. (The relation between cost and production is based on the underlying physical relationships between inputs and production.) We diagram our cost curve in Figure b. Because the fixed cost of land is not included in our set of costs, we identify the costs in this diagram as variable costs.

Figure b   As Variable Costs Increase, the Rate of Increase in Yield Decreases

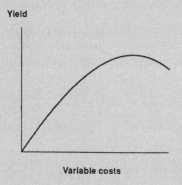

Yield

Variable costs

Notice in Figure b that, although not specifically diagrammed, as yield increases there are diminishing marginal returns to costs, just as there were diminishing marginal returns to seed in Figure a.

It is a convention of economics to draw cost curves with the cost on the vertical axis and the yield on the horizontal axis. So let us redraw Figure b in the conventional way, namely as shown in Figure c. (To see what happens to the cost curve when this is done, you might want to trace Figure b and then flip it over and look at it from the back side so as to get Figure c.)

(continues)

Box 11.2 Continued

With Figure c, instead of thinking about what happens to yield as we increase costs by one unit, we can think about what happens to costs as we increase yield by one unit. If you examine Figure c you will see that we produce under conditions of increasing marginal cost. For each additional unit of yield from our hectare of land, we have to spend somewhat more on our bundle of variable costs. These increasing marginal costs are diagrammed in Figure d.

Figure c   As Yield Increases, Variable Costs Increase at an Increasing Rate

Variable costs

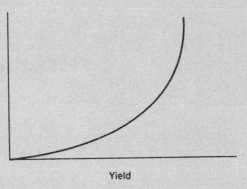

Yield

Figure d   As Yield Increases, Marginal Cost Increases

Marginal cost (vertical scale is expanded from the scale in Figure c)

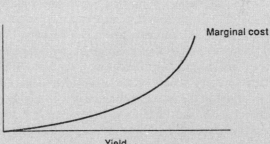

Marginal cost

Yield

Thus we see that we produce under diminishing marginal returns, which results in producing with increasing marginal costs. The two are based on the same underlying physical relationship.

For an individual producer, the marginal cost curve (Figure d) is the price schedule at which he is willing to produce various amounts of goods for the market. He is willing to produce up to the point where the price

(continues)

Box 11.2 Continued

equals his marginal cost of production. If he is producing at this point and we want to motivate him to produce more, barring a shift in technology or a reduction in the costs of some of his inputs, we will have to pay him more. This is represented in Figure e as shifting production from A to B, which is motivated by an increase in price from P_1 to P_2.

Adding up the marginal cost curves (individuals' supply curves) for all the individual producers yields the supply curve for the industry. Increasing the price of the product will motivate the industry to produce more.

Figure e   Increasing the Price of a Product Makes Possible Increased Production

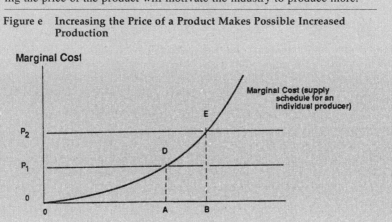

Many analysts are more optimistic about future yields. The FAO projects cereal yields will grow at 1.4 percent per year between 1990 and 2010, compared with a 2.2 percent growth rate between 1970 and 1990. A World Bank Study estimates that grain yields will continue to grow at a 1.5–1.7 percent annual rate. An IFPRI report on food supply and demand in the year 2020 presents a base scenario in which yields continue to grow at the rate observed in the late 1980s and early 1990s. For a criticism of these projections, see WorldWatch Press Release, May 1, 1996. For an FAO defense, see *Food Outlook,* May/June 1996. For an analysis of the debate about future yields, especially focusing on China, see Crosson (1996a).

The optimistic beliefs cited above are based on several observations. A European study (see Penning de Vries et al. 1995 for a description) concludes that potential yields of cereal crops are close to 10 metric tons per hectare, compared to current yields of about 3 metric tons per hectare. Some dramatic reports about new technological breakthroughs have been published. A "super rice" developed in 1994 by the International Rice Research Institute promises yields that are 25 percent higher than current yields. A new cassava strain promises yields that are 10 times higher than current yields. Some experts believe that genetic engineering will provoke a new spurt in yield growth. A recent report estimates that adding or removing deoxyribonucleic acid (DNA) from plants could increase yields by 25 percent over the next 30 years—amounting to an annual increase of 0.7 percent per year.

■ POST-PRODUCTION FOOD LOSSES

Before leaving the subject of food production, we should recognize that food consumption theoretically can be increased *without* increasing food production—if we can reduce losses between the field and the consumer. (See FAO WFS Background Papers Nos. 4 and 8.) These losses are estimated as high as 30 percent (Erlich & Erlich 1991). In developing countries, post-harvest food losses have been attributed to pests (Angé 1993), poor facilities for storage and transportation (James & Schofield 1990), and on-farm handling (FAO WFS Background Paper No. 8). One might think that post-harvest food losses would decline as countries develop economically, because of improvements in roads, credit, and information. However, a study in the United States estimates that over 25 percent of food is lost in retailing, restaurants, and at-home consumption. So in rich countries there may be less food lost to pests and poor storage facilities, but more food is wasted by consumers or thrown away by restaurants.

□ 12

Agricultural Production and the Environment

The previous chapter identified the pace of technology as one of the great unknowns in predicting future food production. A second unknown is the degree and significance of environmental damage; in this chapter, we explore that issue. The issue has two faces: (1) Environmental quality is an important determinant of agricultural output; and (2) agricultural output has significant impact on the environment. We deal first with the interaction between agricultural production and the local environment (the environment in the vicinity of agricultural production). We then discuss the interaction between agricultural production and the global environment—particularly global warming.

■ AGRICULTURAL PRODUCTION AND THE LOCAL ENVIRONMENT

Agriculture uses natural resources—soil and water—to produce food. This can lead to deterioration in the quality of natural resources and their ability to support food production.

□ Land Degradation

The environmental issue with the greatest potential for influencing future food production is land degradation. Land can become unsuitable for agricultural production in the following ways (UN, POPIN 1995):

- Soil can disappear from land through erosion
- Soil can become chemically unsuitable for agricultural production
- Land can become physically unsuitable for agricultural production

Erosion. Wind or water can pick up soil particles from one area and move them; this can harm agricultural production in four ways: (1) The eroded soil may contain nutrients needed for plant development; (2) the remaining soil may be so dense that it is difficult for plant roots to develop; (3) erosion may reduce the capacity of the soil to retain water needed for plant growth; (4) finally, erosion may result in uneven terrain that makes cultivation more difficult.

Soil erosion is to a degree caused by agricultural production: Land used for agricultural production may be bare of vegetation for months at a time; the absense of roots to hold soil in place makes it more easily erodible; plowing of soil in preparation for seeding exposes it to wind and rain and increases the rate of erosion; and irrigation can contribute directly to water erosion.

Chemical characteristics of the soil. Land may become chemically unsuitable for agricultural production for several reasons. The nutrients in the soil may be depleted because of past agricultural production, especially if the same crop is grown year after year. *Salinization* of soil occurs when the salt content of the soil increases to levels unsuitable for agricultural production. Salinization can be caused by irrigating land with water that contains low levels of salts, which are left on the soil when the water evaporates. In some areas, this problem occurs because irrigation depletes the naturally occurring fresh groundwater, and causes seawater to intrude into the groundwater system. A third chemical problem with soil is *acidification*. This can occur when too much fertilizer of certain types is applied, or when drainage problems occur in certain soils. Finally, other pollutants such as oil or excessive use of pesticides can reduce the soil's ability to support agricultural production.

Physical characteristics of the land. Agricultural land can also become unsuitable for production because of changes in the physical characteristics of the land. Soil can become less porous through compaction—when heavy machines or animals pack the soil down—or through the action of raindrops that seal the soil; nonporous soil can prevent or stunt the germination of seeds. Waterlogging occurs when water sits in the root zones of plants; this impedes their development. Waterlogging is caused by poor drainage or overirrigation.

The extent and impact of land degradation worldwide. The Global Land Assessment of Degradation, or GLASOD, study by the UN (ISRIC/UNEP 1991) estimated that 22 percent of agricultural land worldwide (and 38 percent of cropland) has been subject to one or more of the kinds of degradation described above. Of the 2 billion hectares of degraded land, according to this study, 83 percent was degraded by erosion, 12 percent by chemical degradation, and 5 percent by physical degradation. Seventy million hectares are so badly degraded that the damage cannot be repaired. Other studies report the amount of degraded land increases each year by an additional 5 to 10 million hectares (Scherr & Yadav 1997). Pimentel and colleagues (1994) estimate that "Each year, more than ten million hectares (24.7 million acres) of once-productive land are degraded and abandoned." These statistics bear directly on how much land can be devoted to agricultural production in the future. However, as we saw in the last chapter, agricultural land has increased steadily despite these reports of degradation.

A related possibility is that land degradation will reduce yields per hectare. This can occur for two reasons. First, when land becomes so severely degraded that it is no longer capable of supporting agricultural production, new land may be added to take the place of the degraded land. The new land is likely to be of relatively poor quality—otherwise, it would already have been in use. Second, when the land is degraded, but remains in agricultural use, yields on that land drop.

Agricultural scientists disagree about the severity of the drop in yields attributable to land degradation. Pimentel and Giampietro show evidence that corn yields are about 20 percent lower on severely eroded lands in many parts of the United States. Mitchell and colleagues (1997:54) cite other studies estimating that soil erosion was responsible for yield declines of 3 to 4 percent over 100 years. Scherr and Yadav (1997) report yield losses of from 5 to 15 percent attributable to land degradation. See Crosson (1996b) for a review of the debate.

☐ **Water Quality**

In the last chapter, we discussed the importance of water in agricultural production, and cited one report predicting that expanded irrigation will become a substantial source of increased food production in the future. Expanded irrigation requires a supply of usable water—but agricultural production can lead to degradation of water.

Irrigation is the main culprit. In China and India irrigation has caused water tables to drop significantly. In coastal areas, depletion of groundwater reserves can cause saltwater intrusion into the groundwater system. In some soils, irrigation leeches certain salts from the soil and carries them into the groundwater, thus contaminating it and making it unsuitable for future irrigation. Irrigation or rainwater runoff can also carry residues from fertilizers and chemical pesticides, which also creates water-quality problems. In addition, as we have noted, irrigation can contribute to land degradation through erosion waterlogging, salinization, and acidification.

☐ Problems Associated with Agricultural-Input Use

We have already discussed how agricultural chemical use can lead to land degradation or water pollution. In addition, chemical use can create health problems for farm workers. The manufacture of agricultural chemicals can also create environmental hazards. The 1984 explosion at a chemical plant in Bhopal, India, provided a tragic example of this. The poison gas released by the explosion is used primarily for production of insecticides; thousands were killed and tens of thousands were seriously injured (Baylor 1996). In laboratory experiments, some pesticides have been shown to affect hormone levels—which could cause cancer, abnormalities in newborns, or reproductive problems. Evidence is weak, however, that this effect can be found outside the laboratory (Kamrin n.d.).

As the use of mechanization and petrochemicals increases in agriculture, concerns may arise that energy use in agriculture will become an environmental problem. However, Chen reports that agricultural production accounts for only 3.5 percent of commercial energy use in developed countries and 4.5 percent in developing countries (Chen 1990). In developed countries, food processing and distribution uses more energy than does food production.

☐ Other Environmental Problems

Water quality is important in other areas, too: Reduced water quality can directly harm public health. Of special concern here is the possibility that water could become contaminated with pesticides—chemicals that are developed to be toxic. Rachel Carson's *Silent Spring* pointed out the impact agricultural chemicals could have not on only humans, but on birds, fish, and other wildlife. Water contamination from runoff containing animal wastes has been implicated as a source of problems for commercial fisheries in the United States.

A second environmental concern associated with agricultural production involves genetic diversity. For example, with the increasingly widespread use of improved varieties of cereals, scientists worry about the possible loss of genetic material contained in traditional varieties. For instance, in 1949, 10,000 wheat varieties were used in China; by the 1970s only 1,000 remained in use. The loss of genetic diversity can make the food supply more susceptible to disease, and may foreclose the option of future technological improvements based on genetic characteristics of the "lost" varieties.

☐ Environment and Future Prospects
for Agricultural Production

Are these interactions between the environment and food production likely to create critical constraints on future food production? Some ecologists are alarmed about this possibility. (See Cohen [1996a] for a review.) David Pimentel of Cornell University states that the world's resources can support a high standard of living for fewer than 2 billion (compared to today's actual population of nearly 6 billion). This pessimistic view of the future is based on the belief that the world has already expanded agricultural production into areas that cannot sustain it, and has achieved yields per hectare by using production methods that cannot be continued indefinitely. Pimentel cites studies that show the absence of chemical fertilizers in agricultural production will result in cereal yields of between 0.5 metric tons per hectare (in semiarid regions with no fertilizer) and 2 metric tons per hectare (in humid regions using animal manure for fertilizer) (Pimentel & Giampietro 1994). Compare these projections to the average current yield of about 3 metric tons per hectare worldwide, and over 5 metric tons per hectare in the United States.

☐ Technology and the Tradeoff Between Production and the Environment

If David Pimentel represents one extreme in the debate about how many people the world can feed, Julian Simon represents the other. He describes a commercial vegetable farm in Illinois, and uses that as a basis for his optimistic calculations:

> In DeKalb, Illinois, Noel Davis's PhytoFarm produces food—mainly lettuce and other garden vegetables—in a factory measuring 200 feet by 250 feet—50,000 square feet, one acre, 0.4 hectares, 1/640 of a square mile—at a rate of a ton of food per day, enough to completely feed 500 or 1000 people. . . . At the current efficiency of PhytoFarm, the entire present population of the world can be supplied from a square area about 140 miles on a side—about the area of Massachusetts and Vermont combined, and less than a tenth of Texas. . . . PhytoFarm techniques could feed a hundred times the world's present population—say 500 billion people—with factory buildings a hundred stories high, on one percent of present farmland (Simon 1996:chap. 6).

Simon's attitude reflects an enormous confidence in the ability of technology to solve problems. Technological progress is all about getting more from less, and a good deal of agricultural research since the mid-1980s has been devoted to the problem of maintaining or improving agricultural yields while doing less damage to the environment. For example, new plant varieties are being developed that are naturally resistant to pests and thus require fewer pesticides. Tilling and landscaping methods that reduce soil erosion have been widely adopted in parts of the world. "Drip irrigation," which delivers water directly to the plant roots, reduces the amount of water used in irrigation without reducing its effectiveness. The new technology of aquaculture has made "fish farming" a rapidly growing source of food, as Table 12.1 shows. Nonmarine fish production has more than quadrupled during the period shown. The enormous increase during the 1980s and 1990s reflects in part the introduction of aquaculture. (Table 12.1 also shows a source of environmental concern: Natural ocean—or marine—fisheries have increased production to such a degree that they are in danger of being so overfished that the breeding stock is depleted and the total ocean fish population falls.)

Another purpose of agricultural research is the development of technology that relaxes the constraints of environment on agricultural output. For example, scientists are working to develop plants that can survive in brackish water: "Researchers have transferred a gene for salt tolerance from an Old World ice plant into three plants lacking salt tolerance . . . all of which then displayed significantly increased capability to grow with their roots exposed to salt. . . . This . . . will contribute to the effort to engineer plants with improved ability to withstand adverse growing conditions such as under-seawater irrigation" (National Science and Technology Council n.d.). Other ways technology can relax the environmental constraint to agricultural production are the development of chemicals that increase the ability of soils to retain moisture and of seed varieties that are more resistant to drought.

■ **AGRICULTURAL PRODUCTION AND THE GLOBAL ENVIRONMENT**

Agricultural production also interacts with the environment on a global scale, and especially on global warming. *Global warming* refers to the phenomenon by which water vapor, carbon dioxide, methane, and other trace gases in the atmosphere trap heat on the earth's surface. As the quantities of these gases (the so-called *greenhouse gases*) in the atmosphere increase, the

Table 12.1 **Fish Production Worldwide, 1961–1995 (in metric tons)**

	Marine Fish	Nonmarine Fish	Total
1961	30,790,980	8,814,170	39,605,150
1965	39,178,090	10,584,380	49,762,470
1970	52,775,150	12,433,080	65,208,230
1975	51,469,020	13,990,790	65,459,810
1980	55,440,610	16,606,770	72,047,380
1985	64,633,800	21,935,630	86,569,430
1990	69,291,760	28,636,380	97,928,140
1995	69,951,420	38,801,180	108,752,600

Source: FAOSTAT Statistical Database, 1998.

amount of heat trapped increases, and so the average temperature of the earth increases. On these matters we see a high degree of consensus among scientists. There is some disagreement, however, about the extent to which global warming has already occurred, and about the extent to which human activities are responsible for the buildup of greenhouse gases.

☐ The Impact of Agriculture on Global Warming

Agricultural production is a significant source of greenhouse gas emissions worldwide. The three greenhouse gases that are means by which human activity may cause global warming are carbon dioxide, methane, and nitrous oxide. Carbon dioxide comprises nearly 80 percent of greenhouse gases; nitrous oxide, 15 percent; and methane, 6 percent. Carbon dioxide is created when carbon atoms released from plants (as the plants decompose or burn) join with oxygen atoms. Deforestation in tropical areas is thought to contribute about 25 percent of the human-made carbon dioxide released into the atmosphere (FAO Factfile 1997). Methane is created by cattle when they digest food. In addition, paddy rice production is believed to be a major source of methane emissions as decomposing fertilizer reacts with crop residues. Scientists estimate that of methane generated by human activity, 15 to 25 percent is attributable to animal agriculture and 10 to 30 percent to rice production (Neue 1993; Lashof & Tirpak 1990). Release of nitrous oxide into the atmosphere can be increased by use of nitrogen fertilizers.

The lesson here shows that agricultural production creates greenhouse gases; if agricultural production grows to keep pace with food demand, it will add to the greenhouse gas problem. Furthermore, any realistic program to reduce greenhouse gas emissions must address the agricultural component; and an unavoidable tension stands between raising agricultural output and reducing greenhouse gases. Perhaps this tension can be reduced by technological innovations; but for now it remains.

☐ The Impact of Global Warming
on Agricultural Production

Obviously, when the average temperature in an area changes, the agricultural capacity of the area changes—it may become better for some crops and worse for others. However, global warming—if it does become a real problem—is not expected to result in a gradual increase in temperature in every area of the globe. Some areas may become much warmer; some only a little warmer; possibly, some colder. And the global climate change (if and when it occurs) will not simply mean changes in temperature; it is almost certain to change rainfall patterns, making some areas drier and some wetter. It will also change the incidence of severe weather, making some areas more susceptible to hurricanes, tornadoes, and droughts.

Many uncertainties remain concerning future climate change. Will the changes be dramatic or almost imperceptible? Even if the *average* global temperature increases significantly, what will that mean for climates in different geographical areas? A variety of opinions flourish among scientists regarding the impacts of global warming on agricultural production. The debate has centered on two questions: (1) Will global warming cause flooding of coastal areas and loss of agricultural land? (2) What will the impact of climate change be on average crop yields worldwide?

If the average temperature of the earth increases, the volume of water in oceans will increase. This happens not primarily (as the popular belief has it) because of melting polar ice caps, but because the volume of water expands as its temperature increases. Rosenzweig and Hillel (1995) report that the sea level is likely to rise from 4 to 20 inches by the middle of the next century. The danger from higher sea levels is not only flooded land, but increased drainage problems and sea water intrusion into freshwater sources. However, Rosenzweig and colleagues (1993) point out that in some areas, global warming may result in arid land becoming *suitable* for agricultural production due to an extended growing season or changes in rainfall patterns. General agreement prevails that rising sea levels would be an enormous problem in some geographical areas (see Parry et al. 1992; Ibe & Awosika 1991). But what will the impact be worldwide? On the one hand, Pimentel (1993) reports estimates that global warming will reduce cropland by 10 to 50 percent. On the other hand, Wittwer (1995:165–166) concludes that "Although important for localized regions, [cropland loss from rising sea levels] would be relatively insignificant on a worldwide basis."

Global warming can affect crop yields in a variety of ways (Rosenzweig & Hillel 1995):

Increase in atmospheric carbon dioxide (recall that is about 80 percent of the greenhouse gases) increases the efficiency of photosynthesis and thereby boosts plant growth. Wheat, rice, and soybeans are particularly responsive to increased atmospheric carbon dioxide. High carbon dioxide levels also significantly increase water-use efficiency. This may even increase demand for irrigation water when farmers discover that irrigation has a larger impact on yields. In addition, high carbon dioxide levels increase plants' resistance to salinity and drought, and increase nutrient uptake. Finally, noxious weeds are (for the most part) less responsive to carbon dioxide than are crops (Wittwer 1995).

Higher temperatures will increase the length of the growing season. Thus agricultural production may become feasible in areas (closer to the north and south poles) that are currently too cold. Soils in some of these areas (Canada and Russia) are less fertile than other soils; thus bringing these lands under cultivation could cause a drop in average yield. In addition, some crops (notably rice) show yield declines when the temperatures are too high. Finally, increased temperatures cause plants to mature faster. But plants that mature faster have lower food yields. Conversely, faster maturation combined with longer growing seasons may extend the areas in which double or triple cropping is feasible.

Extreme meteorological events, such as hurricanes, tornadoes, heavy rainstorms, or droughts, disrupt crop production and lower yields.

Pests and diseases thrive in higher temperatures; thus, global warming may increase pests and disease and lower yields.

Scientists disagree about the overall impact on yields. An important determinant of this is the extent to which farmers adapt their production decisions to the new climatic conditions. For example, suppose we are analyzing production in an area where rice is the predominant crop. Suppose, further, we conclude that global warming will result in a 30 percent drop in rice yields in this area. A simplistic analysis would conclude that food production would also drop by 30 percent in the area. A more sophisticated analysis would recognize the likelihood that many of the affected farmers

---

Box 12.1 El Niño and Food Production

Every few years, the surface of the Pacific Ocean becomes warmer. Peruvian fisherman named this phenomenon "El Niño" (the boy-child) because it coincided with Christmas (or the coming of the Christ-child). In 1997, the warming was especially large, and this has caused worldwide changes in weather patterns. In Washington, D.C., for example, the winter of 1997/98 was exceptionally mild, with virtually no snowfall. In Los Angeles, rainfall in early 1998 was nearly twice the usual level. The winter also saw March blizzards in the Midwest, and icestorms in New England that left people without electricity for days. The United States was not the only country to feel the effects of El Niño. South America and East Africa experienced heavier rainfall than usual; parts of South Asia were unusually dry.

Because of this "weird" weather, 37 countries were facing food emergencies in early 1998. But the problems are limited to certain areas. Worldwide, cereal production for 1997/98 is projected to be slightly above the record levels of 1996/97. FAO scientist Rene Gommes concludes, "It is important not to minimize risks but also to remember that there have been El Niños without any catastrophes and catastrophes without any El Niños."

will stop growing rice, and will switch to some alternative crop. The actual drop in production may be much less than 30 percent, depending on the alternative crops available, and the extent to which farmers change their cropping decisions.

Rosensweig and colleagues (1993) estimate that if temperatures increase by 2 degrees centigrade, wheat and soybean yields will increase from 10 to 15 percent, and maize and rice yields will increase about 8 percent. However, if temperatures increase by 4 degrees centigrade, yields would decline. (According to a UNEP Fact Sheet, climate models predict an increase of from 1.5 to 4.5 degrees centigrade over the next 100 years.) Wittwer believes that these estimates may underestimate the yield growth from global warming because they ignore possible benefits from increased levels of atmospheric carbon dioxide.

Other prognoses for crop yields show less optimism. For example, UNEP (1990) reports: "Mid-latitude yields may be reduced by 10–30 percent due to increased summer dryness"; although it admits, "higher yields in some areas may compensate for decreases in others." Pimentel (1993) reports: "Under the projected warming trend in the United States, farmers can expect a 25- to 100-percent increase in losses due to insects, depending on the crop. . . . U.S. crop losses due to weeds are projected to rise from 5 to 50 percent. . . . In North America, projected changes in temperature, soil moisture, carbon dioxide, and pests associated with global warming are expected to decrease food-crop production by as much as 27 percent." However, Pimentel sees some reasons for hope. He projects that yields in North Africa may improve from 10 to 30 percent as a result of global warming.

Finally, it should be noted that if global warming causes agricultural production to shift from one geographical area (say North America) to another (say North Africa), there can be problems in establishing the institutions and infrastructure needed to move the food from the production areas to the consuming areas. "While the overall, global impact of climate change on agricultural production may be small, regional vulnerabilities to food deficits may increase, due to problems of distributing and marketing food to specific regions and groups of people" (Rosenzweig & Hillel 1995).

□ **The Ozone Layer**

Depletion of the ozone layer permits more ultraviolet radiation to reach the earth. This in turn can affect agricultural production. Pimentel (1993) reports a potential drop in soybean yields of 30 percent due to this. (Soybeans are particularly sensitive to ultraviolet radiation levels.) Wittwer reports studies that also show substantial yield declines as a response to increased ultraviolet radiation. However, in studies that simultaneously increased both carbon dioxide levels (the greenhouse gas effect discussed above) and ultraviolet radiation levels, yields were basically unchanged.

□ 13

Health-Related Causes of Undernutrition

All infectious diseases have direct adverse metabolic effects.
—Scrimshaw, Taylor & Gordon 1968:12

Complex interactions among diet, disease, and physical characteristics determine the health and nutritional status of people, which in turn affects their enjoyment of life and ability to work.
—Bouis 1991:1

■ THE SYNERGISMS BETWEEN NUTRITION AND HEALTH

A healthy person has a good appetite, likely has a good diet, digests his food well, and makes efficient use of it in his body. A well-nourished person can keep his immune system functioning at a high level and is likely to be healthy.

A sick person is likely to lose her appetite, have a poor diet, digest her food poorly, and use some of her nutrients to fight infection. A poorly nourished person suffers a weakened immune system and is susceptible to infections.

We see a positive feedback loop: Good health promotes good nutrition; good nutrition promotes good health. But when you look at it the other way around—poor health leads to poor nutrition and poor nutrition leads to poor health—you are more likely to call it a vicious circle.

Just as there are strong synergistic relationships between health and nutrition, infection exacerbates malnutrition and malnutrition exacerbates infection. This interrelationship is so important that the definitive review of the literature (Scrimshaw, Taylor & Gordon 1968:267) concludes:

221

"Where both malnutrition and exposure to infection are serious, as they are in most tropical and developing countries, successful control of these conditions depends upon efforts directed equally against both."

■ INFECTION EXACERBATES MALNUTRITION

Infection increases the potential for and severity of malnutrition. Most common Third World infections have a heavy impact on nutritional status in three important ways: (1) through loss of appetite or intolerance for food (e.g., vomiting); (2) through cultural factors (e.g., relatives of the sick individual substitute less-nutritious diets for the regular diet and administer purgatives, antibiotics, or other medicines that reduce absorption of specific nutrients); and (3) through loss of body nitrogen (protein).

This last pathway to malnutrition through infection (loss of nitrogen) is complex enough that it deserves separate discussion. What happens is that protein tissue in the body is used up to fight the infection. To manufacture such disease-fighting materials as interferon, white blood corpuscles, and mucus, the body needs amino acids, which it acquires in part by breaking down previously existing protein—chiefly from the muscles. This borrowing of muscle tissue for fighting infection is one of the reasons you feel so weak following a serious illness. It might seem reasonable to try to keep up the body's supply of protein during an illness through pushing food, but this is usually impracticable. Sick people often have little appetite. During convalescence, with an appropriate diet, the lost body protein is usually replaced.

□ Infection Promotes Dietary Deficiency

A reasonably healthy person who is presently on the borderline of nutritional deficiency may not show clinical signs of nutritional difficulties. But, owing to the above problems associated with infection, an illness can increase his nutritional deficiency, and he can then develop any one or more of a number of conditions caused by dietary deficiency (Scrimshaw, Taylor & Gordon 1968:265):

- Keratomalacia (a softening and ulceration of the eye's cornea) caused by a shortage of vitamin A; if the shortage continues long enough and is severe enough, xerophthalmia (a dry, thickened, lusterless condition of the eyeball resulting in blindness) may ensue
- Scurvy (spongy gums, loosening of the teeth, and a bleeding into the skin and mucous membranes) caused by lack of ascorbic acid (vitamin C)
- Beri-beri (inflammatory or degenerative changes of the nerves, digestive system, and heart) caused by lack of thiamine (vitamin B1)

- Pellagra (a condition marked by dermatitis, gastrointestinal disorders, and disorders of the central nervous system) resulting from insufficient niacin (one of the B-vitamins)
- Macrocytic anemia (anemia associated with exceptionally large red blood cells) caused by a deficiency of vitamin B12 or folic acid (one of the B-vitamins)
- Microcytic anemia (anemia associated with exceptionally small red blood cells) caused by a shortage of iron

In addition to the above, a number of studies show that low-birth-weight babies suffer more health problems as adults than do normal-birth-weight babies. These problems include high blood pressure, too much cholesterol and sugar in the blood, cardiovascular disease, and diabetes. Also, cataracts were significantly less likely to develop in elderly people who took vitamin supplements (or beta-carotene, or of riboflavin and niacin). There is also evidence that undernutrition can increase the possibility that a person who is HIV-positive will graduate to full-blown AIDS. A study that followed HIV-positive men for seven years found those who consumed three to four times the RDA of niacin and vitamin A had a 40 to 50 percent lower chance of developing AIDS (Tang et al. 1993).

☐ Diarrhea and Nutrition

The serious conditions noted above result from a specific dietary deficiency exacerbated by infection. But the most common instance of an illness seriously affecting nutritional status is that of undernutrition induced or exacerbated by a gastrointestinal infection (gastroenteritis) that causes diarrhea or, in its more extreme form, dysentery. An outstanding feature of kwashiorkor, for instance, is the frequency with which it is precipitated by an attack of acute diarrheal disease (Scrimshaw, Taylor & Gordon 1968:27).

For the world as a whole, diarrhea is not as ubiquitous as the common cold, but in many Third World localities it comes in a close second in frequency of occurrence. Diarrhea particularly affects children under five years old, and childhood fecal matter is a main source of the infective material. Food and water are key transmission routes. Children often make their first contact with diarrheal disease organisms through weaning foods (Martorell, pers. comm.). In fact, an outstanding feature of diarrheal disease in the Third World is the concentration of cases among children during and immediately after weaning (Durand & Pigney 1963), illustrated in Figure 13.1.

In a Third World setting, the onset of diarrhea at weaning time (so common that it has sometimes been called by the special name of *weanling diarrhea*) is typically acute and rapidly progressive, with liquid or semiliquid stools, varying from three to as many as twenty a day. About one-fourth of

Figure 13.1 Third World, Age-Specific Diarrheal Morbidity Rates

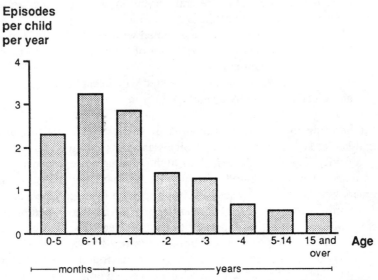

Source: Adapted from de Zoysa et al. 1985:8 using data from Snyder & Merson 1982.

patients have blood or mucus in the stools and, frequently, pus. Fever may be absent, but low-grade fever is usual, along with malaise, toxemia (buildup of toxic substances in the blood), intestinal cramps, and tenesmus (a distressing but ineffectual urge to evacuate the rectum or bladder). The usual clinical course runs four to five days. Repeated episodes can result in a month or more total time spent fighting diarrhea during a year's time (Figure 13.2). In malnourished children a low-grade indisposition often continues for a month or more, sometimes as long as three months, with irregularly recurring loose stools, a progressively depleted nutritional state, and occasional recurrent acute episodes (Scrimshaw, Taylor & Gordon 1968:220).

Although there are some 25 different organisms (bacteria, viruses, and parasites) that can cause diarrhea, all cases result in a shortage of water and salts (electrolytes) in the body. This dehydration of the body can be the most serious consequence of diarrhea. By the time a weanling child is seriously dehydrated from diarrhea, it is lethargic; its eyes are dulled and when it cries there are no tears; its skin is wrinkled like an old man's; it stops urinating; the fontanel (soft spot at the top of an infant's skull) is sunken. If you pinch the child's skin, it only slowly returns to the normal conformation (Goodall 1984). At best this dehydration stands in the way of a quick recovery from the diarrhea. At worst (if the child loses more than

Figure 13.2   Diarrheal Illness, Developing Regions and Selected U.S. Sample

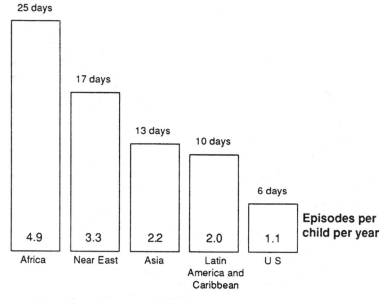

Average number of days per year with diarrhea

Source: Adapted from de Zoysa et al. 1985:11.
Note: An average episode of diarrhea is expected to last five days.

15 percent of his body fluids) it is fatal. A baby may well die within 24 hours of the arrival of these signs of serious dehydration. Some 60 to 70 percent of the 5 million annual diarrheal deaths are caused by this associated dehydration (WHO 1985c:6).

For generations it was thought that the only way to replace these electrolytes was through intravenous injection (IV). Oral replacement using the salts alone simply did not work. In the late 1960s researchers in India and what is now Bangladesh found that merely adding common cane sugar to the missing salts produced a formula that worked by mouth. Called *oral rehydration therapy* (ORT), this simple technology was first used to fight cholera (the most virulent form of dysentery) in an epidemic in India in 1971. Since then it has become a Third World public health mainstay and is being vigorously promoted by both the United Nations Children's Fund (UNICEF) and WHO. UNICEF (1987:8) has called ORT the cheapest and most effective health intervention that can be implemented in the home to decrease childhood mortality. UNICEF estimates that 1 million deaths per year are prevented by ORT. A brief explanation of how it works is provided in Box 13.1.

Box 13.1 Oral Rehydration Therapy (ORT)

Roger M. Goodall

The discovery that sodium transport and glucose transport are coupled in the small intestine so that glucose accelerates absorption of solute and water was potentially the most important medical advance this century.
—Lancet 1978, no. 2:300

In the normal healthy intestine, there is a continuous exchange of water through the intestinal wall. Every 24 hours, up to 20 liters of water is secreted and very nearly as much is reabsorbed. This mechanism allows the absorption into the bloodstream of the soluble breakdown products of digestion.

In a state of diarrheal disease, this balance is upset and much more water is secreted than is reabsorbed, causing a net loss to the body that can be as high as several liters in a day. If more than 15 percent of the body's fluid is lost, death occurs.

In addition to water, sodium is lost. The body's store of sodium is almost entirely in solution in body fluids and plasma. By contrast, 98 percent of the body's total potassium is held within cells.

For the proper functioning of the body, the concentration of sodium in the blood has to be held to within close limits (which perhaps correspond with the salinity of the archaic seas from which our evolutionary ancestors emerged eons ago). This sodium concentration is normally precisely controlled by the kidneys. However, in a state of dehydration water is conserved by the reduction or even complete absence of urination, and the kidneys cannot do their normal job of regulating sodium concentration. Continued diarrhea causes rapid depletion of water and sodium.

Simply giving a saltwater solution by mouth has no beneficial effect because, in the diarrheal state, the normal mechanism by which sodium ions are absorbed by the healthy intestinal wall is impaired, and if the sodium is not absorbed, the water cannot be absorbed either. In fact, excess salt in the intestinal cavity causes increased secretion of water into the intestine (through osmotic pressure), and the diarrhea worsens!

If glucose (also called dextrose) is added to a saline solution, a new mechanism comes into play. The glucose molecules are absorbed through the intestinal wall—unaffected by the diarrheal disease state—and in a process called cotransport coupling, carries sodium through the wall at the same time. This occurs in a one-to-one ratio; one molecule of glucose cotransporting one sodium ion. Glucose does not cotransport water. Rather it is the now increased relative concentration of sodium across the intestinal wall that pulls water through.

It was the discovery of the mechanism of cotransport of sodium and glucose that Doctor Kathleen Elliott, in an editorial in the prestigious British medical journal *Lancet,* described as potentially the most important medical advance of this century. *ORT is, in fact, the practical realization of this potential.*

While common table salt and ordinary white sugar are the dominant constituents of the recipe for oral rehydration salts (ORS) recommended jointly by WHO and UNICEF, two other constituents are included: potassium chloride and sodium citrate.

(continues)

Box 13.1 Continued

Although 98 percent of the body's potassium is held within the cells, prolonged diarrhea will result in a loss of potassium. The loss of potassium from repeated diarrheal attacks over a period of time causes muscular weakness, lethargy, and anorexia. The typical distended abdomen of a chronically undernourished child is caused by loss of muscle tone in the abdominal wall largely attributable to chronic depletion of potassium.

Potassium is not involved in any way in the sodium-glucose cotransport mechanism. But restoring a potassium deficit promotes a feeling of well-being and stimulates the appetite. Although potassium is not absorbed as dramatically as is sodium during ORT, the effectiveness of the recipe is enhanced by its inclusion, especially for a child who has suffered repeated diarrheal attacks.

The loss of body salts and fluid leads to an inappropriate pH level in the blood, called acidosis, that is corrected by the addition of a base such as sodium citrate to the recipe. When account is taken of the different molecular weights of glucose and sodium and the needs of the body for the depleted salts, the completed recipe typically comes out as:

Sodium chloride	3.5 grams
Sodium citrate	2.5 grams
Potassium chloride	1.5 grams
Glucose	20.0 grams

The above to be dissolved in one liter of clean drinking water.

Research is going on at many centers around the world to develop new and improved versions of ORS. Other effective recipes are now in use. Some, for instance, substitute starch for sugar. In the intestine, starch is metabolized to glucose and therefore has the same properties of enhancing sodium absorption. However it has the added advantage that it has less osmotic effect (through this process sugar has some limited tendency to pull water back into the cavity of the intestine).

Although diarrhea always produces at least some dehydration, some of the more than 25 pathogens that cause it may strip the tips of the villi from large patches of the intestinal wall, leaving the inside of the intestine looking rather like a piece of velvet that has lost its nap. This decreases the surface area and can lower by more than 50 percent the specific absorptive capacities of the intestine. The result is malabsorption, which can cause or exacerbate undernutrition, most especially in a child already nutritionally compromised by repeated previous attacks of diarrhea.

Withholding food, even for one or two days, greatly exacerbates the undernutrition. This, coupled with anorexia, caused partly by chronic potassium depletion, results in a vicious circle: diarrhea causing undernutrition and undernutrition causing ever more frequent and severe diarrhea.

More detail on this subject is available in Goodall 1984. Roger Goodall was formerly senior advisor on oral rehydration therapy and essential drugs to UNICEF. He is currently an independent consultant.

■ MALNUTRITION EXACERBATES INFECTION

Malnutrition often amplifies the impact of infection. An example from the Philippines is illustrative. Severely undernourished children admitted to a hospital for acute respiratory infection are found to be 13 times as likely to die from the disease as children whose nutrition is normal (see Figure 13.3).

Malnutrition is almost always synergistic with intestinal diseases caused by worms or protozoa and with any disease caused by bacteria (Scrimshaw, Taylor & Gordon 1968:263–264). That is, malnutrition aggravates the course of the disease, and the disease, in turn, intensifies the malnutrition.

A wide variety of nutrients have been demonstrated to have an impact on the competency of the body's immune system (Gershwin et al. 1985: 2; Phillips & Baetz 1980). The impact of nutrition on infection begins at birth and lasts throughout life. Not only is breast milk loaded with the appropriate nutrients for an infant's diet, but it carries with it a load of

Figure 13.3   Acute Respiratory Infection Mortality by Nutritional Status, Philippine Hospital Cases

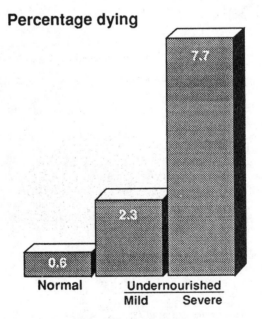

Source: Adapted from Galway et al. 1987:23 using data from Tupasi 1985.

substances that help protect the infant against disease: immunoglobulins, macrophages, lymphocytes, neutrophils, components of the complement system, and so on (Rivera & Martorell 1988). (The complement system involves a set of more than 11 proteins normally found in the bloodstream. These proteins act in conjunction with the blood's antibody system in fighting infection, complementing the work of the antibodies.) Undernutrition increases the duration of infections, especially diarrhea. Unequivocal evidence shows that the immune response is reduced in severe undernutrition, and some evidence suggests a diminished immune response in moderate undernutrition, particularly in wasted children (Rivera & Martorell 1988).

Worldwide, malnutrition is the most common cause of deficiencies in the immune system, even among adults. Two examples will help to illustrate this point: (1) Nutritional supplements given to the elderly have been found to improve their response to the influenza virus vaccine; and (2) among individuals given a vaccine to protect them from tuberculosis, a positive correlation between better nutrition and resistance to the disease was observed (Chandra 1988). Malnutrition interferes with various bodily mechanisms that attempt to block the multiplication or progress of infectious agents (Figure 13.4). The list of ways it can do this is long, but

Figure 13.4   Protective Factors Instrumental in Health Maintenance

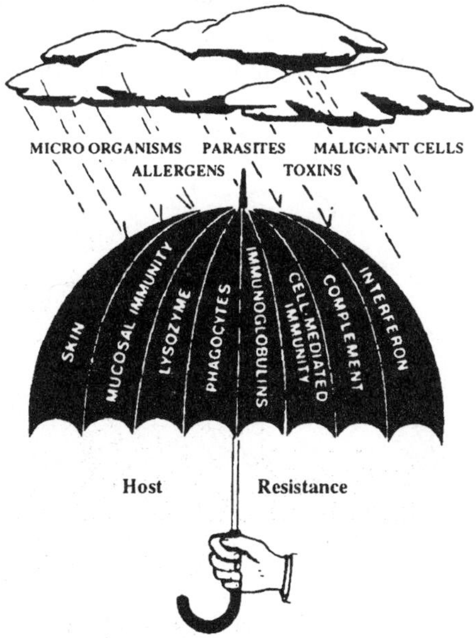

Source: Adapted from Chandra 1980.

significant among them are a decrease in the response and activity of white blood corpuscles; a reduction in the production of interferon; a decrease in the integrity of the skin, the mucous membrane, and other tissues that serve to bar the entrance of infection; and interference with normal tissue replacement and repair (Scrimshaw, Taylor & Gordon 1968:263–264).

The exploration of the mechanisms of how undernutrition affects the immune system has only just begun, but already we have enough information to provide interesting clues as to what is happening. For instance, the mucous membrane not only provides a physical barrier against the entrance of foreign particles that might cause infection (bacteria, viruses), but provides a chemical barrier as well. Mucus contains a variety of biochemical and immunological disease fighters, one of which is an enzyme called *lysozyme,* which has the capacity to attack the cell walls of invading bacteria. Colombian children suffering from protein-energy malnutrition were found to be producing reduced levels of lysozyme. In a process called *cell-mediated immunity,* T-lymphocytes play a key role attacking disease-causing microbes. Children with PEM are also likely to suffer an atrophied thymus, the organ primarily responsible for the "education" and proliferation of T-lymphocytes, and at the same time to produce fewer of these lymphocytes than expected when their bodies are challenged with invading disease organisms (Sherman 1986).

A final point we must remember: Not only does malnutrition reduce resistance to infection, but it decreases stamina, which in turn decreases the capacity to cope with life and to perform on the job, making it more difficult to earn money to pay for transportation to health care centers, to pay for the services themselves, and to pay for appropriate drugs for combating infection.

■ PART 3

POLICY APPROACHES TO UNDERNUTRITION

In Part 2, we looked at the causes of undernutrition—vehicles by which undernutrition is delivered to families—and identified economic, demographic, agricultural, environmental, and health factors. The central activity of Part 3 is to explore public policy alternatives of interest to nutrition planners.

☐ 14

Philosophical Approaches to Undernutrition

In the next section of the book, we consider policies that can be adopted to reduce the degree of worldwide hunger. Before proceeding, we spend a few pages exploring philosophical approaches to the issue. What motivates governments, societies, individuals, or groups of individuals to concern themselves with the issue of undernutrition?

■ FROM THE STANDPOINT OF A MORAL PHILOSOPHER

☐ Charity or Concern for the Poor and Hungry

Our first chapter opened with a reference to starving Ethiopian babies—babies with bloated bellies, spindly arms and legs, and bodies too weak to sit up. The device is a standard technique for grabbing the attention of people attuned to Western culture and making them stop to think about the world food problem.

Those who live in the Western world are exposed to repeated appeals to conscience, asking them to join the battle to end hunger. In 1980, the Presidential Commission on World Hunger urged that the United States "make the elimination of hunger the primary focus of its relations with the developing world." Commenting on this in a paper written for a religious audience, M. McLaughlin (1984) said that "The moral and humanitarian reasons for such a policy seem self-evident."

A common argument in favor of studying and solving the world hunger problem is the moral dictate that each of us should help individuals who are less fortunate than ourselves. The Pope's statement to the World Food Summit, for example, contains the following:

233

In the analyses which have accompanied the preparatory work for your meeting, it is recalled that more than 800 million people still suffer from malnutrition and that it is often difficult to find immediate solutions for improving these tragic situations. Nevertheless, we must seek them together so that we will no longer have, side by side, the starving and the wealthy, the very poor and the very rich, those who lack the necessary means and others who lavishly waste them. Such contrasts between poverty and wealth are intolerable for humanity.

It is the task of nations, their leaders, their economic powers and all people of goodwill to seek every opportunity for a more equitable sharing of resources, which are not lacking, and of consumer goods; by this sharing, all will express their sense of brotherhood. It requires "firm and persevering determination to commit oneself to the common good; that is to say, to the good of all and of each individual, because we are all really responsible for all" (Sollicitudo rei socialis, no. 38). This spirit calls for a change of attitude and habits with regard to life-styles and the relationship between resources and goods, as well as for an increased awareness of one's neighbour and his legitimate needs.

This is a matter of religious conviction or personal ethics. The motivation comes from within the individual. I may believe that I "owe" compassion to the hungry, but that debt is a product of my beliefs, something generated from within myself. In that regard, it is quite different from the debt I owe to the government as taxes.

☐ Food as a Right

This distinction (between being motivated by personal ethics and being motivated by an obligation to society) is important as we consider a second type of moral argument about why we should be interested in the problem of world hunger. That is the issue of "food as a right." Some 85 countries have endorsed the International Covenant on Economic, Social and Cultural Rights (adopted by the United Nations General Assembly in 1966) which defined and formalized the right to food as a basic human right. The right to food was widely discussed in preparation for and during the World Food Summit of 1996 (Pinstrup-Andersen, Nygaard & Ratta 1995; Alston 1997).

If food is a right, then hunger is a violation of that right, and we have a second ethical motivation to be concerned about hunger—the moral requirement that we seek justice and oppose violations of rights. There is a difference between the "charity" motivation (we have an ethical obligation to help the hungry) and the "justice" motivation (food is a right). That difference is illustrated by the following:

- If you accept the view that there is a fundamental right to food, then you are motivated to address the hunger problem even if you do not believe that you have a moral duty to help the poor and hungry.

Your motivation here is simply to ensure the protection of that fundamental right.

- If you believe that you have a moral duty to help the poor, then you are motivated to address the hunger problem even if you do not believe that there is a fundamental right to food. Your motivation here is your duty to be charitable.

To illustrate this difference, consider the right to religious freedom. A Christian who embraces the concept of this right could simultaneously believe (1) that people have a right to worship as a Jew or Muslim; and (2) that nobody ought to exercise that right, because those religions deny the divinity of Christ. Or consider the right to "free speech." A person might simultaneously believe (1) that people have the right to read pornographic books, and (2) that nobody ought to exercise that right.

The assertion that people have a right to food is in this sense stronger than the assertion that people have a moral responsibility to help the poor and hungry. The latter is an assertion of a principle that will guide the speaker's behavior, and a plea to others to adopt the same principle. The former is an assertion that other people have a responsibility to help the poor and hungry even if those people do not choose to adopt the moral principle that would motivate that behavior. In other words, a coercive element is embedded in the "rights" assertion that is absent from the "moral principle" assertion.

The assertion that food is a right (or that people have a fundamental right to food and other necessities or "basic needs") is highly controversial. Let us consider some of the sources of controversy by means of analogies.

Consider a right that we accept as fundamental in the United States: the "right to remain silent" or the right not to incriminate oneself. We accept the existence of the right even when we disapprove of its exercise. For example, if a kidnapper refuses to tell where he has hidden his victim, we may doubly abhor the kidnapper for his silence as well as his violence. Furthermore, we do not seriously argue about whether we should adopt rules permitting police to torture suspects. The widespread acceptance of "the right to remain silent" sets this issue beyond the reach of political debate. It simplifies decision making; we don't need to consider the pros and cons of any action, we need only to answer the question, "does the action violate the right?"

This may explain why activists have pushed to have the right to food accepted as a fundamental right. They may hope to eliminate debate over the costs and benefits of various programs; the existence of the right trumps all other arguments. The FIAN fact sheet on "12 misconceptions about the right to food" states that "governance is negotiable; rights are not." A panel of constitutional experts supporting the concept of economic rights stated: "Fundamental needs such as social welfare rights should not be at the mercy of changing governmental policies and programmes, but must be defined as entitlements." The intention of advancing the "right to food" concept is to force acceptance of more active government programs to combat world hunger without having to justify those programs economically. (See the next section of this chapter.)

The strongest objection to the concept of food as a right is that unlike traditional civil rights, which require government *not to act* in certain ways, economic rights appear to require the state *to act* in certain ways. Traditional civil or political rights do not require government to act. Consider the right to religious freedom, or the right to worship as one chooses. This right imposes on the state the restriction that it cannot pass laws or take actions that interfere with an individual's right to worship. Suppose you want to attend a Zoroastrian temple for weekly worship; but suppose the nearest such temple is in Chicago, and suppose further that you cannot afford to travel to and from Chicago each week. Does the government have any obligation to buy a weekly plane ticket for you? No, at least not as the right to religious freedom is interpreted in the United States.

Economic rights do not only require the government to avoid actions that would interfere with any individual's ability to obtain food; they additionally require the government to take actions to increase the ability of hungry people to obtain food.

The most extreme objections to the concept of economic rights assert that these rights are immoral themselves because they require government to limit the freedom of some members of the society. It is hard to conceive of any effective assertion of economic rights that does not require extensive redistribution of income from rich to poor. If we accept the argument that government limits on freedom are immoral, then any taxation is immoral, since the taxation itself is coercive, restricting individual liberties. But isn't taxation required to guarantee other civil rights? To ensure the right to be free of "cruel and unusual punishment," the government must use tax revenue to build new prisons. As long as it is costly to guarantee individuals their civil rights, some element of government coercion through the taxation system is necessary.

The word *rights* in the traditional sense refers to entitlements that are in most applications absolute. The U.S. government cannot censor a newspaper, or ban a religion, because those rights are absolute. Of course, it is easy to find examples of ways in which "absolute rights" are not absolute. The right of free speech does not extend to cover the right to yell "FIRE" in a crowded theater. The right of freedom of association (the right to choose your own friends) does not mean that an employer has the right to hire individuals of only one race. Absolute rights become limited only when the exercise of the right interferes with another person's exercise of his or her rights. The false yell of "FIRE" interferes with other people's right to congregate safely in a theater. Racial discrimination interferes with employees' rights to be free of discrimination. When one right conflicts with another, as in these cases, it is impossible to guarantee both rights absolutely.

On the one hand, what makes the concept of economic rights so controversial is that economic rights inevitably conflict with other rights because economic rights require government expenditures. On the other hand, the assertion that food is a right gives those who favor government intervention an important argument to use against libertarians. The civil libertarian argues: "The government cannot take my money (through taxes) to buy food for a poor person because I have a right to control my own property." (Notice how the assertion of a right is used to trump other arguments about whether a policy is a good or bad idea.) The hunger activist can respond: "You have a right to property; but the poor person has a right to food. This is a conflict of rights and the government has an appropriate role in settling that conflict."

Further, because economic rights are in inevitable conflict with rights to property, economic rights can never be absolute. So a "right to food" does not mean that as long as a single hungry person exists in the world, the United States cannot devote any government expenditures to defense, or student loans, or drug interdiction, or civil rights enforcement. We have competing social goals that must be pursued with limited resources.

Who decides the priorities for these competing social goals? In the United States, conflicts between rights are typically resolved in the court system, not by democratically elected representatives. This raises the additional question of whether we have a fundamental right to control the level of taxation through a political process. If we have no such right, then courts could require higher and higher taxes to ensure economic rights. If there *is* such a right (to a social contract on taxes), then this right must be balanced against economic and other civil rights.

If we maintain the current system of establishing priorities through a political process, we impose a severe limit on economic rights. The process of simultaneously "guaranteeing" economic rights and property rights is really no different that the process of setting policy goals and balancing competing interests.

■ FROM THE STANDPOINT OF AN ECONOMIST

The last section started as a discussion of moral imperatives, moved on to the notion that the assertion of a right makes economic policy analysis unnecessary, and ended by raising the question: How should we allocate scarce resources to accomplish competing objectives? This question covers familiar ground for economists. Whether the tradeoffs are made by courts, legislatures, or administrators, the economic rule for policy decision making is *maximize total benefits minus total costs* (Posner 1986).

☐ Benefit-Cost Analysis

If we lived in a world of perfect knowledge, perhaps we could make a number of comparisons between costs and benefits from various programs and come up with an allocation where the economists' ideal is met: The last dollar spent on one program gives the same benefit as the last dollar spent on any other program.

We do not live in a world of perfect knowledge, but the concept is useful in thinking about how to allocate public resources among competing programs (such as, say, highway construction, rural electrification, nutrition intervention, education, family planning, and tax reduction). Below we discuss how economics can help us understand the motivation for public policies to fight undernutrition.

☐ Costs and Benefits from Food Consumption

Let us look first at how benefits and costs change as food consumption increases in an impoverished household. For this household, the cost of each extra unit of food is the same—the household can buy more food without affecting the price. In Figure 14.1, the cost per unit of energy is shown as constant (a horizontal line) as food purchases increase.

The benefits from additional calories are more complex to describe. Without a certain minimal level of food, life ends. When there is enough food to sustain life, benefits from small additions are great: prevention of disease; increased amounts of work accomplished; hunger satisfied. But as food intake increases, the benefits from additional amounts decline. The additional energy will fuel activities with fewer benefits, such as recreation and social interaction, and if the process continues far enough, eventually additional energy will end up as excess fat, which can be detrimental to health (a negative benefit).

Social benefits may accrue to low levels of food consumption. To an extent, deaths from undernutrition are part of the earth's "self-regulating" mechanism for two reasons. First, high infant and child mortality slows population growth; and children that survive to the reproductive years are the healthiest and toughest. The impact on population growth is especially high where social attitudes favor boy babies over girl babies. In these communities, scarce food is allocated disproportionately to boys, and girls are more likely to succumb to infection and undernutrition (Cassidy 1987: 309). This results in a situation in which women of childbearing age make up a small percentage of the population. The second way in which undernutrition is part of a self-regulating mechanism is through stunting. In a

Figure 14.1   Marginal Benefit and Marginal Cost of Energy Intake for One
Household

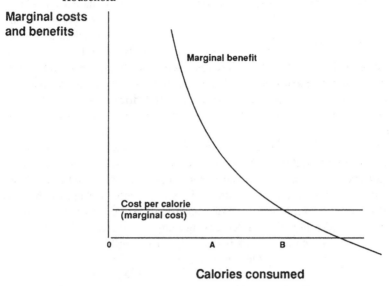

Calories consumed

population where undernutrition is prevalent, those who survive to adulthood tend to be stunted. But small people need less food. David Seckler
(1982) has gone so far as to propose that Third World children who are
"stunted but not wasted," to use the Waterlow classification described in
Chapter 4, have probably not been particularly stressed, but rather are
"small but healthy." This argument has met with considerable criticism
among nutritionists (Martorell 1989).

Conversly, reducing undernutrition also creates social benefits by breaking the cycle of poverty. An example from our Chapter 7 discussion on demographic transition illustrates this point. Suppose that a husband and wife
calculate that they need one child who survives to adulthood to help them
in the fields and care for them in their old age. But because the family is
poor and unable to afford sufficient food, there is a high probability of their
children dying from malnutrition. Therefore, the couple has several children
in the hope that at least one will survive to adulthood. If we could reduce the
childhood mortality attributable to malnutrition, we would actually need less
food (only five years of child nutrition), because less food would be given to
children who ultimately do not survive. Several other ways in which undernutrition exists in a cycle of poverty and undernutrition follow:

- Undernutrition leads to poor productivity in agricultural workers,
  which leads to lower levels of food production, which leads to food
  shortages, which leads to undernutrition.

- Undernutrition leads to increased infant and childhood mortality, which leads to increased birth rates, which leads to increased food demand, which leads to food shortages, which leads to undernutrition.
- Undernutrition leads to poor productivity which leads to low incomes and persistent poverty; persistently poor households are never able to save sufficient resources to accumulate a critical mass to invest in activities (such as education) that would move them out of poverty; the poverty leads to undernutrition.

☐ Declining Marginal Utility of Income

Above, we discussed the principle that as food consumption increases, unit by unit, declining marginal benefits (or "decreasing marginal utility") accrue from adding an additional unit. Many economists accept the hypothesis that this principle can be extended to cover the consumption of all goods taken together: thus, a decreasing marginal utility of income.

A direct implication of this is that a dollar is worth more to a poor person than to a rich person. On the one hand, the idea is that a couple more dollars to a poor person will be spent on "necessities"—items that are fundamental to life. On the other hand, taking a couple of dollars away from a rich person will cause that person to consume fewer frivolous things. Therefore this transfer from rich to poor increases the "common good." This may explain why governments are motivated to adopt programs that have the effect of redistributing wealth from the rich to the poor.

The practical problem is that the declining marginal utility of income hypothesis implies that appropriate policy is total and complete equality of income distribution. If one person in the country (or the world) earns slightly more than another, then dollars should be taken from the former and given to the latter. Most people reject this policy prescription. That rejection raises questions about whether this is the true explanation for policy concern about the poor and hungry.

☐ Basic Needs

An alternative (attributable to Arnold Harberger) to the decreasing marginal utility of income explanation is that we all (or at least many of us) suffer when any person in the world (or country or ethnic group or family) suffers from undernutrition or failure to meet "basic needs." When a hungry person is fed, a direct benefit goes to that person (which benefit is reflected in the market transaction), but also an indirect benefit goes to me, because I care about human suffering. This indirect benefit is external to the market. Because such a reduction affects my happiness, I would be willing to pay to see the incidence of hunger reduced or eliminated. The reduction of hunger is a good: The more it happens, the better I feel. But there is no market on which I can purchase this good. This is a case of missing markets, or *externalities*. Private action is unlikely to solve this problem. Because I know others also care, I may wait for *them* to take actions to reduce hunger, in which case *I* get the good (reduced world hunger) free of charge. Government action may be justified in creating an artificial market by collecting money from each of us who derives satisfaction from reductions in hunger, and using that money to reduce hunger.

The difference between the externality argument and the declining marginal utility argument in their policy implications is that the government should spend money only on actions that have this external benefit. Therefore the government policy might well be to support hunger reduction programs, but not to support programs that would allow a poor person to buy a television.

■ FIVE WORLDVIEWS ON THE WORLD FOOD PROBLEM

From the above discussion we see a number of approaches to the world food problem. In two seminal papers on toddler malnutrition, anthropologist Claire Cassidy (1980, 1987) brings order and clarity to this subject by identifying and describing various worldviews of the hunger problem. Cassidy begins her classification by postulating three general interpretations of the universally observed fretfulness, crying, frequent illnesses, and even deaths that are associated with Third World weaning children who are at risk for undernutrition: (1) the activist position; (2) the adaptor position; and (3) the acceptor position. These interpretations lead to five worldviews of the hunger problem: (1) altruism; (2) intervention economics; (3) bioecology; (4) social cohesion; and (5) status quo. Her scheme is shown in condensed form in Figure 14.2.

The activist believes that there is a problem: Children are undernourished and something should be done about it. The activist has difficulty seeing any benefits to undernourished children. Activists come in two categories, the altruist, who would like to see every child in the world nourished properly but who is less conscious of the economic cost of programs that would accomplish this goal than is the economist (who would intervene in the socioeconomic system in such a way that the last dollar spent in each of the alternative social welfare programs yielded an equal return).

The adaptor is not so sure that there is a problem: He notes that benefits accrue from adapting persons to the existing situation. The adaptor is fully aware of scarce resources. He knows that there are times when, for the benefit of the group, it makes sense to feed adequately the more productive members of the family (the working adults) and to slight the less productive (the children and old people), even if in the process, some must

Figure 14.2   Five Worldviews Relevant to the World Food Problem

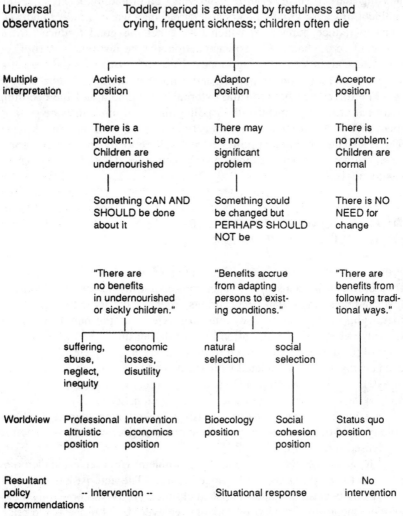

Source: Adapted from Cassidy 1987:297.

die. Those who note that the natural selection happening here tends to adapt the genetic material of the group to the harsh conditions under which they live are said to be taking the bioecologist's position. Those who note the benefits to society from lower birth rates (from preferences shown boy babies over girl babies), or who note the economic savings (food savings) to society from a stunted population, are said to be taking the social cohesionist's position.

The acceptor does not think there is a problem. To him, children who show symptoms that biomedical specialists call undernutrition are behaving normally. Children have always behaved in this way. Following traditional ways has, in the past, assured the survival of the group, and therefore why change now? The acceptor therefore goes with the status quo.

To the activist, intervention in the system is required. To the adaptor, intervention may be required, depending on the situation. The adaptor would question saving infants' lives without the assurance of adequate resources to properly raise the children saved. The acceptor sees no need for any intervention.

Although most people will find value in more than one of the above positions, most of us side more heavily with one or the other. Westerners (and we) tend to take the activist position. Low-income Third World people tend toward the adaptor position, or in some cases even the acceptor position. These differences in worldview can, at the least, lead to difficulties in communication between aid givers and aid recipients and at worst can lead to rejection and failure of aid programs (see Box 14.1).

Box 14.1
Worldview Conflicts and Change Agent Dilemmas

Claire Monod Cassidy

Western humanitarian philosophy focuses on the individual, views the child as of prime importance, and uses activism to solve problems. In contrast, many nonindustrialized peoples focus on the importance of the group, view the productive adult as of prime importance, and use consensus to address problems. These philosophical differences mean that customs Westerners interpret as damaging are, to many non-Westerners, plausible, reasonable, acceptable, normal, or even benevolent.

Persons holding such different perspectives use different decision modes and, in a nutrition intervention setting, may have considerable difficulty communicating. The stage is set for conflict—and for intervention failure—if these differences are not understood and adjusted for.

The intervention economist, typically Western-trained, sees the societal costs of hunger and sickness as measured mainly in material terms of money and goods, and is concerned with the disutility or inefficiency of the systems that foster malnutrition. Solutions tend to be activist and material, emphasizing, for example, improved commodity exchange or production, or income generation and redistribution.

In contrast, the intervention altruist, also typically Western-trained, sees costs mainly in terms of the social-spiritual quality of individual human lives (especially those of infants and children) and worries about suffering

(continues)

Box 14.1   Continued

and social distribution programs for the needy, and educational and outreach (nonmaterial) aids that are intended to change behavior and decrease inequity.

Of these two activist positions, the intervention altruism approach focuses primarily on the individual, while the intervention economics approach focuses on impersonal abstractions such as the sector, region, or market. Neither focuses on the society, and thus both effectually, if unintentionally, deemphasize the importance of the community or familial context in which suffering occurs. However, it is precisely this social context that has value for most of the activists' target populations.

The activist child-survival focus is a short-range type of future orientation; some present lives are saved, but little emphasis is placed on providing long-term supportive social, educational, or economic contexts for those lives. For example, ORT is popular because it can both cheaply and relatively easily prevent toddler and infant deaths from diarrhea. Most often, however, its use is not linked to efforts to maintain the child once it survives diarrhea, or to prevent recurrent bouts. UNICEF's four-part plan to save 20 million preschool lives a year by encouraging use of vaccinations, breastfeeding, growth charts, and ORT does provide a larger context for ORT. But it is not a maintenance context, for the plan does not address the linked, long-term problems of underemployment, poverty, inequity, lack of educational facilities, or rapid population growth.

In their enthusiasm for the position, altruists may be tempted to assign pejorative labels to nonaltruists: "ignorant" if circumstances suggest that the nonaltruist has not had the opportunity to learn altruistic behaviors, and perhaps "inhumane," "abusive," "racist," or "neglectful" to those who have apparently rejected components of the altruistic worldview.

Additionally, activists frustrated by being unable to promote change as fast as they would like to, summarize their perceptions of the "traditional" client populations' attitudes as if they were a mirror image of the activist position. Thus, where the activist finds abnormality, this traditional "acceptor" is assumed to find normality; where the activist loves change, the acceptor is supposed to abhor it; and where the activist recommends intervention, the acceptor wants none.

Although there is no doubt that individual villagers sometimes think in this rigid acceptor manner, I do not know of modern ethnographic sources that describe any groups of people whose thinking would conform to this model. Rather, most Third World villagers tend to think like adaptors.

There are two adaptor positions, the bioecology and social cohesion positions. The first summarizes a position of evolutionary and ecological biologists, few of whom are directly involved in delivering development aid. The second represents the position of many Third World rural and poor urban populations. Both adaptor positions emphasize the context in which an organism finds itself, and both ask how an individual organism relates to the larger context. Thus questions of "good" are typically phrased in terms of group continuity rather than of individual life, and it is often recognized that what damages an individual organism may paradoxically help maintain the larger group. Also, adaptors measure time in years or generations

(continues)

Box 14.1 Continued

rather than in the months characteristic of activist thinkers. Thus adaptors find that short-term individual survival is relatively unimportant unless those who survive grow to adulthood and take their proper places as productive members of the community.

Another reason adaptors tend not to think in utopian terms is that they assume that scarcity exists and that there is never enough to provide an ideal environment for all organisms. Consequently, some competition for resources is inevitable and "normal." Together, these values mean that adaptors measure the desirability of change against their own twin realities of scarcity and competition, and express good in terms of long-term group continuity.

The social cohesionist realizes that one means of coping with scarcity is to maintain a high ratio of producers to nonproducers, and one way to do this is to deny resources—at least in a relative sense—to those perceived as less productive. The most productive members of such societies are adults. Among the less productive members are children. Many customs and behaviors that activist interveners have associated with poor child health and lowered chances for survival can be interpreted as societal efforts to decrease the resources devoted to child rearing. This approach might not make sense where food is abundant or most children live to school age, but where food is scarce it does.

It is important to note at once, however, that societal efforts to be frugal are typically unrelated to whether or not parents love their children. Numerous ethnographic studies show that, with few exceptions, poor and village parents do love their children and that the quality of their love is no different from that which altruistic parents may offer their children.

Children who survive resource competition in a family of extreme scarcity enjoy steadily increasing social value as they mature and become productive. A four-year-old who can carry and look after a younger sibling is already productive and proportionately more valued. In asking the young child to work, its parent is perhaps acting out of economic necessity but is also, and more importantly, drawing the child closer to valued adult groups and expressing approval and trust.

The worldview differences contrasted here can lead to miscommunication in intervention settings. Where the altruist focuses on individuals, physical health, and longevity, the social cohesionist focuses on group robustness. Where the social cohesionist fears scarcity, the altruist hopes it is not true, and the activist claims we can change the world so as to eliminate what we fear. Where the activist orients toward children, the social cohesionist orients toward adults. Worse, when both focus on children they want to raise them quite differently. Consider again the case of the four-year-old toting its younger sibling. An altruistic thinker might find that requiring such a child to work devalues it and might attempt to re-rig the system so as to eliminate this custom. Yet in the village context, relieving the child of its physical burden is equivalent to relieving it of some part of its social value and of its sense of belonging.

Worldview conflicts like those summarized here have seriously eroded the effectiveness of the well-meant programs of donor activists. How can

(continues)

Box 14.1   Continued

we resolve the dilemma that worldview differences weaken the effectiveness of donor programs? It is obvious that interveners have three basic
choices:

1. They can see the activist and adaptor positions as mutually exclusive
and withdraw from further intervention work, feeling it to be useless.
2. They can see the two positions as mutually exclusive and be so convinced of the superiority of their own ethic that they interpret their mission
as one of replacing the worldview of their clients.
3. They can recognize the validity and cogency of both positions and
seek commonalities that will permit true communication between intervener
and client. The aim is to help clients to engage in ameliorative design (by
their definition) of their own cultures.

Based on my assumption that most interveners are impelled by a sin-
cere desire to help, and can recognize the rights of others to believe and behave differently from themselves, I suggest that most professional interveners will aspire to the third of the three possibilities.

For a more in-depth treatment of worldview conflicts and change agents see Cassidy
1980, 1987.

To the reader, the next part of this book will appear heavily freighted
with the attitudes of the intervention economist. We will be examining and
evaluating policies to improve health and reduce fertility rates. We will
also be examining and evaluating policies and programs designed to increase the income of the poor and reduce the inequality of income and
wealth (of which food supplementation, mentioned in this chapter, is only
one of a number of alternatives). But in addition to the above intervention
economist approaches, we will borrow from other worldviews when we
examine programs for famine relief (altruism) and when we stress the existence of Third World resource scarcity and the importance of taking a
long-term view of the good of the community (adaptor).

☐ 15

Policies Aimed at Health-Related Causes of Undernutrition

If we could increase the health spending in the developing countries by only $2 per head, we could immunize all their children, eradicate polio, and provide the drugs to cure all their cases of diarrheal disease, acute respiratory infection, tuberculosis, malaria, schistosomiasis and sexually transmitted diseases.
—Hiroshi Nakajima, director-general of WHO, in WHO 1989:1

■ THE ECONOMIC EFFICIENCY OF PUBLIC HEALTH PROGRAMS

In Chapter 13 we noted the positive feedback loop between good health and good nutrition. Good health promotes good nutrition; good nutrition promotes good health. In recent years experts have said that, by and large, it is cheaper to maintain good health than it is to make people well after they get sick. This idea is coloring many of the current health care developments in the Third World, which are emphasizing low-cost delivery of health services to the poor. We see "barefoot doctors" in China, "nutrition huts" in the Philippines, and "health huts" in Haiti.

Actually, we have known of the economic efficiency of public health programs for a long time, and, despite the emphasis in many Western countries on private health care, governments have been sponsoring public health services in the West for many years. Modern engineering principles were applied to water-borne sewage disposal systems in the West during the 1840s. By the early 1900s it was common for local governments in the Western world to consider the supply of drinking water properly within their purview. In this century public programs promoting the iodization of salt and the fortification of flour with vitamins have become routine in the

West. (The history of such programs in the United States is outlined in Box 15.1.) Third World countries now sponsor parallel public programs for drinking water, sewage, food fortification, and salt iodization (see Box 15.2).

The present emphasis on publicly sponsored, low-cost primary health care for the poor is relatively recent. Most common Third World illnesses can be successfully treated in the field by paramedical workers using simple equipment and a limited range of medicines. Thus a strong argument de-

---

Box 15.1   A Brief History of Food Fortification in the United States

Richard Ahrens

The leading cause of draft deferment in the United States during World War I was the swelling of the thyroid gland called goiter. One problem associated with goiter was that boys who had the condition could not fit into the tight collars of the military uniforms. In 1923 the Harding Commission, appointed by President Warren Harding, recommended a voluntary program for the iodization of salt to combat goiter. A gentlemen's agreement was worked out between the salt companies and the executive branch of the government that there would be no price difference charged between the iodized and uniodized product.

During Word War II a bill was introduced into Congress that would have made it mandatory that all table salt be iodized, but the bill was defeated in committee when a number of medical doctors testified that there were probably some people in the United States who were sensitive to iodine and who would have skin problems as a result of being unable to obtain iodine-free salt.

Fortification of flour arose at the start of World War II, after President Franklin Roosevelt asked the National Academy of Sciences (NAS) to evaluate the nation's readiness for war. As one of their recommendations, the NAS came up with a proposal to ask flour millers to fortify wheat flour with iron, thiamin, riboflavin, and niacin. The flour fortification program became policy in 1940 and was looked after by the U.S. War Department. Later it became the province of the U.S. Department of Health, Education and Welfare, and now it is the province of the U.S. Food and Drug Administration.

A recommendation to increase substantially the iron fortification of enriched flour and bread came out of the 1969 White House Conference on Food, Nutrition and Health, and in 1973 the Food and Drug Administration proposed to triple the iron-enrichment level in flour. Several experts recommended against this proposal because doing so would exacerbate a problem of iron toxicity (hemochromatosis) among some 100,000 people, and by 1977 the idea of upping the iron level in flour was dropped.

Richard Ahrens is professor of nutrition at the University of Maryland and teaches a course on the history of nutrition.

Box 15.2   Food Fortification in the Third World

Eileen T. Kennedy et al.

Countries in which a single grain product supplies a disproportionate share of the total dietary intake consistently show a higher prevalence of micronutrient deficiencies. Fortification intervention schemes have been put into effect in order to alleviate this problem.

Fortification is a process whereby nutrients are added to a food to maintain or improve its quality; protein, amino acids, vitamins, minerals, and fat are all fortifications that can be added to a food. In order for fortification to be feasible and effective, a carrier for a particular fortificant must be consumed regularly and in sufficient quantity. As such, staples such as grains, sugar, salt, monosodium glutamate (MSG), and other condiments have been used as carriers in fortification interventions.

To serve as carriers, however, these staples must pass through the market. Thus, fortification of staples produced for consumption on the farm is not usually feasible, and malnourished members of semisubsistence farm households cannot usually be reached by this approach.

Microlevel fortification interventions have been regarded as a relatively easy method of alleviating some forms of malnutrition among food-purchasing households, since micronutrients can be added to food with a minimum of change in the diet and at a relatively low cost.

Vitamin A, iodine, and iron-folate are the three most common micronutrient deficiencies in developing countries. As a result, fortification programs have been focused on these three nutrients.

The most dramatic results have been obtained by the addition of iodine to salt. Iodization of salt has almost completely eliminated goiter and cretinism in the United States and some parts of Latin America and Asia.

The results of vitamin A and iron-folate fortification programs are less clear-cut. Results from a sugar fortification project in Guatemala and an MSG fortification program in the Philippines indicated that serum vitamin A levels were increased as a result of these interventions. The MSG fortification also showed a reduction in the clinical signs of vitamin A deficiency.

A limited number of iron-folate supplementation programs have been successful in improving hematological status in pregnant women. Results of iron-folate supplementation for preschoolers, however, have been less successful. In Tanzania, iron supplementation of the diets of children 5–14 years old failed to improve hematological status; the prevalence of malaria was then diagnosed as the primary cause of the anemia rather than simply dietary iron deficiency.

Source: Extraced from Kennedy et al. 1983:42–46.

velops for placing increased emphasis on preventive medicine carried out by lower-level technicians in clinics close to people's homes, contrasted with curative medicine carried out by highly trained physicians surrounded by a hierarchy of staff in expensive urban hospitals.

Development programs that lean toward emphasizing human capital development (which would include primary health care and public health programs) not only serve to improve people's productivity, especially at the bottom end of the income distribution, but may also raise per capita income faster than programs that emphasize physical capital investment (industrialization). So although we are now discussing policies aimed at health-related causes of undernutrition, keep in mind that these policies not only serve to improve simultaneously health and nutritional status, but they also serve to accelerate income growth among the poor and help to reduce income inequality, both of which, in turn, help to reduce Third World undernutrition.

One highly effective means of delivering primary health services where costs are very low relative to the benefits is through maternal and child health care centers.

■ SUBSIDIZING MATERNAL AND CHILD HEALTH SERVICES

Providing public subsidies for expanding and improving maternal and child health services is entirely consistent with promoting better nutrition in the Third World and can be done within the framework of modestly trained field health technicians working outside the hospital. The success of programs to immunize children against common diseases demonstrates this point.

In 1974, less than 5 percent of children in the developing world were immunized against six common, vaccine-preventable childhood killers— measles, tetanus, diptheria, pertussis, tuberculosis, and polio. Today, that number is 80 percent. This enormous increase is due in large part to government policies—in particular the World Health Organization's Expanded Program on Immunization. UNICEF estimates that over 9 million lives per year are saved by immunization. However, the work is not finished. About 25 million infants worldwide are not immunized each year (WHO 1996).

The World Bank (1993 World Development Report) urges public health officials to promote immunization with a new vaccine—for hepatitis B and yellow fever—and recommends that this be combined with supplements of vitamin A and iodine, saying such a combination "would have the highest cost-effectiveness of any health measure available today."

In areas where the childhood diet is short on vitamin A, a program for its distribution would be an appropriate activity for maternal and child health centers. This idea is supported by an interesting controlled experiment that was conducted in Ache province in northern Sumatra, where vitamin A deficiency may well be the most severe in the world. During a one-year period, some preschoolers in Ache were given one capsule containing

200,000 International Units (IU) of vitamin A every six months. Others were given no vitamin A supplement. The vitamin A supplement was shown to reduce dramatically both the risk of xerophthalmia and the death rate (Sommer et al. 1986; Gopalan 1986). Vitamin A pills such as those used in this experiment can be manufactured for less than five cents (U.S.) each. The cost of distribution far exceeds the cost of the pills. The presence of an ongoing maternal and child health care center permits the cost of a vitamin A supplementation program to be shared among the costs of other health delivery programs.

Such other health delivery programs appropriate to maternal and child health care centers include promoting growth monitoring of preschoolers, providing family-planning services, and promoting the use of oral rehydration salts for the control of diarrhea.

And, of course, maternal and child health care centers are logical vehicles for gaining health and nutrition benefits through promoting breast-feeding. The sanitary and educational conditions prevalent in low-income Third World homes can easily lead to a diarrhea disaster for a bottle-fed infant (see Box 15.3). But there are other problems when low-income Third World mothers substitute the bottle for the breast. To such mothers, commercial infant bottle-feeding formula can seem exorbitantly expensive. So mothers tend to overdilute the mixture with water or even to mix it with white flour or sugar (after all, it looks very much the same). These practices can lead to marasmus. Even in relatively well-off Third World households, the knowledge regarding nutrition can be such that substituting the bottle for the breast can lead to marasmus (see Box 15.4). Breast milk also contains anti-infective properties not present in infant formula. Furthermore, lactation prolongs postpartum amenorrhea (the lack of menstruation that reduces fertility following birth). The contraceptive protection from lactation declines with each month of breast-feeding following birth, and about 7 percent of women conceive during this period without having resumed menstruation (World Bank 1984:116). Nevertheless, lower fertility during lactation does reduce the chance that another pregnancy will follow too closely upon the recent birth, and increases the physical, emotional, and economic resources the mother has available for care of her infant.

■ PUBLIC HEALTH MEASURES TO INTERRUPT THE TRANSMISSION OF DIARRHEA

Programs to interrupt the transmission of diarrhea are among the important activities that public health services can undertake to promote better Third World nutrition. Leading measures to take here include better handling of

Box 15.3   The Difficulties of Preparing Baby Formula in a Third World Low-Income Household

Michael Latham

The reasons for the contamination of baby formula, or milk, in a baby bottle are numerous. Milk is a good vehicle and culture medium for pathogenic organisms. It is incredibly difficult to provide a clean formula, let alone a sterile one when:

1. The family water supply is a ditch or a well, contaminated with human excrement (and few households in developing countries have their own safe supply of running water).
2. Household hygiene is poor and the home environment is characterized by flies and feces.
3. There is no refrigerator or other safe storage place for a mixed formula.
4. There is no turn-on stove and in order to sterilize the bottle or boil some water, someone has to gather fuel and light a fire on each occasion.
5. There is no suitable equipment for cleaning the bottle between feeds or when the bottle used may be a cracked and almost uncleanable soda bottle.
6. The mother, with little access to education, lives in the pre-Pasteur era, having little knowledge of hygiene and no knowledge of the germ concept of disease.

Source: Extracted from Latham 1984:60.

fecal wastes, especially those of children; programs to teach cleanliness, especially washing of hands before cooking or eating; improving case management, especially through promoting ORT; promoting breast-feeding; increasing the rate of measles immunization; and improving the local water supply.

Not only do breast-fed infants have a lower morbidity rate from diarrhea, but breast-feeding protects against death from diarrhea. Infants who receive no breast milk are about 25 times more likely to die of diarrhea than those who are exclusively breast-fed (Feacham & Koblinsky 1984).

Measles-associated diarrhea is more severe and is more likely to lead to death than other diarrheas. One estimate suggests that up to a quarter of diarrheal deaths among preschoolers could be prevented by an effective measles immunization program (Feacham & Koblinsky 1983).

Box 15.4   Marasmus in a Newly Rich Urbanized Society

Peter Pellett

I was long of the opinion that infantile marasmus would be essentially eliminated when social and political change were accomplished such that abject poverty no longer existed. However, recent experience in Libya, a rich but still developing nation, has caused me to reconsider somewhat this view.

The Libyan Arab Republic was formed in 1969 by a coup d'état led by Colonel Muamar al-Qaddafi against the king. During the eight years between then and 1977, real incomes for ordinary workers in Libya increased fourfold. In 1977 the major food items (flour, rice, tomato paste, meat, olive oil, coffee, tea, and sugar) were subsidized by the government, and baby foods were tax-free. Both gross poverty and inadequate housing were largely eliminated and phenomenal social progress was accomplished.

Despite this, in 1977 infantile marasmus in Libya remained a widespread problem. As elsewhere in the developing world, breast-feeding had declined.

In a study in Tripoli, the capital city of Libya, we compared the family backgrounds of 50 marasmic infants with the backgrounds of 50 essentially healthy infants of similar age. Total income was similar in both sets of families, and major consumer items such as TV sets, cars, and refrigerators were widely present in both groups. However, families with marasmic infants had less-literate mothers who tended to breast-feed for shorter periods and to feed purchased pureed baby foods more frequently. We concluded that the causal factor for marasmus in most of these instances was probably unhygienic infant feeding, despite the availability of clean water and modern kitchen facilities.

Although there were no statistical studies to back them up, some local hospital staff members were of the opinion that the rapid decline in breast-feeding and the accompanying rapid increase in bottle-feeding and in the use of purchased pureed baby foods had combined to increase mortality rates for children during the early period of the very rapid rise in per capita income!

For more information on the topic see Pellett 1977; Mamarbachi et al. 1980.

Improving the local water supply in rural areas can involve something as simple and effective as technical assistance and encouragement for the construction and use of rainwater-gathering vats. Use of such vats provides not only a clean but a convenient source of household water. When a mother does not have to walk so far to get her household supply of water she has more time available for other activities, including child care.

Providing an ample supply of clean water to the poor in a Third World city can be a political as well as an engineering problem. Port-au-Prince (in Haiti) during 1976 provides an extreme example. A shortage of water outlets promoted a substantial and profitable private market for what was, ostensibly, a publicly provided city service (see Box 15.5).

Box 15.5   The Political Economics of Drinking Water

Simon M. Fass

An in-depth examination of one small segment of the public service sector in Haiti, specifically water distribution management in Port-au-Prince, highlights the severe consequences which deficient administration can bring to bear upon a relatively large number of people.

In Port-au-Prince, in 1976, about 50 percent of the water input leaked out of the municipal water system. For the most part the loss was due to breaks and leaks in pipes, but much of it occurred because connections to reservoirs in homes and establishments were not equipped with automatic shut-off valves, or sometimes any valves at all. When such reservoirs, including swimming pools, were full, the overflow spilled into the streets. Since there were no metering devices or enforced penalties for not having valves, and the water tariff was on a flat-rate basis, subscribers had little incentive to invest in appropriate valves. The United Nations estimated that control mechanisms at private connections could have reduced losses to a more reasonable rate of 30 to 35 percent.

Individuals installed reservoirs because of irregular distribution and pressure of water flows. Heavy demand fluctuations, variations in rainfall, limited public storage capacity, and high distribution losses caused the irregularities. Subscribers had to be prepared for periods of several days, sometimes weeks, between deliveries through the pipes.

The 30,000 legal and clandestine private connections in 1976 provided direct service to only about 150,000 residents. The remaining 490,000 residents were in theory serviced by the 36 officially designated standpipes [public water outlets employing multiple spigots] that were supposed to exist at the time. In reality only 27 standpipes functioned. The others had long since been destroyed. The total outflow from the operating standpipes on any given day did not exceed 1.4 million liters. Thus under the best of circumstances their total supply could not provide more than 2.8 liters per person each day for the 490,000 residents presumably dependent on them. To put this in perspective, a single flush of a modern toilet facility requires 19 liters.

The extreme scarcity caused by the municipal distribution system led the city's population to adapt in a number of ways. There were a number, something on the order of 40,000, who relied on leaks and breaks in the pipes. It was common to knock a hole in a pipe, if necessary digging into the street to find one, plugging it with a wooden spike when not in use, and attaching a short rubber hose from the hole to a bucket when drawing water from it. Since penalties for this practice could be quite severe, this method of obtaining water was not widespread.

(continues)

Box 15.5   Continued

A more common practice, providing water to some 95,000 residents, was sharing among neighbors. In a number of areas, high, middle, and low income homes are located side by side. In such neighborhoods, the proportion of families with connections tend to be relatively high, and so the number of individuals requesting water from a particular subscriber on any given day, usually in the form of a request to a household servant, is low, typically less than 10 or 12.

The majority of nonsubscribers, however, some 300,000 low income residents who lived in downtown areas with relatively few private connections, were obliged to buy water from fixed and mobile vendors. The shortage of water outlets had in effect given rise to a rather substantial private market for a publicly provided service.

The Private Water Market, 1976

The private water market in 1976 contained three principal sets of vendors. The first set were tanker truck operators who drew water from the fire hydrants and transported it to industrial and commercial establishments and to about 1,200 higher income homes located in areas without piped service or with very irregular service. Charges for truck supply varied between U.S. $3.00 and U.S. $6.00 per m^3. The gross revenues of truckers, who paid nothing for water, either in the form of user charges or in the form of license fees, amounted from these consumers alone to an average or $2,700 per day, $980,000 per year, and an annual return of $39,000 per truck.

There were substantial profits to be made, and often truckers were known to break pipes in order to create demand for transported water over the extended periods required to locate the breaks and repair them.

The second set of vendors consisted of some 2,000 households which had connections to the system and sold water in lower income areas to neighboring consumers and/or to mobile sellers who would transport it further afield. The common method was to sell water by the bucketful (about 18 liters per bucket).

The minimum price, in effect during the rainy season if water was flowing in the pipes, was two cents a bucket, or about $1.10 per m^3. In the dry season the typical price would be ten cents, equivalent to $5.60 per m^3. During drought periods, as happened in 1975 and 1977, unit prices could reach anywhere from $10.00 to $20.00 per m^3 for several months at a stretch.

The third set of vendors were mobile vendors who bought water from connected households and transported it to consumers. They numbered 14,000 or about 4.5 percent of the urban labor force.

The margin charged by the vendors in ordinary circumstances was one cent per bucket, or two if the transport distance was long. These were margins on top of whatever the vendors themselves paid to connected families. For 1976, the aggregate net earnings of mobile vendors came to $930,000, or approximately $5.50 a month for each vendor.

(continues)

Box 15.5   Continued

Total expenditures by consumers in the private water market thus amounted to about $3.8 million a year, a quarter being paid largely by a very small group of high income residents and the balance by some 300,000 low income families. By contrast, [the municipal water authority's] total annual revenue from the sale of water was $650,000 during the same period.

Impacts on Low Income Families

At a price of $2.30/m^3 a typical family of five would have to spend about $4.00 a month in order to consume 11 liters of water per day. In 1976 about 40 percent of urban families had incomes of $20 per month or less.

Given all the various daily demands placed on the use of money, many of these families found it impossible to spend a fifth of their income on water. They responded in a number of ways.

The poorest of them, with incomes of less than $10 per month, used purchased water only for cooking and drinking. They used surface run-off for cleaning themselves. They might also launder and wash less often. A major hazard was that of illness caused by contaminated water or by residence in areas with disastrous sanitary conditions, susceptibility to which was aggravated by the extra energy expended by already malnourished bodies to trudge 20 kilogram buckets of water several kilometers each day. With the risk of illness came the possibility of seriously compromising the capacity to generate income streams. Curative medical services would require such families to curtail other expenditures further, to dig into savings, or to incur heavy debts.

Source: Extracted from Fass 1982.

☐ 16

Policies Aimed at Demographic Causes of Undernutrition

One result of [population/resource] projections and their use in public discussion of population policy has been a shift in concern toward future generations. In China, as in most traditional societies, childbearing decisions were shaped by a desire by parents to be looked after in old age. By emphasizing future population/resource relationships in shaping family planning programs, government officials have shifted the focus of childbearing from the well-being of parents to the well-being of children.
—Brown 1983:38–39

Rapid population growth makes the task of education more difficult, thins out the supply of capital per person, puts upward pressure on the price of grain, and tends to decrease equity, all of which exacerbate Third World undernutrition. In addition, as we saw in Chapter 5, undernutrition tends to be concentrated among the youngest children of large families. Thus, we have both indirect and direct ways through which reducing the tendency toward large family size will improve Third World nutrition.

The theme of this chapter is the examination of policy alternatives for lowering the fertility rate. We should note at the outset that, worldwide, fertility rates are already falling. The demographic policy problem for the nutrition planner in countries with high fertility and high undernutrition rates, then, is how to accelerate the downtrend, or to put it in other words, how to hasten the demographic transition.

We begin with a review of the causes for the downtrend in fertility rates, which has proceeded furthest, of course, in those countries that have completed or almost completed the demographic transition. Those variables that have contributed to the slow but substantial fertility decline in the high-income, industrialized countries provide, at the least, interesting prospecting ground for policies to reduce fertility in the Third World.

■ ONGOING REASONS FOR THE FALL IN FERTILITY RATES

Over the years, research has produced increasingly reliable and convenient methods of contraception, thus making it easier to limit fertility. But at the same time many other things have been happening that have lowered human fertility rates (Caldwell 1983; Pullum 1983). It is a widely observed phenomenon, for example, that high income yields lower fertility, at least after the initial stages of extreme poverty are overcome. In Figure 16.1 and Table 16.1 this relationship is illustrated.

When very poor families experience an increase in income their initial reaction is often to have more children. (The increased income, for instance, may enable a marriage that otherwise might have been postponed for want of adequate dowry. Or the increased income might motivate the substitution of bottle-feeding for breast-feeding, with its consequent increase in the mother's fertility.) But as incomes rise, other factors mitigate to reduce fertility. Higher income is usually associated with better education, and with more education parents tend to trade child quantity for child quality. They spend a greater proportion of their child-rearing resources on

Figure 16.1   Relationship Between Fertility and per Capita Income

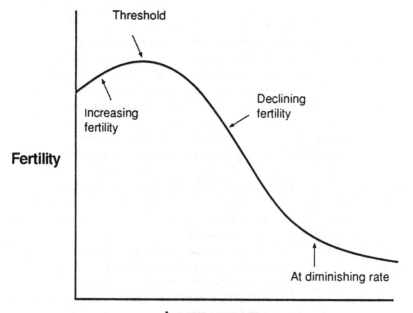

Source: Adapted from World Bank 1984:109.

Table 16.1 Population Growth, Birth Rates, and Death Rates for Selected Country Groups, 1995

	GNP per Capita 1995 ($)	Population Growth 1990–1995 (percent)	Total Fertility Rate (births per woman)	Crude Birth Rate (per 1,000 total population)	Crude Death Rate (per 1,000 total population)	Annual Rate of Natural Increase (percent)	Life Expectancy at Birth
Africa	651	15.71	5.8	41.3	13.0	2.84	54.9
Asia	2,413	9.30	2.9	24.4	7.9	1.65	65.2
Latin America	3,274	9.30	3.1	25.9	6.7	1.92	68.9
Developing countries	1,090	10.55	3.5	27.7	8.6	1.91	63.6
Developed countries	24,930	2.72	1.6	11.9	10.3	0.16	74.3
World	4,880	8.76	3.1	24.4	8.9	1.55	65.7

Source: GNP per capita: World Bank, World Development Report, 1997. Other data: World Resources Institute (1996), World Resources, 1996–97.

their children's health and education, with correspondingly smaller resources left over for raising more children. As income continues to rise, alternative uses of family resources open up: travel, more education, more leisure-time activities, for example. These, in turn, further compete with child-rearing resources in family decisionmaking, putting more downward pressure on fertility.

As education, income, and health improve, a decline in infant and child mortality rates normally occurs. After one or two generations of low infant and child mortality rates, people are less inclined to produce large numbers of children to ensure that at least some offspring will survive to maturity. Very high levels of income lead to a proliferation of private pension programs, or even government-sponsored social security programs, all of which lessen the pressure to have children to provide someone to take care of you in your old age.

The education of women is particularly significant in reducing fertility. Educated women are more likely to postpone marriage in order to enter the work force, more likely to delay having children in order to remain in the work force, and are more likely to know about and use contraception than are uneducated women (Anon. 1988). The relationship between education and fertility for selected countries is shown in Figure 16.2.

Increased employment of women outside the home lessens their dependence on men (who sometimes are less motivated to limit family size than are women) and increases their tendency to make decisions in favor of using contraception; at the same time, it is inclined to change women's images of themselves. As women gain more and more equality with men in the work force and elsewhere in society (gaining the right to vote, to inherit property, to own land, to participate in the choice of a husband, etc.) they move away from thinking of themselves primarily as wives and mothers

Figure 16.2   Total Fertility Rate by Education of Wife, Selected Countries

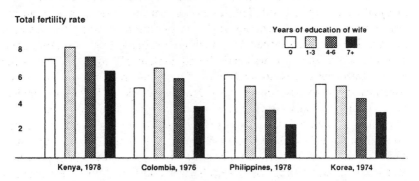

Source: Adapted from World Bank 1984:110.

and toward thinking of themselves as playing multiple roles in life. And as they do this, they tend to have fewer children.

■ PUBLIC MEASURES TO ACCELERATE THE DEMOGRAPHIC TRANSITION

The phenomena we have been discussing will continue to put downward pressure on worldwide fertility rates. But in some regions of the world the advantages of lower fertility rates are so great that governments want to accelerate the downward movement.

Most countries have a set of pronatalist public policies left over from the days when wars, famines, and high mortality rates from uncontrolled infectious diseases, such as smallpox and the bubonic plague, regularly decimated their populations. Pronatalist policies include tax deductions in proportion to the number of children in the family (common throughout much of the world), unlimited subsidized maternity leaves sponsored by government or private industry (again common throughout the world), and child care subsidies during the first several years of a child's life (found only in certain high-income countries, e.g., Canada, France, Australia). For countries with such policies, a first task in the direction of reducing fertility is to modify these policies so that they favor small families.

□ Economic Incentives and Disincentives

Economic incentives to reward low fertility and economic disincentives to discourage high fertility can both be used to motivate lower fertility.

One of the more imaginative incentive schemes was set up on three tea estates in India. By law, the tea estates are required to provide substantial maternity and child care benefits for their workers (tea pickers are usually women). The benefits include hospitalization and medical care for the mother and infant as well as long-term food, clothing, schooling, and medical care for the child. The tea estates set up a "savings account for family planning." Each woman employee of childbearing age is offered a savings account, the proceeds of which are available to her on retirement, and into which the firm will pay the equivalent of one day's wages for each month that she is not pregnant. If a woman becomes pregnant, the company suspends payments for one year. For third and more pregnancies, the company not only suspends payment for a year, but also reclaims part of its past payments into her account to help pay for its legally mandated maternal and child care expenses. Women thus have a choice: maternity and child care benefits for more children, or a better retirement program. Many women are opting for fewer children and more retirement benefits (Brown 1974:169; World Bank 1984:126).

Economic incentives for lower fertility are attractive, but they are expensive. In Bangladesh a program was proposed that would provide a 12-year bond with a maturity value of around $350 for women of child-bearing age who had only two or three children and who underwent sterilization. Attached to the proposal was a scheme whereby couples who signed certificates to delay their first birth for three years after marriage, or who delayed their second and third births for at least five years, would be given $20 on presentation of their certificates after the agreed time, provided they had kept their pledge. It was estimated that to cover the entire population with both schemes would require about 10 percent of the annual government budget (World Bank 1984:126).

Not only are incentive payments for low fertility expensive, but they waste a certain amount of public resources, as people who would have had fewer children despite the program go ahead and claim its benefits.

While economic incentives involve payments provided to delay or limit childbearing, economic disincentives usually involve the withholding of social benefits from those couples who produce more than some targeted number of children.

In the early 1980s a series of economic disincentives to large families was in use in Singapore. The system (which was dropped subsequent to a decline in birth rates) included incentives to have two children but disincentives for more than two. The system was summarized by a Draper Fund report (Salaff & Wong 1983:16) as follows:

- Paid maternity leave for the first two children, but not for third and subsequent children
- Preference in the choice of primary school given only to the first two children, with highest preference to the two children of a parent who has undergone sterilization before age 40
- Removal of the large-family priority in the allocation of subsidized housing; only families with three or fewer children are allowed to rent rooms in public housing units
- Escalating delivery fees in public hospitals for higher-order births, as well as fees for prenatal care (fees are remitted if sterilization follows delivery)
- Full tax relief only for the first two children, and none for fourth or subsequent children

During this same period a somewhat more draconian set of rewards and punishments, using "Glory Certificates" to promote the one-child family, was in place in China (see Box 16.1).

The government can also influence infertility indirectly by adopting policies that reduce benefits to parents having more children, and raise the costs of child rearing. For example, policies described by the catch-phrase "empower-

---

Box 16.1   The Chinese Glory Certificate System

Lynn Landman

To stimulate acceptance of the one-child family, the Chinese have instituted a system of incentives. Those who contract to limit their families to one child receive "Glory Certificates." Such couples are widely publicized and held up as models for their countrymen, as are the rewards they earn. In general, these may include free and priority medical care for the child; priority admission to nurseries, kindergartens, and primary schools; allotment of larger housing accommodations; bonuses for city workers and increased work points, as well as large private plots and larger housing, for peasants. All these benefits remain in effect until the child reaches 14.

If holders of "Glory Certificates" renege on their commitment, they must return all the benefits and, in addition, their annual income may be reduced by 5 to 15 percent for varying lengths of time. Those who already have two children and go on to have a third must pay all the expenses associated with childbearing, and will not be entitled to paid maternity leave. Salaries are reduced and the usual subsidized grain allotment is not provided for the third child, obliging parents to purchase it on the open market at higher prices. Job promotions may be withheld for a time and mothers sometimes are fired from their jobs.

In a country where per capita annual income is only about $235, where housing is in short supply and schooling and jobs are not guaranteed, these incentives and disincentives may be presumed to carry considerable clout.

Note: The 1989 World Population Data Sheet of the Population Reference Bureau gives the total fertility rate for China as 2.4. While this is remarkably low for a Third World country, it is more than double China's target total fertility rate of one.

Source: Landman 1983:9.

---

ing women" work to reduce fertility in a variety of ways. First, as women feel that society and culture give them greater permission to participate in childbearing decisions, the costs to women of childbearing and child rearing are more fully taken into account. Second, as women become better educated, they become more aware of birth control techniques. Third, as women become better educated, their value as workers increases; thus they see higher costs of foregone earnings or production as they devote time and attention to childbearing and child rearing. Fourth, as women become more socially accepted in the labor market, their value as workers increases. Fifth, better education of women is likely to lead to reduced infant and child mortality rates, so that fewer births are necessary to achieve the desired number of surviving children. Sixth, better educated women are more likely to want a good education for their children. This reduces children's availability to the labor force, and therefore reduces the economic benefits and raises the costs of having children.

☐ Moral Suasion and Regulation

The average age at marriage for women in Bangladesh is 16. Half the women in South Asia and sub-Saharan Africa are or have been married by the time they are 19. The younger a woman is when she marries, the longer she is exposed to the risk of conception. So, to reduce fertility it seems reasonable to try to persuade people to postpone marriage. Minimum marriageable age legislation is commonly used to attempt to encourage support for later marriage. Of those countries that have tried it, China seems to have been most successful. In 1980 the government of China raised the legal minimum age at marriage to 20 for women and 22 for men.

India has long promoted a vigorous advertising campaign to encourage the small family, with government-sponsored advertisements appearing on billboards, buses, at movie theaters, in magazines and newspapers, and on radio and television. (India's total fertility rate in 1986 was 4.4. By 1990–1995, it had fallen to 3.8.)

Some countries have tried intense community pressure on couples of childbearing age to limit their family size. Examples of such efforts in Indonesia and China are described briefly in Box 16.2.

Box 16.2   Community Pressures to Lower Fertility

Rodolfo A. Bulatao

Pressures can be exerted by the community, or by major sections of it, to promote lowered fertility. Two cases will illustrate group pressures: *banjars* in Bali and production teams in China.

Banjars—traditional units of local self-government, which serve as centers for mutual aid and cooperative work—consist of all the male household heads in a hamlet or subvillage. The form is centuries old. The traditional head of a banjar is democratically elected but has no official standing. Instead, the banjar also has a second, official head, who may be appointed and may have charge of more than one banjar (Hull 1978).

Banjar meetings may be held every month (or 35 days), usually with perfect attendance (there is a system of fines for absence or lateness) and typically discuss development of the community and religious affairs (Astawa 1979).

Since 1974 these meetings have also included discussion of the family-planning status of each family. Each member is asked what he and his wife are doing about family planning. A register is kept, and a color-coded map of the community indicating eligible couples and their contraceptive status is prominently displayed in the banjar hall (Meier 1979).

The decline in marital fertility in Bali of about 30 percent in less than a decade has been dramatic enough to be labeled a "demographic miracle" (Hull et al. 1977). How much of the change has been due to the community

(continues)

Box 16.2 Continued

pressures exerted through the 3,700 banjars is a difficult and probably unanswerable question. Other elements of the Balinese situation, such as acute pressures on the land, the penetration of modern influences (through such means as consumer goods, communication, and transportation systems, Western-style schooling and tourism), and cultural factors like the relative independence of young couples—which may facilitate contraceptive decisions—may encourage the decline in fertility. Furthermore, the effective logistical system of the family-planning program and creative uses of native art forms to communicate family-planning messages, and a stable, supportive government, may be influential.

Production teams in China, which are usually the effective unit in rural areas for production and income sharing, consist of 30 to 40 households in a small village, within which kinship ties may be strong. Production teams assume important responsibility for the fertility of their members. As part of the national *wan xi shao* campaign (named for the reproductive norms of later marriage, longer birth spacing, and fewer births), the production teams were responsible for deciding which couples could have births, in line with the reproductive norms and with team quotas set from above (Chen & Kols 1982). The team birth-planning leadership group (the leaders all being local residents) might call all eligible couples to a meeting, at which their individual birth plans could be scrutinized and allocations made. Under the one-child campaign, which replaced the wan xi shao campaign in 1979, community birth planning still takes place, although allocation of birth quotas follows different norms. As couples become familiar with the system, the time-consuming meeting to adjust birth plans may be dispensed with, and the leaders may simply notify couples of their decisions. Adherence is in theory voluntary, resting on persuasion and education. Such elements as adult study groups and visits from birth-planning delegations maintain the peer pressure (Chen 1981).

As with the Balinese banjars, it is not possible to determine the specific impact of the social pressures exerted through production teams, which are only one element in the Chinese population program.

For greater detail on local control of fertility see Bulatao 1984a.

☐ Subsidizing Family-Planning Services

Use of contraceptives among married women of childbearing age varies widely in the Third World, from less than 10 percent in sub-Saharan Africa to around 40 percent in Latin America to as high as 70 percent or more in China and Singapore (World Bank 1984:128). Controlled experiments conducted in Mexico, India, Bangladesh, Korea, and the Philippines have all demonstrated that the provision of family-planning advice, technology, and materials significantly reduces fertility.

In a 31-country study, Bongaarts (1982) looked at determinants of fertility decline as it proceeds from rates well above six to rates close to two. The difference in total fertility was almost five children. He found that, in the countries studied, higher age at marriage reduced total fertility by 1.4 children. Increased use of contraception reduced fertility by 4.5 children. More induced abortion accounted for a reduction of 0.5 children, for a total reduction of 6.4 children. Reduced breast-feeding, of course, works the other way around, and accounted for an increase in fertility of about 1.5 children. On the bottom line of Table 16.2, these data are expressed as percentage contribution to reduction in fertility decline. Data for selected individual countries are also shown in Table 16.2.

In most Third World countries a substantial gap exists between women who would like to limit their fertility and their access to modern contraceptive methods (Table 16.3). In the conclusion to a major National Research Council survey of how specific program elements contribute to the effectiveness of Third World family-planning programs, Simmons and Lapham (1987) note that family-planning programs increase the availability of contraception and the level of contraceptive use and that they lower fertility, but that their impact varies with programmatic and environmental factors. For instance, the availability of multiple public and private channels for the delivery of services increases the effectiveness of national programs. A wide choice of methods is more effective than a narrow choice,

Table 16.2 Accounting for Fertility Decline in Selected Third World Countries

Selected Countries and Years	Total Fertility Rate			Percentage of Reduction by Contributing Factor				
	Initial	Final	Differ-ence	Higher Age at Marriage	Reduced Breast-feeding	More Use of Contra-ception	More Induced Abortion	All Other Factors
India (1972–78)	5.6	5.2	.5	41	−58	114	—	3
Indonesia (1970–80)	5.5	4.6	.9	41	−77	134	—	2
Korea (1960–70)	6.1	4.0	2.2	50	−38	53	30	4
Thailand (1968–78)	6.1	3.4	2.7	11	−17	86	16	4
Composite of 31 countries (long term)	>6	<3	5	28	−29	90	10	1

Sources: Composite of 31 countries: Bongaarts 1982; all other data: Bulatao 1984b:38.
Note: — = not available. The composite of 31 countries' data account for the decline in total fertility typical of countries that started their fertility decline with rates around six (the predecline phase of fertility rates) and ended rates below three (the postdecline countries). The difference in pre- to postdecline rates among these countries amounts to almost five children.

because diverse groups of clients have different needs. Good leadership and positive political support also increase the effectiveness of such programs.

Table 16.3   Percentage of Married Women, Age 15–44, Who Do Not Want to Become Pregnant and Who Use Contraception

Region, Country, and Year of Survey	Percentage Who Do Not Want a Birth During the Next Year	Percentage Who Do Not Want Any More Births	Percentage Who Use a Modern Contraceptive Method
Africa			
Benin 1981–82	70*	8	1
Botswana 1984	76	31	19
Cameroon 1978	—	—	1
Ghana 1979–80	65*	11	6
Ivory Coast 1980–81	41*	4	1
Kenya 1984	77*	35	10
Lesotho 1977	—	14	3
Mauritania 1981	54*	14	0
Nigeria 1981–82	33*	4	1
Senegal (rural) 1982	78	7	0
Sudan (north) 1978–79	—	18	4
Zimbabwe 1984	76	22	28
Near East			
Egypt 1980	74*	53	23
Jordan 1983	86	42	21
Morocco 1983–84	—	41	22
Syria 1978	—	36	15
Tunisia 1983	86	67	35
Yemen, Arab Republic 1979	27*	19	1
Asia			
Bangladesh 1979–80	71*	48	9
Fiji 1974	84*	51	36
Java and Bali 1976	—	42	24
Republic of Korea 1979	81*	76	43
Malaysia 1974	90*	43	26
Nepal 1981	55	42	7
Pakistan 1975	—	42	4
Philippines 1978	—	58	17
Sri Lanka 1982	91	65	32
Thailand 1981	89	66	56
Latin America and Caribbean			
Barbados 1980–81	—	52	45
Bolivia 1983	89	74	11
Brazil (northeast) 1980	90	58	29
Brazil (south) 1981	87	49	52
Colombia 1980	84	69	43
Costa Rica 1981	84	53	57
Dominican Republic 1983	88	72	43
Ecuador 1979	91	59	27
El Salvador 1978	93	53	32
Guatemala 1983	79	40	21
Guyana 1975	—	62	32

(continued)

Table 16.3   Continued

Region, Country, and Year of Survey	Percentage Who Do Not Want a Birth During the Next Year	Percentage Who Do Not Want Any More Births	Percentage Who Use a Modern Contraceptive Method
Haiti 1983	78	59	4
Honduras 1981	92	76	24
Jamaica 1983	97	54	49
Mexico 1979	88	65	34
Panama 1979–80	90	63	57
Paraguay 1979	84*	31	25
Peru 1981	92*	74	18
Trinidad and Tobago 1977	—	56	49
Venezuela 1977	—	57	38

Source: Galway et al. 1987:43.

Note: Percentages not wanting a birth are adjusted to exclude the percentage undecided or not stated. Modern methods of contraception include voluntary sterilization, oral contraceptives, intrauterine devices (IUDs), condoms, injectables, and vaginal methods (spermicides, diaphragms, and caps).

*Only fecund married women are included.

■ THE COMPLEMENTARITY OF
FERTILITY REDUCTION POLICIES

Fertility reduction policies often complement each other. For instance, providing subsidized family-planning services not only makes the technology available for reducing fertility but sends a message to the community that government supports the idea of fertility regulation. Joel Cohen (1996b) recommends, as part of any population control policy, "doing everything at once."

However, fertility reduction policies are often also complementary with other programs that help to reduce undernutrition. For instance, successful promotion of prolonged breast-feeding not only reduces fertility but improves childhood nutrition and health. Persuading couples to marry later in life not only reduces fertility but, as women remain in the work force longer as a result, raises per capita income, improving nutrition. Increasing the educational level of women not only decreases fertility but increases their future productivity and undoubtedly improves the quality of the child care they deliver. Cohen (1996b) quotes economist Robert Cassen as saying, "virtually everything that needs doing from a population point of view needs doing anyway."

☐ 17

Policies Aimed at Reducing Inequalities and Raising the Income of the Poor

The advent of high-yielding varieties, increased reliance on chemical pesticides and fertilizers, control over irrigation water, and the multitude of ways in which urban-dominated agricultural policy can countermand any nominal gains from better land-use opportunities, all combine to render—in many instances—land ownership quite irrelevant. There are so many factors that impinge upon the economic environment of a newly landed peasant that the legal and/or economic relations of that person to the land resource may be quite beside the point. Land cannot be considered important in either a policy or a political context when it is often so irrelevant in the ultimate reckoning of a peasant's economic position.

—Bromley 1981:399

In Chapter 9 we argued that inequality of income, in and of itself, contributes to undernutrition. Programs that reduce the income gap (and therefore reduce the size of the Reutlinger triangles) will reduce the tendency of the rich to bid food away from the poor, and thus improve the nutrition of both groups.

In this chapter we examine a set of policies and programs that are commonly advocated for reducing income inequality, either by increasing the income of the poor or by transferring income or wealth from the rich to the poor.

A related set of policies aimed at lowering the price of food will be left for discussion in the next chapter. Food-linked income transfer programs include famine relief programs, food consumption subsidies, and selling in the Third World at below-market prices, food obtained on concessional terms from the developed countries (e.g., the PL480 Food for Peace Program). Such programs are usually intended to lower the domestic price of food. It therefore seems appropriate to consider them, together with other policies aimed at lowering food prices, in a separate chapter.

■ LAND REFORM

Land reform is one of the most common ways of attempting to redistribute wealth and the income associated with it. Since 1960 virtually every country in the world has passed land reform laws (De Janvry 1981:385). Land reform can mean many things, but typically it means at least one of the following:

1. *Redistributing the ownership of private or public land in order to change the pattern of land distribution and size of holding:* At the one extreme this might mean creating small plots from large blocks of land and allocating these small plots to the poor. At the other extreme it might mean nationalizing all agricultural land and assigning it to large, state-owned farms.
2. *Changing the rights associated with land:* For instance, tenant farmers or sharecroppers can be made owners of the land they work. Lenders, too, can be prohibited from taking land from smallholders for lack of payment of debt.

Land reform can mean other things, such as consolidation of individual holdings, that is, regrouping fragmented holdings into contiguous blocks of land (World Bank 1975:2–21). In this case there is no objective for wealth redistribution, but only productivity considerations. In most cases of land reform the hope is that the twin objectives of accelerated growth and increased equity can be accomplished.

□ The Hope for Land Reform

The land reform program carried out by the U.S. military government in Japan following World War II is widely credited with helping significantly with the reconstruction of Japanese agriculture at the time. Similarly, a land reform program in Taiwan at about the same time is credited with stimulating greater productivity in Taiwanese agriculture.

Given the tendency for land distribution to be skewed in such a manner that relatively few owners control very large shares of this valuable productive resource, land reform presents an attractive tool for redistributing wealth.

In Figure 9.4 we saw the Lorenz curve for the skewed land distribution in 1968 and 1981 for the Indian village we have looked at from time to time in this book. In Table 17.1 the same data are presented in a different form.

In 1981, 20 percent of the households owned 76 percent of the land. This, by the way, was after a land reform program that limited farm size to a maximum of 50 acres in India (De Janvry 1981:386). The situation in this village is representative of much of the agriculture of the Third World, where landownership typically is concentrated and where a third of the families, more or less, typically own no land. But in some places, concentration of ownership is more intense.

Before Algerian independence from the French in 1962, the good farmland in that country had become concentrated into large estates. In 1960, 6,000 French colonists owned one-third of all the agricultural land (the best land) while 2 million Algerian peasants owned the other two-thirds (the marginal land) (Aron et al. 1962). In other words, 0.3 percent of the farmers owned one-third of the land. This situation was certainly one of the most dramatic instances of a skewed landownership pattern. (The French-owned farms were nationalized in a land reform program initiated in 1962.)

During the 1960s and 1970s, Latin America became notorious for concentration of landownership in the hands of the few. A 1988 study found that, in Colombia, the top 10 percent of owners control more than 80 percent of the total farmland (Stevens & Jabara 1988:272–273). Gini coefficients for land concentration in Latin America run very high. A 1975 collection of such coefficients listed Colombia at 0.86 and Peru, the highest, at 0.95 (World Bank 1975:26).

In Figure 17.1 land distribution in Wisconsin is compared to that in Brazil. Over half of the farmers (and over half of the farmland) in Wisconsin are on farms of between 100 and 500 acres. In Brazil, over three-

Table 17.1   Acres of Land Owned, by Ownership Group, Bagbana Village Households, 1968 and 1981

| | Land Owned | | | |
| | 1968 | | 1981 | |
Quintile	Land Owned	Percentage of Total	Land Owned	Percentage of Total
Highest	202.6	73	192.0	76
Second	54.2	19	43.8	17
Third	19.6	7	15.6	6
Fourth	1.5	1	1.3	1
Lowest	0	0	0	0
Total	277.9	100	252.7	100
Gini ratio	.7142		.7388	

Source: Fishstein 1985:74.

Figure 17.1   **Agrarian Ownership Structure in Wisconsin and Brazil, 1980**

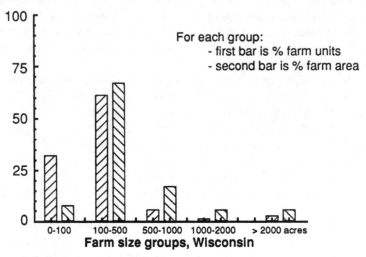

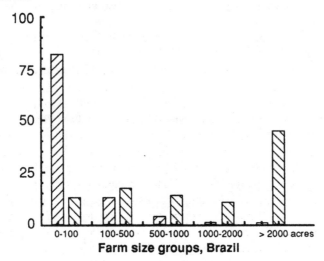

Source: Adapted from Carter 1989:1.

fourths of the farmers are on holdings of less than 100 acres whereas almost half of the farmland is in holdings greater than 2,000 acres in size.

In the late 1990s, a major land reform program is being considered in Zimbabwe. In 1997, President Mugabe proposed a plan that would seize

10 million acres of farmland owned by about 1,500 large commercial farmers and redistribute it. The land reform initiative is a response to land-ownership patterns that were established during colonialism when blacks in Zimbabwe (then called Rhodesia) were legally prohibited from owning some of the best farmland. As a result, "Whites make up 2 percent of Zimbabwe's population but own 70 percent of the nation's best land" (Duke 1998).

Not only is land reform attractive as a means of wealth redistribution, but it has compelling logic for productivity. Remember in Chapter 11 we pointed out that production per unit of land in the Third World is typically higher on smaller farms (Figure 11.1). This suggests that dividing up large landholdings should result in increases in productivity.

But we see another compelling productivity argument. Farmers with limited capital typically operate their farms on shares, splitting a share of the harvest (typically around 50 percent) with the landlord. A share tenant who receives only half of the returns from his last hour of labor on the farm is presumably less motivated to work long hours than would an owner. Because tenant farmers normally operate on a short-term lease, often on a year-to-year basis, the insecurity of tenure discourages them from spending on land-associated capital investments such as fences, irrigation, or fruit trees (Herring 1983:253). These arguments suggest increased productivity from transferring landownership from the landlord to the tiller.

☐ Disillusionment About Land Reform

Despite the compelling nature of the equity and productivity arguments for land reform, many oppose the concept. The history of the twentieth century is replete with instances where land reform failed to live up to its promise. The Communist Revolution in China brought with it an agrarian reform that eliminated private ownership of land in the early 1950s. The move to communal ownership initially spurred agricultural production; but by the late 1950s agricultural production had stagnated. During the 1980s, laws were changed to permit leasing and sales of agricultural land, thus returning agricultural land to private ownership. A World Bank paper describes the effects: "Gradual reform in rural areas lifted agricultural production and income and controlled poverty. In the early stages of reform inequality also lessened, although it has increased in recent years. (The Gini coefficient—which measures the inequality of income distribution, with 0 to signify absolute equality and 100 absolute inequality—increased to 30.7 in 1993, from 27.4 in 1978 and 21.5 in 1984)" (Ying 1996).

But not only the grand socialist experiments with collectivized agriculture have experienced major disappointments. Various other types of reform have produced unforeseen consequences, some of which made the supposed beneficiaries worse off than they might have been without the reform. A few examples will illustrate some of the common difficulties.

One of the most pressing goals of the 1962 Algerian land reform was to provide employment for as many workers as possible. Yet it did not take the self-management committees on the newly nationalized large estates long to realize that fewer workers on their farms meant more returns per worker, and an early study of the situation showed employment on the farms actually decreasing after reform (Foster & Steiner 1964). A later study of the ongoing land reforms in Algeria (Pfeifer 1985:81) concluded that the reform "promoted, rather than curtailed, the class differentiation of agricultural producers into successful commercial farmers and propertyless wage workers." Pfeifer goes on to observe rather caustically that "in this, the 'agrarian revolution' in Algeria in the 1970s seems to have completed the historic task begun by the French intruders in 1830."

An agrarian reform law passed in Peru in 1969 was intended to do something about the skewed landownership in that country. An important principle of the reform legislation was "land to the tiller." By late 1978 ownership of 8.6 million hectares had been transferred, and some 370,000 families had benefited from the reform (Alberts 1983). But the benefits went largely to the rich. Reforms carried out on the sugar estates, for instance, mainly benefited the permanent workers. The families living outside the sugar plantations received no benefits at all. In a detailed study of the reform, Alberts (1983:47, 49, 141–142, 175, 226) concluded that "the poor majority of Peruvian peasants has only received land, credit and technical assistance to a minor extent." According to Alberts, "the agrarian reform did not accomplish a radical and lasting improvement in the degree of equity within the agricultural sector. The economic policies implemented by the military government were not conducive to agricultural growth nor did they accomplish anything toward reducing the urban-rural income gap."

In the early 1950s Burma undertook an economic development program that included a land reform component designed to provide land to the tiller. All agricultural landholdings in excess of 50 acres were subject to confiscation, and those up to 50 acres were also subject to confiscation unless the entire 50 acres were worked by the owner and his family. To retain their lands, absentee owners began working the land themselves, forcing their former tenant farmers off the land and making landless laborers of them. The former tenants usually stayed on as laborers, but they no longer enjoyed some of the benefits that had been theirs as tenants (Walinsky 1962:137, 294).

This same Burmese economic development program undertook to protect farmers from losing their land to banks and moneylenders when they defaulted on their loans by making it illegal to foreclose on mortgages on agricultural land. This not only denied landowners the opportunity to use their land as collateral to raise capital for farm investments, but the diminished security for the lender meant that the farmer-borrower had to pay higher interest rates for his money. Thus the protection afforded the cultivator came at a high cost (Walinsky 1962:504–505).

In 1972 a land reform law in the Philippines gave permanent tenure rights to those who had sharecropped a piece of land for three or more years. Sharecropping had traditionally been a way for the young landless worker to get started in farming, but after passage of this law it became next to impossible for a landless worker to gain access to land through sharecropping. Landowners were too worried about becoming disenfranchised again.

The disillusionment with land reform comes not only from the multiplicity of disappointments in real-world attempts to implement it, but from a growing realization that who owns a piece of land is only one, and sometimes only a minor one, of the variables that affect the productivity of the workers and of the land they work. After all, some form of tenant farming (renting, sharerenting, sharecropping) in the highly productive U.S. corn belt is, in places, the predominant pattern. As was noted by Bromley (1981), availability of low-cost purchased inputs, attractive farm-gate prices for farm produce, appropriate technical assistance, paved farm-to-market roads, and so on often turn out to be more important in determining farm productivity than who owns the land.

With so many botched cases of land reform on the record, people are asking whether land reform can even be expected to do a creditable job of redistribution. De Janvry (1981:389) makes this observation: "With agriculture well advanced on the road to modernization . . . any drastic land redistribution is likely to nullify past technological achievements and imply shortfalls in production, at least in the short run. Where the population is increasingly landless and urbanized, the social cost of higher food prices [because of the inefficiencies resulting from land reform] may be more widespread than the welfare gains of land redistribution."

Critics of land reform ask if the inequality in the ownership of land is any greater than the inequality in the ownership of oil wells, or ships, or factories, or radio stations, or automobile plants. And if concentration in these sources of wealth turns out to be greater than that in land, they ask, why should these sorts of concentration not be shared among the people along with the land?

An important problem associated with land reform, or even the threat of land reform, is the chilling effect it may have on investment in agriculture relative to investment in other productive activities. Landowners who fear that land reform may be in the offing are understandably hesitant to invest heavily in productive improvements for their farms. In this view, land reform is part of a number of antiagricultural policies collectively referred to as *urban bias,* about which we will have more to say in Chapter 19.

■ PROGRESSIVE TAXATION

Taxes that take a greater percentage of income or wealth from the rich than they do from the poor are called *progressive.* Progressive taxation is one way of transferring income or wealth from the rich to the poor. In developed countries the income tax is usually designed to be progressive, and the same features can be incorporated into the tax structure of the Third World, as they often are.

Taxes that take a greater percentage of income or wealth from the poor than they do from the rich are called *regressive.* Sales taxes have a reputation for being regressive. In the developed world the poor spend a greater proportion of their income compared to the rich, who save a greater proportion of theirs. However, in the Third World the poor are not generally as well integrated into the market economy as are the rich. The poor are much more likely to barter and exchange goods and services and to raise some of their own food. All these activities escape the sales tax. So in the Third World a sales tax is generally progressive and can therefore be recommended as another method of reducing income disparity.

Income and sales taxes are attractive alternatives to land reform because they transfer income from the rich to the poor across all sectors of society. We must bear in mind, however, that the method of spending the money in the government tax till can have distributive effects just as surely as does the method of collecting it. Spending public money on programs to increase agricultural production can do much to improve the nutritional status of the poor through the impact of such expenditures on lowering the price of food and increasing employment (see Chapter 20). Conversely, a mere transfer of purchasing power from the rich to the poor may prove less effective as a way of improving the nutrition of the poor. For example:

> To take a simple case within a developing country, say India. If one rupee of purchasing power is taken away from a person in the top 5 percent of the income distribution, that will cause a reduction, in constant prices, of 0.03 rupee in foodgrain consumption. That same rupee provided to a person in the bottom 20 percent of the income distribution will provide increased demand for 0.58 rupee of food grains. The one-to-one equality of financial transfers is matched by a 19-to-one inequality in the material transfers. Thus, a marginal redistribution of income is profoundly inflationary in driving up food prices. In this case, what the left hand of society gives to the poor, the right hand of the market takes away (Mellor 1988:1003).

Taxing land according to use-value is another attractive alternative to land reform. Through a properly executed land-use survey, farmland can be classified according to its value associated with its use-potential. Often Third World land taxes on good farming land are so low that large land-holders can afford to keep their holdings while farming them inefficiently. By raising taxes and keeping them proportionate to land use-value, farmers who are making poor or inefficient use of their land will be forced to sell out to those who would farm the land better. The beauty of this system is that it readjusts resource use by weeding out the bad farmers without up-rooting the good farmers, who may be doing a fine job for society.

■ MINIMUM-WAGE LAWS

It is frequently, and often emotionally, argued that minimum-wage laws are an effective way to improve the income of the poor. There is no question that, for those workers covered by minimum-wage legislation and whose wages are higher than they would otherwise be, minimum-wage laws yield a higher level of living. However, effective minimum-wage legislation, as it raises wages at the bottom end of the scale, motivates entrepreneurs to substitute capital for labor. This drives labor out of the economy covered by minimum wage and increases unemployment in the economy generally (Mincer 1976). If credit subsidies are available, the motivation to substitute capital for labor is even greater.

Minimum-wage laws are more easily enforced in urban than in rural areas. So one result of effective minimum-wage laws is an increase in the wage differential between the country and the city. In the Third World the difference in wage rates between farm and city has resulted in mass migrations of rural population to the city in search of jobs. Although the probability of an unskilled rural migrant's obtaining an urban job may be small, the decision to migrate may be rational because some, in fact, do get good urban jobs (Todaro 1980). The waiting may take months, years, or even a lifetime; but if enough get jobs, then by and large for most people the wait seems worth it.

Effective minimum-wage legislation increases the ultimate reward from waiting for an urban job. It simultaneously increases the number of people in the queue, increases urban unemployment, wastes labor resources, and increases the number of family members accompanying unemployed migrants who may be subjected to undernutrition.

■ ECONOMIC GROWTH

There is no doubt that broad-based economic growth is one of the most effective antipoverty programs. Economic growth creates jobs and raises the incomes of the poor. To a limited degree, government projects can contribute directly to economic growth; but in general governments do not create jobs very efficiently. Developing countries must rely on growth in the private sector for their economic prosperity. A comprehensive literature deals with prerequisites and policies concerning economic growth. Here we give a brief synopsis.

Economic growth comes from three main sources:

- High savings leading to increased capital stock
- High labor productivity
- Adoption of new technology

This translates into four broad policy recommendations:

- Promotion of savings and investment through good macroeconomic policy
- Promotion of labor productivity through education, health, and antipoverty programs
- Market orientation to promote appropriate incentives to economic decisionmakers
- Promotion of development and increased productivity in the agricultural sector

☐ Macroeconomic Policy

Good macroeconomic policy, based on the experience of East Asia, where growth has been extremely rapid in a number of countries for a long period up to the 1997 "Asian crash," should have the following three objectives: (1) low inflation; (2) low budget deficits; and (3) stable exchange rates.

Low inflation contributes to growth by encouraging savings. Suppose you could earn 5 percent a year interest by leaving your money in a savings account, but that during the year, all prices increase by 20 percent. At the end of the year, you have $1.05 for every dollar saved, but the $1.05 does not buy as much at the year's end as the $1 bought at the year's beginning. In this way, high inflation discourages savings. As inflation becomes lower, individuals are more confident that their savings are not going to be eaten up by inflation, and therefore saving increases. This makes more money available for lending to businesses and entrepreneurs who can buy new equipment (which increases economic production) and start new business (creating new jobs). The principal cause of high inflation is rapid growth of the money supply. In many countries the size of the money supply (the amount of currency in circulation) is under the control of a central bank. Experience in different countries shows that inflation is lower in countries where the central bank is independent of the political process. In the United States, for example, the Federal Reserve determines the size of the money supply. The chairman (and other policymaking officers) of the Federal Reserve are appointed for seven-year terms, and are subject to confirmation by the Senate. The length of the term, and the checks and balances of Senate confirmation, make the Federal Reserve independent from the political process.

A government budget deficit occurs when the amount of spending by the government exceeds the government's income from taxes and fees. Low budget deficits contribute to growth in the following ways: First, one way governments finance the budget deficit is through printing extra money to pay their bills. This increases the money supply and causes inflation, creating problems discussed in the previous paragraph. A second way to finance budget deficits is to borrow the money to pay the bills. This uses savings that would otherwise be invested in private businesses. For example, think of a number of people who have some savings and are considering whether to buy government bonds or bonds from a private company. If they buy government bonds (lending their money to the government), the money will be used to finance the budget deficit. If they buy bonds from a private company (lending their money to the private company), the money will be used to buy capital equipment for the business. In this way, the high government deficits discourage economic growth. (It should be noted that not all government expenditures are nonproductive. If the government is investing in projects that yield a higher return than the projects of the private company, the running of deficits would actually improve economic growth.)

Finally, stable exchange rates contribute to economic growth by attracting foreigners to invest in the country. Exchange rates are also determined largely by money supplies in each country, and therefore are in the hands of the central banks.

☐ Investments in Human Capital: Education, Health, Improved Nutrition, Antipoverty

The second general policy recommendation is the improvement of labor productivity through programs aimed at education, health care, and nutrition. Education improves labor productivity in an obvious way—by making workers better able to do their jobs. In addition to training directly related to job performance, general education gives workers better ability to learn new jobs, and therefore improves average labor productivity as workers are able to move from industry to industry with relative ease. Improved health care and nutrition leads to improved labor productivity by making workers healthier, by giving them additional physical strength and endurance, and by improving their mental capacities.

☐ Market Orientation and Appropriate Economic Incentives

A third general policy for growth, *market orientation,* allows prices determined in free markets to be used as a means of organizing the production, distribution, and consumption within an economy. Relative prices provide incentives to producers and consumers: A high price sends the message "produce more, consume less"; a relatively low price sends the message "produce less, consume more." In economies where market prices are severely distorted by government programs and interventions, the signals being sent are distorted as well, and the activities undertaken in response to those signals are likely to be suboptimal.

Market-determined prices provide reasonably good indicators of desirability and scarcity of goods. The kinds of policies that promote market orientation include: openness to free trade and world markets; assignment of property rights to give individuals the right to buy and sell goods, resources, and services; the discouragement of price setting by administrative fiat; and the encouragement of government regulation that operates through the price system rather than by command and control.

☐ Agricultural Development

The economies of almost all developing countries are dominated by the agricultural sector. One of the most important stimulants to economic growth and increased employment in these economies is increased agricultural production. This is important not only because increased agricultural production increases farm employment but because increasing the quantity of food supplied lowers its price.

Food is a wage good (Mellor & Johnston 1984). That is, the cost of food can substantially affect the wage rate. Consider two developing countries that are competing in the international marketplace to sell a labor-intensive product such as shoes. In country A the price of food is high, and in country B it is low. Even though a shoe manufacturer in country B pays lower wages than his competitor in country A, the workers in the shoe factory in country B can live as well as those in country A because they can buy food more cheaply. Low food prices stimulate employment.

As low food prices make possible low wage rates, employment is stimulated not only in the export sector but in the domestic sector of the economy. Local manufacturers can compete more successfully with importers to manufacture goods. Low food prices reduce the proportion of the household budget that all people, middle- and upper-income people as well as low-income people, must allocate to food, and thus release purchasing power for nonfood items. This raises the demand for nonfood goods and services and further increases employment.

Stimulating Third World agricultural production will involve making policy shifts away from the large number of production disincentives now in place and toward production incentives. There are other avenues to stimulating increased agricultural production, such as government sponsorship of agricultural research and educational services. The main policy alternatives available in that direction are outlined in Chapter 20.

■ HUMAN CAPITAL–INTENSIVE PROGRAMS FOR REDUCING INEQUALITY

Government spending on education can do much to improve the productivity and thus the income of the poor, and simultaneously reduce the distance between the rich and the poor. The rich in the Third World do fairly well at seeing to it that their children get a good education. But the poor must depend on government-sponsored educational programs, and improving both the quality and quantity of these programs, especially at the primary and secondary levels where so many of the poor presently drop out, is important for reducing inequalities.

In designing increased educational opportunities for the poor it is vital to take into account the special importance of nutrition in providing equal educational opportunities for girls. Women with some education are more likely to be employed in a wage job than those with no education, and women with more education are likely to earn higher wages than those with less. And the relative earnings of a husband and wife have been found to influence the allocation of resources within a family. A higher wage rate for the wife and mother has a positive effect on the allocation of calories to her and her children and a negative effect on the husband's calorie allocation (Senauer et al. 1988:179).

Methods of improving the income potential of the low-income segment of a population through health care and fertility control programs, already discussed in Chapters 15 and 16, are also important in increasing the income of the poor and in reducing income inequalities.

☐ 18

Policies Aimed at Lowering the Price of Food Through Subsidized Consumption

In developing countries . . . direct government intervention in the production, pricing, and distribution of foods on a massive scale is common. There is a profound distrust of the ability of the market to value and allocate resources. . . . Government intervention gives rise to price distortions in the domestic economy that have serious allocative and efficiency effects. In order to defend domestic controls, it becomes necessary for governments also to control border trade. This type of policymaking, thus, has a lock-step nature to it where the implementation of certain policies necessarily requires further controls on other parts of the economy. . . .

The policies of intervention are rooted in a model of development where it is thought desirable, in the interests of growth and development, to skim excess resources from agriculture and direct them toward industrialization; the assumption being that such a diversion of agricultural surpluses does not reduce agricultural output. . . . Only recently have the self-defeating nature of these interventions, in the longer run, and the extent of their generally negative effect on agricultural output been fully understood.

—Bale 1985:abstract and 10–11

In Chapter 8 we argued that lack of purchasing power is one of the leading causes of undernutrition. Purchasing power is a function of both income and the price of the goods and services purchased (see Box 8.2). In Chapter 17 we surveyed policies designed to increase the income of the poor. Food is a major component in the budget of the low-income people most at risk for undernutrition, so in this chapter we survey policies aimed at lowering the food prices paid by consumers.

■ RATIONALE FOR EXPLICIT FOOD SUBSIDIES

There are a number of reasons why food consumption subsidies are so popular. Developed countries have generally followed farm production policies that have led to burdensome agricultural surpluses. Furthermore, large numbers of people are hungry now and it would therefore seem logical to feed people today rather than to sponsor programs, such as enhanced agricultural production research, that may take months or years to produce obvious benefits. Finally, occasional famines dramatize human hunger and make the logic of transferring surplus food from the developed world to the Third World inescapable.

Box 18.1   The Increasing Cost of Increasing Food Consumption Through a Subsidy

Shlomo Reutlinger

If households allocate only an increasingly smaller share of additional income to the augmentation of their energy intake, then the marginal cost of inducing energy augmentation through public intervention rises sharply as higher levels of intake are sought.

As an illustration, consider a nation in which 5 million people have average daily energy intakes of 1,500 calories, 15 million of 1,600 calories, 10 million of 1,700 calories and the remainder of 1,800 calories and more. Let's further assume that, with declining income elasticity of demand as income rises, the additional (annual) income required to increase daily energy intake by 100 calories is $10, $15, and $25, respectively, at the level of intake of 1,500, 1,600, and 1,700 calories. If the goal of the public intervention is to assure the entire population a minimum energy intake of 1,600 calories, 5 million people at very low levels of intake would have to get a total cash transfer of 50 million dollars. If the goal were to assure a minimum of 1,700 calories in the population, an additional 15 dollars per capita would have to be provided to the 5 million people with the lowest energy intake as well as to 15 million more people. The additional cost would be 300 million more dollars. If a minimum energy intake of 1,800 calories were to be assured, the additional cost would be 1,000 million dollars. The marginal cost of raising minimum energy intakes from 1,700 to 1,800 calories is 20 times the marginal cost of raising minimum intakes from 1,500 to 1,600 calories.

The above calculations are illustrative, but not unrealistic, given what we know about the declining marginal propensities of households, at different levels of energy intake and income, to allocate additional income to energy intake. The marginal cost of public interventions to increase energy intake rises sharply as higher levels of intake are sought.

Source: Extracted from Reutlinger 1985.

There are other reasons for the popularity of food consumption subsidies. By and large, rich people prefer to give hungry people food rather than cash (see the discussion of "basic needs" in Chapter 14). Further, particular groups of rich people derive benefits from food distribution programs: These groups include food processors and input suppliers in food-exporting countries; farmers, who see the demand increased for their products; grain elevators, which hope to store the food before shipment; the sea-freight shippers; and finally the private voluntary agencies such as CARE and Catholic Relief Services that assist in distributing surplus food.

In the Third World, political leaders are interested in creating or continuing such programs. Also in the Third World, the groups most likely to influence political power are the military, civil servants, urban labor, and industrial interests. All of these groups are happy to be the recipients of cheap food, and political leaders are generally happy to curry favor among them, even at the expense of the country's rural sector (Hopkins 1988).

Proof of the political popularity of food price subsidies can be found in the morning newspaper. In several countries people have responded to the elimination of these programs by rioting in the streets. For example, in 1996, the International Monetary Fund (IMF) pressured Jordan to cut food price subsidies, with the result that bread prices doubled. In response, angry demonstrators in several Jordanian cities demanded that the prime minister be removed from office (Reuters 1996).

■ MARKETWIDE EXPLICIT SUBSIDIES

In an attempt to reduce food prices, some countries have adopted marketwide food subsidies—that is, subsidies that are available to all, not just to the needy. Some developing countries (for example, China and Brazil) have borne most of the costs of their food subsidies themselves. Other countries (for example, India and Egypt) have shared the costs with foreign donor countries who donate food for the purpose. (Food aid is discussed later in this chapter.)

We will look at experiences with marketwide food subsidies in three Third World countries: Brazil, an upper-middle-income country that bore most of the costs itself; Egypt, a middle-income country that shared the costs with foreign donors; and Sri Lanka, a low-income country that shared a small part of the costs with foreign donors and eventually decided to shift from a marketwide food subsidy to a subsidy targeted at the needy.

□ Brazil

During the period 1966–1982 the government of Brazil attempted to achieve self-sufficiency in wheat production and at the same time provide cheap wheat to its consumers. As part of its attempt to achieve these goals, the government became the sole seller and buyer of both domestically produced and imported wheat. The prices of wheat and wheat products were rigidly controlled throughout the economy. Farmers were encouraged to increase wheat production through a price-support subsidy, and millers were provided with wheat at a price substantially below that paid to the producer, with the government making up the difference out of the general tax till.

In their study of the Brazilian wheat policy, Calegar and Schuh (1988: 9–10, 43–45) determined that 86 percent of the subsidy went to consumers. That means only 14 percent of the subsidy costs went to administration or were lost through slippages such as manipulations by the millers. Even so, only 19 percent of the total subsidy went to the true target group, the low-income consumers. Furthermore, gains in consumer welfare were slightly biased toward the high-income population groups (they bought more bread per capita than did the low-income groups). Calegar and Schuh conclude that the marketwide wheat consumption subsidy was not an effective policy for redistributing income and suggest that a preferred policy would be to target the food subsidy specifically at low-income groups.

☐ **Egypt**

The Egyptian government has a history of intervening in the food-marketing system that dates back to Biblical times when Joseph, interpreting the pharaoh's dream, recommended storing grain during seven fat years to prepare for the seven lean years that he prophesied were to come (Genesis 41). Since the mid-1970s, the Egyptian government has taken on a substantial burden of public expenditures for food subsidies, with the share of the government expenditures for this purpose running as high as 17 percent (Alderman & von Braun 1984:12).

Additional costs of the Egyptian food subsidy have been borne by North American and European governments, which have provided substantial quantities of food at below-market prices. Indeed, the availability of such programs may be one of the reasons that Egyptians embarked on such an ambitious marketwide food subsidy.

As of the late 1980s the Egyptian government was handling the major share of the sales of bread, flour, pulses, sugar, tea, and cooking oil in the country, making these commodities available to householders at prices significantly below world prices. Farm-gate prices (prices the farmer receives at the farm gate, before paying transport costs to market) deviated less from world prices than did retail prices (Table 18.1), but both sets of prices demonstrated a priority goal of Egyptian policy: Cheap food for all.

The policy is widely credited with keeping the Egyptian rate of undernutrition to a minimum. Average calorie consumption was above standard

Table 18.1   **Farm-Gate and Retail Price of Selected Agricultural Commodities, Egypt, 1982**

	Price as Percentage of World Price	
	Farm-Gate	Retail
Wheat	64.5	36.8
Rice	26.6	17.7
Sugar	46.0	27.3
Beans	75.4	49.0
Cotton	27.2	41.3

Source: Rountree 1985.

even among the poorest 12 percent of the population as a whole (U.S. Dept. of Agriculture 1984:9), although significant numbers of urban households in the lowest-income quartile were found to be calorie-deficient (Alderman & von Braun 1984).

Despite the apparent success of the Egyptian food subsidy, it has been criticized as inefficient. Sources of inefficiency include:

- *Waste:* With bread as cheap as it is in Egypt, farmers purchase significant quantities of it for livestock feed. The resources spent processing the wheat into bread are a dead loss to society when the bread is fed to livestock.
- *Underinvestment in industry:* The more foreign exchange that is spent on a food subsidy the less is available for industrial investment. One study estimated that a 10 percent increase in available foreign exchange would increase industrial investment by 6 percent and industrial output by 4 percent (Scobie 1983). High rates of government spending on imported food could adversely affect industrial employment among the poor.
- *Consumption inefficiencies:* Because of the depressed price of wheat, Egyptians eat more wheat than they would if they were paying the world price. A loss to Egyptian society associated with this overconsumption results because government paid more for the last tons of wheat it bought at world market prices than Egyptian citizens would have been willing to pay for them. The amount of this cost above worth is represented by triangle 1 of Figure 18.1.

☐ Sri Lanka

When a general food subsidy is substantial, the costs of the program become so high that it becomes necessary to limit access through a system of rationing. This is illustrated by the experience of Sri Lanka. During World

Figure 18.1   **Cost Above Worth and Producer's Surplus Lost Due to a
Marketwide Explicit Subsidy**

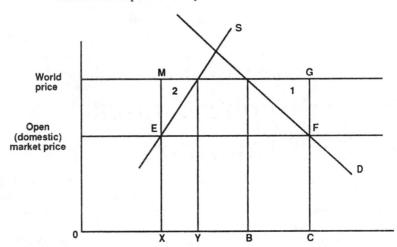

Cost above worth: Suppose that D represents the demand curve for wheat, and that amount OC represents the wheat consumed, given the domestic market price. If BC quantity of wheat is imported, then the area of the triangle 1 is a loss to society since government paid more for this wheat than it was worth to consumers.

Producer's surplus lost: Now suppose that S represents the supply curve for wheat, assuming no concessionary sales were available. Quantity OX represents wheat produced in Egypt given a depressed, domestic market price. Quantity XY represents wheat imported that would have been produced locally had the local price of wheat been equal to the world price. The area of triangle 2 is a loss to the Egyptian farmer because it is a producer's surplus he could capture were he getting the world price, but which he now misses out on. Notice that the consumer would not care whether he paid the world price to the farmer or to a foreigner. But the Egyptian farmer cares because he can produce that quantity of wheat with fewer resources than can the foreigner. And the economy cares, too. Triangle 2 is a loss to the Egyptian economy.

War II, when rice supplies were limited, the government instituted a program under which rice was sold at a subsidized price, but the quantity to each consumer was rationed (Edirisinghe & Poleman, 1983).

In 1953, the costs of the rice program became too high, and price increases of nearly 300 percent were announced. A massive protest stopped the price increases and forced the resignation of the prime minister. From 1954 to 1966, Sri Lankans could buy rice at prices substantially below the market price, but, through rationing, access was restricted to four pounds per week (equivalent to about 1,000 calories per person per day) (Edirisinghe 1987:12–13). In 1966, the basic weekly ration was cut in half, but issued at no charge. Two things were significant here: (1) Because government did not need to purchase as much rice overseas, substantial foreign exchange savings accrued; and (2) there were no food riots.

In 1978, the ration system was targeted to the lower end of the income range through a means test. A year and a half later, food stamps were substituted for the ration cards. Food stamps carry a fixed rupee value; therefore their purchasing power declines with inflation, resulting in an automatic reduction of the costs of the food subsidy with no further government action. In 1985, targeting was restricted further, so that only the poorest quarter of the population was eligible for food stamps (Sahn & Edirisinghe 1993). The policy reforms reduced government costs: Food subsidies amounted to 23 percent of government expenditures in 1970, 19 percent in 1978, and 4 percent in 1984.

■ SUBSIDIES TARGETED TO THE CHRONICALLY NEEDY

The Sri Lankan experience (as it had evolved by the 1980s) illustrates a second category of food price subsidies: those targeted to the poor or chronically undernourished. *Targeting* means that a person receives the food subsidy only if he or she meets certain criteria. Common criteria involve some measures of undernutrition and economic status. For example, a study of the Philippines advised a two-step procedure for targeting: (1) Identify target villages with high concentrations of underweight preschoolers; (2) within the selected villages, identify households containing preschoolers whose anthropometric measurements indicate they are at high risk for undernutrition (Garcia & Pinstrup-Andersen 1987:78). In other cases, a maximum income or wealth level is established, and individuals must fall below that level to participate in the subsidy. It is difficult to enforce these targets. For example, the Sri Lankan program in 1978 restricted participation to households with annual incomes below Rs 3,600 (about $240). A survey of household income indicated that only 7.1 percent of the population lived in households below this eligible income level. Yet, almost half the population managed to qualify for the program (World Bank 1986:93).

Targeted subsidies can be administered in a number of ways. For example, they can be targeted geographically: Limit the programs to regions where large numbers of undernourished live. To some degree, donors of food aid choose recipient countries based on this criterion. Other methods of targeting include self-targeting, direct distribution, rationing, food stamps, and food-for-work.

□ Self-targeting

The easiest way to target a food subsidy is to subsidize foods with negative income elasticities of demand: the inferior goods, to use the economists' jargon that we adopted in Chapter 8. Inferior foods vary from culture to culture but are typically starchy staples such as cassava, yams, maize, sorghum, or millet. As income increases, people usually eat less of these products (review Figures 8.2c and d).

The government of Bangladesh experimented with this idea in one area by subsidizing sorghum consumption, but the experiment, although supposedly successful, was not implemented countrywide (Karim, Majid & Levinson 1984; Ahmed 1988:226).

☐ Direct Distribution

Affluent countries are familiar with direct food distribution programs carried out through school lunch programs or by soup kitchens set up in low-income urban areas. In the Third World, direct distribution of food is more likely to take the form of supplemental feeding programs targeted at the groups most vulnerable to undernutrition: pregnant and lactating women, infants, and preschoolers. Despite the popularity of such programs, the results have been disappointing (Kennedy & Knudsen 1985).

Beaton and Ghassemi (1982) found that in the eight supervised feeding programs and 13 take-home food programs for which they had data, the net increase in food intake by the target recipients ranged from 45 to 70 percent of the food distributed, with one program showing a net effect of only 10 to 15 percent. Some of the reasons for these disappointing results are discussed in Box 18.2.

☐ Rationing

A subsidized food-rationing system allows a consumer who holds a ration card to purchase a specific amount of some food or foods in a given time at a price lower than the market value.

A subsidized food-rationing system requires either that the government set up a marketing system of its own, which it operates or licenses to operate parallel to the regular market (which may be declared illegal and is then called a black market); or that the government set up a system for reimbursing commercial retail outlets for the discounts that they give for the rationed food. In either case government must employ auditors to monitor the system to minimize cheating.

A 1983–1984 experiment in the Philippines provides a case study of costs and benefits from a real-world, subsidized food-ration scheme. The experiment was set up so that all households in seven villages, known for a high incidence of undernutrition and poverty, were provided subsidized food. These villages were matched with seven control villages. The program did increase food consumption among the target villages. Although distribution of the extra food within the household favored adults, preschool children also consumed more and showed improvements in their nutritional status. If only weight gains among the undernourished were counted as benefits, the cost of adding one kilogram to the weight of an undernourished preschooler was estimated at $101 per year. (Edirisinghe

Box 18.2   Supplementary Feeding

Eileen T. Kennedy and Per Pinstrup-Andersen

Supplementary feeding programs distribute foods through noncommercial channels to pregnant and lactating women, infants, and preschoolers. These programs are the most common form of nutrition intervention in developing countries.

There are three common forms of delivery: 1) On-site feeding, 2) take-home feeding, and 3) nutrition rehabilitation centers (NRC's). NRC's include both residential facilities and programs in which children are cared for during the day but return home at night.

Data from more than 200 supplementary feeding projects indicate that many supplementary feeding programs have had a significant and positive effect on prenatal and child participants (Anderson et al. 1981; Beaton & Ghassemi 1982). Despite the significant, positive effect, however, the benefits are usually small. Increments in birth weights attributed to the supplementary feeding programs are typically in the range of 40–60 grams. Similarly, the increases in growth seen in preschoolers, although significant, are small.

Several reasons are given for these small but significant effects. First, it appears that only a part of the food given is actually consumed by the target population. "Leakages" occur when the food is shared by nontarget family members or when the food is substituted for other food that normally would be consumed. Other factors, such as the timing of supplementation, duration of participation, nutritional status of recipients, and related services available, all influence the effectiveness of supplemental feeding.

Timing of supplement. Pregnancy and the period from six months to three years of age are the most nutritionally vulnerable times. Studies indicate that it is the last trimester of pregnancy that is the most critical for supplementation. Preschoolers below the age of three are also at special risk. Inappropriate weaning practices, delayed introduction of solid foods, food taboos, and infection all contribute to a higher prevalence of second- and third-degree malnutrition in this group.

Duration. For prenatal women, there appears to be a minimum participation of 13–15 weeks needed to produce significant changes in birth weight. For infants and children, the minimum level of participation needed to affect growth depends heavily on the type of delivery system used.

Nutritional status of participants. Children with second- or third-degree malnutrition exhibit greater benefits from supplemental feeding than do marginally undernourished children. The same is true for pregnant women.

Other services. Inadequate intake of food is only one of several factors that contribute to undernutrition. Undernutrition and infection often occur simultaneously. It is not surprising, therefore, that the most successful supplementation activities have been those with strong ties to primary health care programs.

Source: Extracted from Kennedy & Pinstrup-Andersen et al. 1983:35–40.

[1987:70], in his study of food subsidies in Sri Lanka, found that discrimination against younger family members diminished when the more productive members of the household had at least 80 percent of their energy requirements met.)

The researchers in the Philippine experiment estimated that the cost-effectiveness of the program compared favorably with other programs. Costs were kept low through careful targeting, the cooperation of the local bureaucratic structure in administering the program, and by using existing retail outlets instead of a parallel, government-operated marketing system (Garcia & Pinstrup-Andersen 1987:9, 78–79).

Although the Philippine effort was targeted at rural villages, it has been found that nationwide subsidized ration schemes generally show an urban bias. For instance, the subsidized wheat ration system in use in Pakistan was found to contribute about 11 percent of household income for urban households with incomes below the median. Rural households gained less than 1 percent of their income from the system. The reasons for the difference are that rural households are less likely to participate in the program, smaller quantities of rationed food are available there, and wheat is not sold in many rural areas (Rogers 1988c:247).

☐ **Food Stamps**

Food stamps are somewhat different from ration coupons for purchasing subsidized food. Food stamps have a face value that can be used in any food store to purchase food at the market value. In addition, people are usually expected to purchase their food stamps. Since a food stamp plan does not require government to set up a parallel marketing system for the subsidized food, the system may be cheaper than rationing.

The first food stamp plan ever was introduced in the United States just before World War II, but it is the 1961 revision of the plan that economists like to talk about. In this version eligible families got stamps with a cash value depending on household needs for food. They paid varying amounts for the stamps depending on their income level. This arrangement made it possible to vary the food-linked income transfer according to need and therefore extend the limited government food welfare expenditures to a broader segment of the population.

In his study of the food stamp program in Sri Lanka, Edirisinghe (1987:55) found that the caloric intake response to an additional rupee from food stamps was exactly the same as from an additional rupee of income. Because of decreasing income elasticity of demand as income rises, the cost of providing 100 additional calories through food stamps increases as income increases. Despite this finding, food stamp programs will probably stay around simply because they are more acceptable politically than straight cash transfers.

☐ Food-for-Work

Adding the requirement that recipients of food aid work in exchange for the food-linked income transfer is an interesting twist. Food-for-work (FFW) has the potential to increase the productivity of the region in which it is applied and, at the same time, provide productive activities for recipients who would otherwise be unemployed or underemployed (Mellor 1988:1004). FFW projects typically improve rural infrastructure through building farm-to-market roads, constructing irrigation canals, and so forth. They have also been used in improving squatter settlements or in erecting community buildings (Jackson & Eade 1982:24).

During the early 1980s an FFW project in the Rift Valley of Kenya employed low-income farmers on local public works projects, particularly for erosion control and water-harvesting devices. The project had two positive economic outcomes: A good deal of farmland was improved and its access to irrigation water enhanced; the participating farmers used some of their food-linked income transfers for capital investments on their farms and thus increased their own productivity. In fact, during the second year of the program the farmers devoted fewer hours to FFW activities, apparently in part because of a greater need to tend their own farms (Bezuneh, Deaton & Norton 1988).

This success story is heartwarming, yet at the same time it introduces one of the problems with FFW: The benefits often go mainly to those who possess land. Typically, the recipients of FFW food are not landowners but the landless unemployed and underemployed. If their projects improve the productivity of land owned by others, the inequality of asset distribution in the area could increase. In one FFW tree-planting project in Ethiopia the workers became so resentful that their work was enhancing the private property of already powerful landed people that they planted all the trees upside down (Maxwell 1978a:40).

Another problem stems from the growing number of FFW laborers who are women. The extra time they put into FFW programs may detract from the quantity and quality of child care that they give their children. Typically they leave their infants and preschoolers to be cared for by older siblings (Kennedy, Pinstrup-Andersen et al. 1983:28).

■ FOOD AID AND THE COSTS OF EXPLICIT FOOD SUBSIDIES

Explicit food subsidization is an expensive way of improving nutritional status. This is especially true of food aid—subsidized food sold (or given away) by food-exporting countries (e.g., the United States, Canada, and Europe). In recent years, the magnitude of food aid to the developing countries has declined, but it still remains significant (see Table 18.2). This table shows country-to-country donations, and also includes donations from the World Food Program—a multilateral agency of the UN that is funded by donations from developed countries.

OXFAM, one of the leading voluntary agencies involved in distributing surplus food to Third World countries, commissioned a report on food aid for such purposes as disaster relief, food-for-work, mother and child health, and school feeding programs. Jackson and Eade found that the cost of the sea-freight to the U.S. food aid program came to 53 percent of the value of the food. When the food arrives at a Third World port, there are other costs—warehousing, transportation, and administration as the food is distributed to the needy. The OXFAM report's authors found that the sea-freight plus within-country costs of the U.S. food aid program in one country, Guatemala, ran to 89 percent of the original cost of the food (Jackson & Eade 1982:65).

Jackson and Eade cite a number of disturbing studies that suggest that sometimes ways can be found to improve Third World nutrition more cheaply than with explicit food subsidies. To cite one example, a study in India found that it cost 1.5 times as much to prevent a child's death through supplementary feeding as it would to provide basic medical services, and that "for children aged 1–3 years, nutrition supplementation was

**Table 18.2   Quantity of Food Aid from All Donors, 1977–1996
(in metric tons)**

	Non-cereals	Cereals	Total
1977	528,673	9,991,781	10,520,454
1978	629,300	10,150,010	10,779,310
1979	553,382	9,764,895	10,318,277
1980	582,375	9,685,137	10,267,512
1981	752,693	10,207,130	10,959,823
1982	699,818	10,238,110	10,937,928
1983	687,865	10,978,030	11,665,895
1984	831,092	13,960,320	14,791,412
1985	834,000	11,892,730	12,726,730
1986	988,334	13,773,620	14,761,954
1987	1,261,348	15,123,990	16,385,338
1988	1,461,302	11,884,810	13,346,112
1989	1,182,438	12,139,030	13,321,468
1990	1,318,220	13,399,360	14,717,580
1991	1,038,516	13,577,350	14,615,866
1992	1,955,901	15,132,690	17,088,591
1993	1,981,527	13,006,630	14,988,157
1994	1,671,015	9,442,945	11,113,960
1995	1,197,755	7,742,956	8,940,711
1996	861,761	4,871,807	5,733,568

Source: FAOSTAT, 1998.

up to 11 times more expensive in terms of lives saved than medical services." The study concluded that "even where it has been nutritionally effective, supplementary feeding has not proved to be cost-effective" (Maxwell 1978b:295 fn. 36, 297).

Despite their expense, these programs can provide a solution to the most immediate of Third World nutritional needs, such as famine relief. Note, however, that to be effective, they must be well administered, and this in itself is expensive. Note also that these programs do not become self-sustaining. Long-term, self-sustaining solutions to the hunger problem will have to involve changes in population growth rates, purchasing power of the poor, income distribution, and health.

■ EFFECTS OF EXPLICIT FOOD SUBSIDIES

Explicit food subsidies succeed in transferring income, but they are expensive. Third World governments seldom own the resources to sponsor explicit food subsidies on their own. Therefore, the direction of income transfer through these programs has been mainly from the developed to the underdeveloped world, chiefly through PL480 and the World Food Program (WFP).

These subsidies increase food consumption. Because of the fungibility of the food transferred (commonly grains or grain products) in the Third World setting, the food received is usually treated as the equivalent of cash. Therefore some of the resulting increased purchasing power is spent on nonfood items.

Marketwide subsidies usually benefit urban consumers far more than rural consumers. This is due in part to the difficulty of running a subsidy program in rural areas and in part to the greater political clout of urban special interest groups. In these untargeted subsidies the rich enjoy a greater income transfer than the poor because the rich purchase more food. Even so, the poor may well get a greater percentage increase in income from the subsidy.

In very low-income households the lion's share of the increased food consumed may go to the productive adults unless the subsidy is sufficient to approach food adequacy among those adults.

Even with foreign assistance, explicit subsidies can be expensive to Third World governments, often claiming more than 10 percent of their annual budget expenditures. The question must be raised whether the same amount spent on other programs would accomplish more for the poor. Careful targeting of the subsidy can save considerably on costs.

Food subsidies put downward pressure on wages, which partially offsets the real-income transfer. Still, lower wages may increase employment among the poor.

If the food for an explicit food subsidy is purchased in the same country where it is dispensed, the demand for food is increased, because the poor are now eating more than they otherwise would. This results in higher food prices, which work as an incentive to agricultural production. The U.S. food stamp and school lunch programs thus provide an incentive to U.S. agriculture.

Conversely, if the subsidized food is purchased in a developed country and dispensed in a Third World country, the effect is to raise farm prices in the developed country and lower them in the Third World country. The program thus acts as an incentive to agriculture in the developed country but as a disincentive to agriculture in the Third World country. In the developed world, special interest groups who benefit from food surplus disposal programs are likely to insist that their donated food does not depress Third World farm prices. We find it hard to see how they can claim the incentives to the developed world's agriculture without recognizing the corresponding disincentives to agriculture in the Third World.

If Third World farmers bear some of the costs of explicit food subsidies through the price disincentives described above, those costs are small beside the costs they may incur from implicit food-linked income transfer programs.

■ FAMINE AND DISASTER RELIEF

The subsidies described above are permanent policies aimed at chronic undernutrition. Human disasters (war, civil unrest) and natural disasters (earthquakes, drought, flooding) adversely affect local food availability and provide circumstances for strong arguments for emergency, or nonpermanent, food consumption subsidies. Although shortage of food can contribute to famine, contrary to popular conception, this is not the leading cause of famine. The more likely cause of famine following natural disaster or war is lack of purchasing power (Sen 1981). The farm family whose crops have failed, or the landless worker who is out of a job, are the people who starve during a famine. Reutlinger and his colleagues (1986: 27) list the groups most likely to fall victim to famine:

- Small-scale farmers or tenants whose crops have failed and who cannot find other employment in agriculture (the Wollo in Ethiopia in 1973)
- Landless agricultural workers who lose their jobs when agricultural production declines (Bangladesh in 1974) or who face rapidly rising food prices and constant or declining wages (the Great Bengal famine of 1943)

- Other rural people, including destitutes and beggars, who are affected by a decline in real income in the famine regions (almost all famines)
- Pastoralists who get most of their food by trading animals for foodgrains; their herds may be ravaged by the drought, or animal prices may collapse relative to foodgrain prices (the Harerghe region of Ethiopia in 1974 and the drought-stricken Sahel in 1973)

The authors of the well-documented and detailed OXFAM report (Jackson & Eade 1982) warn that poorly supervised or uncontrolled distribution of food aid can do more harm than good. To quote one example, a field worker helping out in a drought-relief food aid program (where the food handouts were supposed to be free of charge to the recipients) wrote:

> In Haiti we had . . . a problem of theft and mishandling. In [a] town . . . fairly near to us and very badly hit by drought, the magistrate (appointed mayor) was known to sell PL480 food for $7.00 a 50 lb. bag. At other times the CARE food distributors were so desperate that they would just throw bags of food off the truck and drive on so that the food would go to the strong and the swift (p. 9).

When a disaster has created the need for assistance, but the local food supplies are adequate, supplying emergency food relief can be counterproductive. It depresses the local price of food, in turn depressing the income of the local farming community, and may lead to other socially undesirable results (see Box 18.3).

Sometimes famines are the result of political forces operating within a society where those in power attempt to gain control of resources or subdue opposition through programs that result in starvation. The Soviet famine of 1932–1934 provides one such example. During its first five-year plan the Soviet government felt that, to carry out its program of rapid industrialization, it needed to control agriculture. The policy it used was collectivization of peasants' farms. The disruptions growing out of collectivization and the heavy food procurement requirements of central government led to a famine that killed some 5 million people in the Ukraine and nearby regions. The peasants were not interested in joining socialized agriculture, and government used the famine to drive the last diehards onto state or collective farms, or out of existence (Dalrymple 1964).

The Ethiopian famine of 1984–1985 is a more recent example of government-induced starvation. In the Western countries that supplied over $1.2 billion for food aid to Ethiopia during the crisis, the commonly accepted explanation for the famine was that a record-breaking drought was the chief cause. Journalists covering the famine cited official Ethiopian

Box 18.3   When Food Aid Is Not Needed

Tony Jackson and Deborah Eade

Imported food may not be necessary at all, despite a major disaster, and its arrival may do more harm than good. The classic example of this comes from Guatemala where the earthquake in 1976 killed an estimated 23,000 people, injured over three times as many and left a million and a quarter homeless. The earthquake occurred in the middle of a record harvest. Local grain was plentiful and the crops were not destroyed but left standing in the fields or buried under the rubble but easy to recover.

During the first few weeks, small consumer items—salt, sugar, soap, etc.—were in short supply and temporarily unavailable in the shops. Some of these small items, such as salt, were lost when the houses collapsed. People expressed a need for these food items in the short period before commercial supplies were resumed. However, during that year, about 25,400 tons of basic grains and blends were brought in as food aid from the US. A further 5,000 tons of US food aid already stored in Guatemala were released and supplies were also sent in from elsewhere in the region.

Catholic Relief Services (CRS) and CARE both received reports from their field staff saying food aid was not needed. The Director of CARE's housing reconstruction program visited the disaster area soon after the earthquake. In a US Government report he stated:

> Another thing I was really concerned with was whether there was any need to import food or seed. But I saw no indication of that whatsoever. First of all, the earth was not damaged, and there was no reason why the crops couldn't be harvested on time, and I believe it was a good crop that year. Also, in a few places I visited, I asked people if they could pull the food they had in their houses out of the rubble, and they said they certainly could.

CRS field staff objected to the importing of food aid but they were overruled by their headquarters in New York. Two weeks after the disaster, the League of Red Cross Societies asked national Red Cross Societies to stop sending food. As early as February (the same month as the earthquake), the Co-ordinator of the National Emergency Committee of the Government of Guatemala asked voluntary agencies to stop imports of food aid. On 4 March, the Assistant Administrator for the Latin America Bureau of the United States Agency for International Development (AID), the Hon. Herman Kleine, testified before a House of Representatives Sub-Committee. "I should like to add here, Mr. Chairman, that the Guatemalan Government has requested officially to all donors that further contributions not be of food and medicine but roofing and building materials."

Finally, the Government of Guatemala invoked a presidential decree to prohibit imports of basic grains from May 1976 onwards. Yet after this decree, quantities of food aid were still imported in the form of blended foodstuffs. One article refers to these blends as "basic grains in disguise."

Field staff and local leaders identified three negative results. Firstly, they considered that food aid contributed to a drop in the price of local grain that occurred soon after the earthquake and continued throughout 1976. As

(continues)

Box 18.3   Continued

to the need for basic grains, a peasant farmer explained: "There was no shortage. There was no need to bring food from outside. On the contrary, our problem was to sell what we had."

After an extensive survey of towns and villages in the worst-hit areas six weeks after the earthquake, an OXFAM–World Neighbors official reported: "Virtually everyone in the area is selling more grain this year than he does normally. Furthermore, emergency food shipments have drastically curtailed demand for grains. Thus the prices of the farmers' produce have plummeted."

Later, the then Director of CRS in Guatemala was to tell the *New York Times:* "The general effect was that we knocked the bottom out of the grain market in the country for nine to twelve months."

This las view may be overstated as other factors, such as the excellent grain harvest, would usually have led to a fall in prices anyway. Nonetheless, the basic fact remains: $8 million of food aid was sent into a country with plentiful food-stocks of its own. Any food that it was necessary to distribute to earthquake victims could have been bought in Guatemala (as WFP did).

The second negative effect of the continuing supply of free food was to encourage the survivors to queue for rations instead of engaging in reconstruction or normal agricultural work.

Thirdly, it brought about a change in the quality and motivation of local leadership. The OXFAM–World Neighbors official, quoted above, noted:

> Immediately after the earthquake, we tended to see the same leaders whom we'd seen before the earthquake—people [with] a high degree of honesty and personal commitment to the villages. But gradually . . . I began seeing fellas who I knew were totally dishonest. They'd go into the different agencies and . . . say that theirs was the most affected village in the Highlands, and they'd get more food. So largely because of the give-aways, the villages started to turn more to leaders who could produce free things like this, whether they were honest or dishonest, rather than to the leaders they'd been putting their trust in for years.
>
> With larger and larger quantities of free food coming in, there are increased incentives to corruption. . . . Groups that had worked together previously became enemies over the question of recipients for free food.

Source: Extracted from Jackson & Eade 1982:9–11. (Consult the source for copious documentation.)

government explanations of the cause of the famine as a disastrous failure of rain, and their reports were backed up by official reports from UN representatives and other dignitaries who also accepted the Ethiopian government's position.

In retrospect, we find that rainfall was down during and preceding the famine, but that the drought was not much worse than Ethiopian farmers had come to expect as their lot. A study by Clay and Holcomb (1986:192) found that the main causes of the famine were government policies designed to accomplish "massive collectivization of agricultural production and to secure central government control over productive regions of the country where indigenous peoples have developed strong antigovernment resistance." The Clay and Holcomb study in Ethiopia involved hundreds of interviews, including both farm families and representatives of public and private agencies delivering famine assistance. The explanations of Oromo farm families of the decline in productivity in their area is particularly revealing. All respondents reported a decline in agricultural production since 1976. Their average yield in the 1975/76 crop year was 4,600 kilograms, whereas their average yield on the same land in the 1984/85 crop year was only 900 kilograms. When asked the reason for the decline, none of the farmers reported lack of rain. They cited a host of other reasons, all of which had to do with government policies (see Table 18.3).

Clay and Holcomb concluded that, in the case of the 1984–1985 Ethiopian famine, foreign food aid was distributed with very little monitoring by the aid donors and was, in fact, used mainly by the central government

Table 18.3 **Causes of Agricultural Production Declines as Reported by a Sample of 45 Oromo Farmers, Ethiopia, 1985 (Interviewed in Yabuus, Sudan, Factors Mentioned in Combination)**

	Percentage Responding
Lack of rain	0.0
Government programs interfere with food production	
Work required four to five days a week on peasant association collective plots	95.4
Other peasant association obligations	27.2
Required attendance at peasant association meetings and literacy programs	73.4
Disarming populations	63.6
Military conscription	15.6
Imprisonment prevents farm work	86.3
Government policies force redistribution of assets	
Land redistribution	52 2
Forced sale of oxen to pay taxes and "voluntary contributions"	41.0
All products confiscated for taxes (including seed grain)	36.3
Oxen and tools confiscated for collectivization or resettlement	13.6
Oxen given to others in peasant association	6.8
Government "improvement" programs destroy crops	
Government "experts" untrained in farming	13.6
Grass, for erosion control, overtook crops	9.0

Source: Clay & Holcomb 1986:124.

to help suppress resistance groups within the country and probably increased the death rate through starvation (see Box 18.4).

Martin Ravallion (1997) recently completed a thorough review of the economics literature regarding famines. He cites examples of failed policy responses to famine: "The British government's . . . non-intervention in food markets during [nineteenth-century] famines almost certainly made matters worse. . . . At the other extreme, . . . food procurement policies

---

Box 18.4   Politics and the Ethiopian Famine, 1984–1985

Jason W. Clay and Bonnie K. Holcomb

Governments as well as humanitarian assistance agencies have not attempted to systematically understand the causes of the present famine. While their assistance, they claim, feeds the hungry, they fail to address the issue of whether their assistance will eradicate or exacerbate the conditions that led to the present famine. If the West is willing to feed starving Ethiopians without asking how they came to be in that condition or evaluate whether Western assistance programs alleviate those conditions, then they will face a monumental task in the future. The government of Ethiopia is establishing a social and economic system that will produce starving people for generations to come.

Assistance to the government, unless scrupulously monitored:

• Facilitates the uprooting of distinct peoples in one region of the country and the displacement of self-sufficient food producers in another, primarily through the resettlement program.

• Gives hostile Ethiopian government forces access to areas that had successfully withdrawn from the reach of the state and re-established efficient, autonomous agricultural production systems.

• Reinforces transport and communication lines of obvious strategic military importance in areas that the government has not been able to control militarily.

• Supports programs designed by a tiny minority of the region's inhabitants while simultaneously undermining programs that have broad popular support.

• Allows the government to reinforce the programs that lead to the famine as well as intensify programs, such as resettlement and villagization, that will spread the famine to previously productive and fertile regions.

According to our own research and the efforts of numerous other individuals and organizations, Ethiopian government policies have become the major cause of death in the country. The provision of "humanitarian" assistance, with no questions asked, helps the Ethiopian government to get away with murder.

Source: Clay & Holcomb 1986:192–193.

implemented [by] . . . the Soviet Union . . . resulted in severe famine in the Ukraine in the 1930s" (Ravallion:1225). Ravallion draws the following lessons for policies in response to famine:

- *Better governance:* Greater democratization and freer flow of information in a society make it more difficult for a government to ignore famines.
- *Early warning and rapid response:* Policy interventions are likely to be more effective if they take place before famine conditions are firmly entrenched.
- *Increase aggregate food availability:* Policies to increase the total amount of food available in famine areas include food aid, policies to discourage hoarding in private or public storage, policies to encourage domestic food production.
- *Distribution policies:* "Although the case is often strong for increasing aggregate food availability during a famine, food handouts need not be the best form of intervention from the point of view of minimizing mortality. Cash or coupon payments to potential famine victims can provide more effective relief than the usual policy of importing and distributing food" (Ravallion:1230).
- *Stabilization policies:* "An effective but affordable . . . stabilization policy in famine-prone economies . . . will probably combine buffer stocks and . . . a relatively open external trade regime" (Ravallion: 1233). Buffer stocks are programs where the government purchases food in periods when it is plentiful and sells food out of their stocks when shortages occur.
- *Other policies:* Ravallion argues that there are potential synergies between policies to address famines and other policies to spur economic development, including credit programs, improved infrastructure, and assignment of property rights.

□ 19

Policies That Lower the Prices Paid to Farmers: Implicit Subsidies and the Costs of Urban Bias

The most important class conflict in the poor countries of the world today is not between labor capital. Nor is it between foreign and national interests. It is between the rural classes and the urban classes.
—Lipton 1977:13

The last chapter described programs that effectively lowered the prices paid by consumers to below the levels that would have been paid in the absence of the programs. These are programs that are (or can be) implemented without lowering the price received by farmers. In this chapter, we point out that many developing countries have adopted policies that reduce food prices in the economy as a whole—both the prices paid by consumers and the prices received by farmers.

As pointed out in Box 19.1, one of the surprising anomalies of the world food problem is that developed countries (where agriculture is already highly productive and food supplies are abundant) have generally stimulated farm production by engaging in agricultural policies that result in high farm prices, whereas Third World countries (where agricultural production is often marginal and food supplies are scarce) generally have discouraged farm production by engaging in agricultural policies that result in low farm prices. A central idea underlying Third World policies that result in these low farm prices is that they represent an easy way to transfer income. Popular as they are, such pricing policies are not an efficient way of transferring income to the poor.

Recall our discussion about policies that lower consumer prices, illustrated in Figure 18.1 of the last chapter. When a government policy also reduces producer prices, it gains the additional impact of discouraging domestic production. This is also illustrated by Figure 18.1. Because the

---

Box 19.1   Pricing Policies in World Agriculture

Anandarup Ray

Even a casual look at agricultural policies around the world reveals many surprising anomalies. In the United States, for example, the government pays farmers not to grow cereals; in the European Community (EC), farmers are paid to grow more. In Japan, rice farmers receive three times the world price for their crop. In 1985, farmers in the EC received 18 cents a pound (US) for sugar that was then sold on the world markets for 5 cents a pound; at the same time, the EC imported sugar at 18 cents a pound. Canadian farmers pay up to eight times the price of a cow for the right to sell that cow's milk at the government's support price.

In contrast to industrial market economies, developing countries tend to tax agriculture—even those low-income countries that depend critically on agriculture for their economic growth. Some pay their producers no more than half the world price for grains and then spend scarce foreign exchange to import food. Many subsidize consumption to help the poor, but end up reducing the incomes of farmers who are much poorer than many of the urban consumers who benefit from the subsidies.

Most developing countries pronounce self-sufficiency in food as an important objective, while taxing farmers and subsidizing consumers and thus increasing their dependence upon imported food. And in periods of economic adjustment, when shortages of foreign exchange make export promotion urgent, many have increased taxes on agricultural exports and cut producer support programs, while relying on unrestricted food imports to satisfy urban consumers.

Source: Extracted from Ray 1986:2.

---

domestic price of wheat is depressed below the world market price, farmers produce less than they would if they were paid the world market price. This loss of production is represented by triangle 2 in Figure 18.1.

■ IMPLICIT SUBSIDIES TO CONSUMERS/IMPLICIT TAXES ON FARMERS

Third World government activities that result in low (that is, below–world market) farm prices include: noncompetitive procurement of grain from farmers; below-market food prices set by law; foreign trade controls; support of an overvalued domestic currency; and limits on cash cropping. All these activities are carried out in the name of lower food prices, and all of them, in turn, amount to implicit food subsidies to consumers, and implicit taxes on farmers.

Third World implicit food subsidies are almost always paid for by the farm sector through the below-market food prices. The difference between the depressed price the producer gets for his food (depressed because of an implicit consumer subsidy program in operation) and the international price for that food is a hidden cost to the farmer. The farmer's contribution to the food subsidy represents an income transfer from the farmer to the recipient of the subsidized food.

In this way, farmers have sometimes paid the lion's share of a food subsidy. In Table 19.1 we see data on the distribution of costs of food subsidy systems in three South Asian countries—Sri Lanka, India, and Pakistan—during the 1970s. During the years cited, rationed food in these countries was available at about half the market price. In all three countries, but particularly in India and Pakistan (where producers were picking up the tab on over half the cost of the subsidy), part of the heavy burden of price subsidization was shifted to farmers through the use of forced government procurement at below-market prices. Marketing regulations such as administered prices also helped to keep producer's prices below world levels. India and Pakistan set prices in their fair-price ration shops at a high enough level to cover most of their procurement costs, administrative expenses, and possible losses on imports, leaving the rest of the cost of the subsidy to be borne by the farm population (Scandizzo & Tsakok 1985:60–76).

Because of their nature, most implicit food-linked income transfers are marketwide, but some can be and are, occasionally, targeted to low-income groups. We will now examine several commonly practiced programs that result in implicit, food-linked income transfers from farmers to the recipients of subsidized food.

☐ Noncompetitive Procurement

A number of countries have used compulsory procurement to obtain grain from farmers at below-market prices. In India, for instance, the Food Corporation of India (FCI) is empowered to obtain grain from farmers through compulsory means. State corporations often act as agents for the FCI for both procurement and later distribution through the "fair-price" shops. In 1981 in India there were about 280,000 fair-price shops distributing subsidized grain through a rationing program available to some 660 million people. During the 1980/81 agricultural year about 35 percent of the rice and 60 percent of the wheat sold in the market in India was procured by government agencies (George 1988).

Compulsory procurement amounts to a tax on the growers of the commodities procured. One problem is that it may motivate some farmers who have the opportunity, because of climate, soil, and topography, to switch from producing grain to producing nontaxed alternative crops, such as

Table 19.1 Extent and Cost of Food Subsidy Systems for Sri Lanka, India, and Pakistan, 1970s

| | Ration Price as Percentage of Open Market Price 1 | Quantity Rationed as Percentage of Total Consumption 2 | Per Capita Cost (U.S. dollars) 3 | Fiscal Cost of Subsidy to the Economy | | Budgetary Cost as Percentage of Total Expenditure 6 |
				Government's Share of Cost 4	Producer's Share of Cost 5	
Sri Lanka						
1974	48	46	15.01	68	32	17
1975	60	54	10.14	87	13	16
1976	65	53	7.02	89	11	—
India						
1974	47	15	7.88	10	90	—
1975	47	18	4.22	20	80	—
1976	60	13	3.54	10	90	—
Pakistan						
1974–75[a]	44	32	7.19	24	76	13
1975–76	55	27	7.34	45	55	11
1976–77	51	33	5.03	36	64	—

Sources: Ration price as percentage of open market price in Sri Lanka: Edirisinghe 1987:12; all other data: Scandizzo & Tsakok 1985:64.
Note: a. For Pakistan the cost estimate refers to the calendar year; for example, the 1974 estimate appears under 1974–75.

vegetables and fruits. Increasing the quantity supplied and thus lowering the price of vegetables and fruits benefits chiefly the high-income consumer. Low-income consumers do not spend much on these foods.

□ Administered Prices

In many Third World countries, farm-gate and retail food prices have been set by government regulation. An administered price may be fixed substantially below the international price. This ceiling price becomes the highest price that can legally be offered to farmers. When this price is below the market price it may be necessary to dissuade farmers from selling their crops on the black market by making it illegal for anyone but government representatives to purchase or transport the commodities covered by the ceiling price. This requires that government enter the marketing system as an active participant or at least license certain firms to do so.

Malcolm Bale (1985:13) describes how such a system of below-market ceiling prices worked in Pakistan in the decade prior to 1981, after which the administered prices were allowed to rise:

> The government sets a price at which it will buy wheat. Farmers may sell to government agents or private traders. The government buyers resell to ration shops at a fixed (low) price, which essentially sets the upper limit of the open market price. Private middlemen typically pay producers less than the government price because they provide extra services such as credit or transportation to growers. Wheat procured by the government is milled and sold by privately owned ration shops to ration card holders at the same price at which the government sells the flour to them. The ration shop covers costs and profits by selling the gunny bags in which flour is delivered. Until 1981, the government price of wheat was as much as 60 percent below the border price.

Pakistani wheat farmers were implicitly taxed, and Pakistani consumers were implicitly subsidized by the support prices. A similar program kept the price of rice in Pakistan at an average of 35 percent below the border price until the 1980s (Bale 1985).

In Tanzania, where, until recently, the government controlled most aspects of agricultural marketing, government-controlled farm prices were lowered between 1970 and 1984 so that the average of official producer prices declined 46 percent. Rising export taxes and the costs of the government marketing program reduced the farmers' share of final sales value of export crops to 41 percent in 1980. Output of some export crops (cashews, cotton, and pyrethrum) fell drastically in the 1970s. By 1984 the tonnage of export crops moving through the government marketing boards was 30 percent less than it had been in 1970 (World Bank 1986:74–75). The implicit tax on agriculture was a substantial disincentive to agricultural production.

A common aspect of administered prices has been pan-territorial and pan-seasonal pricing—that is, the practice of maintaining identical prices across time and place within the economy. The policy discourages private traders from storing food just after harvest and shifts the burden of storage, together with its costs, to the government. Jamaica practiced pan-pricing when, for several years prior to 1980, it placed a ceiling price on the retail price of wheat flour, all of which was imported. Most of the flour imported into Jamaica is landed at Kingston, and the administered ceiling price made it just barely profitable for supermarket operators in the city and suburbs to stock flour. But the cost of transporting the flour to remote markets in the mountains some distance from the port was greater than the legally allowed marketing margin. In time, the only flour available in many remote locations was black market flour, which sold at a considerable premium. Thus the rural poor ended up paying more for their flour than they would have paid without the government policy, while the urban rich found flour available at reasonable prices in their supermarkets.

☐ **Export Taxes**

Third World governments have placed taxes on the export of agricultural commodities. This not only generates revenue for the government but lowers the domestic price of the commodity, because exporters can pay farmers only the world price minus the export tax they have to pay to the government. The lower price can be a substantial disincentive to production. The government of Ghana set up its own Cocoa Marketing Board and gave it a monopoly on buying, transporting, and exporting cocoa. Then it undertook to raise significant tax revenue from cocoa exports. This combined with exchange-rate manipulations to raise the effective export duty on cocoa from a high of 54 percent in the last half of the 1960s to 90 percent in the last half of the 1970s. Domestic cocoa prices fell to levels far below those in competing cocoa-exporting countries, and Ghana's share of world cocoa exports fell from 40 percent in 1961–1963 to 18 percent in 1980–1982 (World Bank 1986:76).

From 1940 to 1972 the government of Argentina generally maintained a policy to keep agricultural prices low relative to the prices of nonagricultural goods. This was accomplished through a variety of measures that, in general, added up to a high tax on agricultural exports and a tariff on nonagricultural imports. This resulted in an implicit tax on agriculture that is estimated to have amounted to 50 percent of total agricultural output during the period. Among the consequences of this policy were that employment in agriculture declined, agriculture lost resources to nonagriculture, and agricultural productivity grew more slowly. In fact, per capita agricultural production in the 1970s was less than it was before World War II. And this in a country known for its excellent agricultural soils and climate and during a period when per capita world agricultural production was growing (Cavallo & Mundlak 1982:13–14).

☐ Overvalued Domestic Currency

In additon to skimming resources from the agricultural sector through export taxes on farm products, governments of developing countries have also engaged in activities that further tax agriculture through an over-valued exchange rate (Schuh 1988). Here is what typically happens: As economic development proceeds in a Third World country, local demand for attractive foreign goods usually becomes so great that a foreign currency deficit develops. People want lots of foreign currency so they can buy foreign-made goods, which ultimately must be paid for in foreign currency. (To simplify the discussion we will refer to local currency as rupees, a common Third World currency denominator, and to foreign currency as U.S. dollars, the standard currency of world trade.)

As the dollar deficit develops, the value of the rupee falls relative to the dollar. That is, you must spend more and more rupees to buy one dollar. As the value of the rupee falls, the cost (in terms of rupees) of imported goods rises. Government frequently attempts to stop this progression by fixing into local law the price of rupees relative to the dollar. This fixed ratio becomes the official exchange rate. As the free-market value of the rupee continues to fall, government usually defends the exchange rate by discouraging the purchase of foreign goods. It does this by such measures as requiring that approved buyers obtain a license to buy dollars (at the official exchange rate) from the central bank; placing quotas on imports; and placing high tariffs on imports. The limitations on imports serve to protect domestic industry by cutting back on foreign competition and by raising the local price for industrial products. (For the level of protection afforded to industry in selected countries, see Table 19.2.) One result of this, of course, is that prices rise on the inputs that farmers use for increasing their production, such as fertilizers, irrigation pumps, and pesticides, whether foreign or domestic. But perhaps more important to farm profitability is what it does to the prices of farm products that are exported.

Let us assume that rice costs \$0.25 per pound on the world market. And let us further assume that the official exchange rate is Rs 6 to \$1. A dollar will buy four pounds of rice on the world market, and Rs 6 will buy four pounds. The local farmer can therefore export his rice at Rs 1.50 a pound (assuming no export tax).

But let us also assume that, because of the continued deterioration in the free-market value of the rupee, it now takes Rs 10 to buy a dollar on the unofficial market. The value of a pound of rice on the international market is really Rs 2.50 (Rs 10 equals \$1, so four pounds of rice are really worth Rs 2.50 a pound at the market rate). The farmer who exports his rice

Table 19.2   **Protection of Agriculture Compared with Manufacturing in Selected Developing Countries**

	Year	Relative Protection Ratio[a]
Philippines	1974	0.76
Colombia	1978	0.49
Mexico	1980	0.88
Nigeria	1980	0.35
Egypt	1981	0.57
Turkey	1981	0.77
Ecuador	1983	0.65

Source: World Bank 1986:62.
Note: A ratio of 1.00 indicates that effective protection is equal in both sectors; a ratio less than 1.00 means that protection is in favor of manufacturing.
a. Calculated as $(1 + EPR_a)/(1 + EPR_m)$, where EPR_a and EPR_m are the effective rates of protection for agriculture and the manufacturing sector, respectively.

at Rs 1.50 a pound because he gets only the official exchange rate for his rice is being taxed Rp 1 per pound for his exports. Since the export price sets the domestic price, the farmer who sells on the domestic market is also being taxed Rp 1 per pound for his sales. The domestic consumer receives the benefit of the tax when he purchases the rice at Rs 1.50 rather than at the world price of Rs 2.50.

When you combine the implicit tax resulting from the overvalued domestic currency with an explicit export tax and thus force farm prices well below the international market, and when, in addition to this, you throw in the condition that the farmer is required to pay more than the world price for his modern purchased inputs, you have a recipe for a substantial disincentive to agricultural production.

Malcolm Bale (1985:24) studied five developing countries from the point of view of the impact of overvalued domestic currency on agricultural production. He found that

> The extent to which currencies are misaligned in most developing countries is not widely recognized, and certainly its effect on output is not generally appreciated by their policy makers. For example, in the Philippines during most of the 1970s, the exchange rate was overvalued by an estimated 25–30 percent; in Jamaica during the early 1980s by 35 percent; in Colombia in the early 1980s by about 25 percent; and in Nigeria during the past five years by 44 percent. When margins of less than 10 percent determine the outcome of a sale or a profit, the effect of implicit taxes of these dimensions on domestic agriculture can be devastating.
>
> The results of these World Bank studies show that misaligned exchange rates have played the prime role in inhibiting agricultural performance.

In a study of the impact of trade and exchange-rate policies on agricultural production incentives in the Philippines, it was found that a 10 percent rise in the domestic price of imported goods (caused by tariffs, for example) results in a 6.6 percent decline in the domestic price of agricultural export products relative to home goods (Bautista 1987:9).

Thirty-one countries of sub-Saharan Africa, for which data on changes in the degree of overvaluation of domestic currency were available, were examined for the relationship between these changes and agricultural productivity. The countries fell into two groups of approximately equal size, those whose degree of overvaluation was lessening and those whose degree of overvaluation was increasing. Those countries found to be lessening the degree of overvaluation of their domestic currency were found to be increasing their agricultural production, on the average, at 2.4 times the rate of those who were increasing the degree of overvaluation of their currency (Cleaver 1985:18–19).

□ Limits on Cash Cropping

A *cash crop* is one that is produced for sale. The commercial orientation of the crop (regardless of whether it is a food or a nonfood crop) identifies it as a cash crop. An *export crop* is, of course, a particular kind of cash crop: one that is ultimately exported from a country (von Braun & Kennedy 1986:1). In contrast to cash crops, those grown by farm families for their own consumption are called *subsistence crops*.

It is often argued that the growing of cash crops, and in particular, the growing of cash crops for export, limits the local food supply and therefore raises local food prices. So limits on growing cash crops for export from Third World countries are often proposed as a means of forcing a shift in cultivation to food crops, thereby lowering the local price of food.

Lappe and Collins (1977), proponents of this point of view, quote a Colombian government economist as estimating that, in Colombia, "one hectare planted with carnations brings in a million pesos a year; planted with wheat or corn, the same hectare would bring only 12,500." In other words the gross returns from a field of carnations in Colombia are 80 times the gross returns from grain. These authors assume that growing carnations for export will automatically raise local food prices through limiting the local food supply, and observe, rather sarcastically, that, "if the local peasants cannot afford chicken or eggs, perhaps they can brighten their shacks with cut flowers" (p. 266).

The argument that growing cut flowers in Colombia deprives the local peasants of their food supply misses a couple of important points: (1) Colombians can purchase a lot more grain from the United States (the recipient of the cut flowers) in exchange for a field of carnations than they can raise on that field themselves; (2) the cut-flower industry is highly labor-intensive. Regardless of who owns or manages the field of carnations, many more peasants are going to be employed to produce an acre of cut flowers than to produce an acre of grain.

What happens when Third World farmers do expand their production of cash crops? Let us look at the evidence from recent studies.

Kennedy and Cogill (1987) studied smallholders in a low-income farming region in southern Kenya. These farmers were reducing their activities in subsistence agriculture and increasing their commercial sugarcane production. As sugarcane acreage expanded it replaced maize acreage. However, the return to labor for sugar was three times the daily agricultural wage rate and significantly higher than the return to maize. Incomes of the farmers who had joined the cane-growing scheme were significantly higher than those of nonsugar farmers, and the increased income positively affected household calorie consumption. For each 1 percent increase in sugarcane income, household energy intake was found to increase by 24 calories (p. 9). The increase in household calorie intake translated into modest increases in calorie intake among the children (Kennedy 1989:54). The expansion of the sugar industry in the area also increased employment. Typically the sugar mill hired laborers and supplied them to the sugar farmer for such tasks as weeding, cutting the cane, and transporting the cut cane to the mill (Kennedy & Cogill 1987:9).

Bouis and Haddad (1990) studied families in an area of Mindanao, in the Philippines, where a sugar mill had been introduced seven years earlier. Among those who had access to land, all households grew corn but some had switched part of their acreage from corn to sugar. Women were found to be more involved in corn production than in sugar production, contributing 23 percent of the total labor going into corn production, but only 11 percent of the total labor going into sugar production. During breast-feeding, wives in households that grew some sugar spent less time away from home, more time at child care, and less time in field work. The youngest children in sugar households grew significantly taller than the same age group in corn households.

In a study that looked at the household-level effects of cash cropping in rural Guatemala, von Braun and his colleagues (1989) surveyed 400 households, about half of which had recently started raising nontraditional vegetable crops for export. The nontraditional export crops were substantially more profitable than traditional crops and were adopted by even the smallest farmers. Net returns per acre from one of the export crops, snow peas, averaged 15 times those of maize, the most important traditional crop. Returns per unit of family labor for the new crops in general were about twice as high as for maize and 60 percent higher than those for traditional vegetables.

Because the export crop producers produced yields for their subsistence food crops some 30 percent higher than the nonexport crop yields of their neighbors, the export crop producers usually had larger amounts of maize and beans available, per capita, for home consumption. Among the reasons for their higher yields was their purchase and use of fertilizer; thus, their increased incomes helped increase yields on their subsistence crops. Nontraditional export crops enhance local employment, not only on the farm (see Figure 19.1) but also, through backward and forward linkages, off the farm. The farmers purchase locally manufactured sticks and ropes for tying snow pea plants, for instance. And the marketing of the vegetables for export is labor-intensive, requiring such tasks as selection, grading, and packing of the produce (von Braun et al. 1989:11–12, 48).

In a statistical analysis of 78 developing countries that devote at least part of their farmland to cash crops, von Braun and Kennedy (1986:2) did not find support for the hypothesis that the expansion of cash cropping happens at the expense of producing staples. To the contrary, growth in areas allocated to cash crops positively correlated with growth in staple food production. Furthermore, growth in share of cropland allocated to cash crops is generally positively associated with per capita staple food production.

We can reasonably argue that limiting cash crop production may, in fact, limit rural incomes and create adverse affects on nutrition. Unfortunately, the advantages of export crop production in the Third World are often neglected by policymakers (see Box 19.2).

Figure 19.1   Labor Inputs for Traditional Crops (Maize and Traditional Vegetables) and New Export Vegetables (Broccoli, Cauliflower, and Snow Peas), Guatemala, 1985

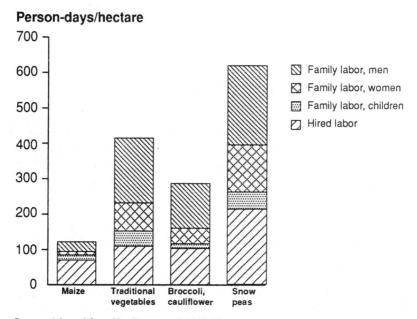

Source: Adapted from Von Braun et al. 1989:49.

Box 19.2   Export Crops and Food Crops

Uma J. Lele

Development debates and government and donor policies have not stressed the critical role of agriculture for the development of the rest of the economy. Instead of promoting policies that support balanced development of the agricultural sector as a whole, they have tended to emphasize the conflict between food and export crop production.

The attainment of food security is of fundamental importance in the farming decisions of small rural households. Assured food crop production releases land and labor for diversification into other higher-value production for domestic use or export. Export crop production, however, helps raise and stabilize household and national income, thereby increasing food security.

Due to labor intensity, export crops tend to generate greater employment than food cropping. Moreover, the production of most export crops tends to be scale-neutral and therefore can be undertaken by farmers with holdings of any size. Despite these features, export crops were neglected by both governments and donors in the 1970s.

Source: Extracted from Lele, n.d.

■ FARM TAXATION VERSUS IMPLICIT FOOD SUBSIDIES

Government must be financed. And the taxation system that finances government should not only be fair, it should be economically efficient. For efficiency and fairness, all sectors of the economy must bear a portion of the total tax burden, and the tax incidence should fall proportionally across all sectors. Of course agriculture should be taxed. The problem in the Third World is how to avoid *excessive* taxation of agriculture.

We have seen that producers are commonly taxed as much as 50 percent or more on farm commodities that are involved in implicit food subsidy programs (see India data, columns 1 and 5 of Table 19.1). Rates of export taxation to the order of 50 to 75 percent for farm products have not been unusual (World Bank 1986:64).

It is inequitable to place such a heavy tax burden on the agricultural sector when other sectors are taxed at a lower rate or even subsidized with protective import measures. And it is inefficient. Placing an unduly heavy tax burden on agriculture steers productive resources away from this sector and slows productivity within agriculture. The resources lost to agriculture would have yielded a higher return to society in agriculture than they will at the margin in a protected industrial sector. The growth rate of per capita income slows, and to the extent that such policies exacerbate unemployment, the poor suffer more than do the rich.

There are explicit tax alternatives to the implicit taxes on agriculture: taxing agricultural land; taxing agricultural income; and taxing agricultural commodities at the point of consumption rather than lowering farm-gate prices. Because these explicit taxes are readily identifiable, they are more likely to be applied equitably relative to other sectors of the economy than are implicit taxes. And because they are not commodity-specific, they do not favor the production of one agricultural commodity over another. For both of these reasons they are more economically efficient than are implicit taxes.

Complaints about the high administrative costs of taxing agricultural land have been used to explain why this method of taxing agriculture has fallen out of favor. Such complaints are hard to justify. It is, after all, fairly easy to determine who has an economic interest in farming the land; the sort of title search that may be necessary during the transfer of landownership is unnecessary for tax purposes. Market prices can be a ready guide to the value of the land, and satellite imagery now provides a cheap means of sorting out which regions have access to irrigation water or are growing which crops. Setting up an equitable system of land taxation today is technically feasible and not unduly expensive.

It is possible to tax agricultural income, especially income from the large agricultural holdings. In Latin America, 1 percent of the population controls over 50 percent of the land, and the operations of these landholders account for more than one-sixth of the gross national product for the area (World Bank 1986:83). The income of these large landholders would be fairly easy to identify for taxation. For large agricultural corporations, the personal income tax can be used to tax employees and the corporation profits tax can be used to tax the business itself. As the tax collection system improves it can be extended downward toward the smaller farmers, as appropriate.

Taxing agricultural commodities at the retail level instead of at the farm gate puts a greater burden on the wealthy than on the poor, because the wealthy are more likely to purchase their food at a retail outlet where the tax is collected.

Shifting from implicit taxes on agriculture to explicit taxes does not have to cause the demise of all food-linked income transfer programs. Such programs can be financed by explicit means using money in the public tax till. This type of financing has the advantage of providing considerable motivation to the framers of the food subsidy to target it carefully toward the most needy.

■ THE COSTS OF URBAN BIAS

When Third World governments adopt policies that lower the price of farm outputs and raise the price of industrial products, they are demonstrating a preference for industrial development over agricultural development. This preference for industry or, more broadly, for the people and resources concentrated in the cities, is sometimes called *urban bias*.

Societies pay a heavy price for urban bias. As governments encourage the substitution of locally made industrial goods for imported goods (the policy is sometimes called *import substitution* for short), the growth rate of the entire economy is inhibited. In a worldwide study of the effects of such policies, Chenery, Robinson, and Syrquin (1986:356–358) found that "economies which pursued export led growth—as opposed to a strategy of import substitution—grew faster, industrialized sooner, had higher rates of total factor productivity growth, and tended to achieve the input-output structure of an advanced economy faster." These researchers showed that shifting away from a tariff-induced import substitution trade policy to a neutral trade policy can account for an increase of as much as one percentage point in annual rate of growth of the entire economy. They further found that export-led economies are more likely to attract capital inflows. This helps to explain the success of such export-oriented economies as Korea and Taiwan.

A common aspect of Third World urban bias is the implicit taxation of grain, which is often the leading agricultural product. Taxing one commodity or set of commodities to the exclusion of others shifts resource use in the direction of the untaxed commodities. When the taxed commodity is grain (the diet of the poor), the tax encourages the production of nongrain foods such as livestock products (livestock can eat the grain before it is taxed), fruits, and vegetables—favorites of the rich. It is hard to make a case that there is any nutritional gain in lowering the price of foods for the rich while limiting the production of the chief foods of the poor.

But perhaps the ultimate problem with urban bias is that, as it slows the growth of the entire economy, it deprives the poorest not only of jobs but of possible income transfers from the rich to programs that would improve the welfare of the poorest.

Urban bias and its accompanying discrimination against the poor has been widely and loudly criticized, but never more eloquently than by Michael Lipton (see Box 19.3).

A five-volume World Bank study (Krueger, Schiff & Valdes 1991) confirmed the policy bias against agriculture in great detail. A synopsis of the findings of that study are found in a 1995 article by Schiff and Valdes. They concluded that (for the 18 countries in their study), compared to non-agricultural prices, agricultural prices were 43 percent lower than they would have been in the absence of policies biased against the rural sector.

Box 19.3   Urban Bias in World Development

Michael Lipton

The most important class conflict in the poor countries of the world today is not between labor and capital. Nor is it between foreign and national interests. It is between the rural classes and the urban classes. The rural sector contains most of the poverty, and most of the low-cost sources of potential advance; but the urban sector contains most of the articulateness, organization, and power.

So the urban classes have been able to "win" most of the rounds of the struggle with the countryside; but in so doing they have made the development process needlessly slow and unfair. Scarce investment, instead of going into water-pumps to grow rice, is wasted on urban super-highways. Scarce human skills design and administer not clean village wells and agricultural extension services, but world boxing championships in showpiece stadia.

The poor—between one-quarter and one-fifth of the people of the world—are overwhelmingly rural: landless laborers, or farmers with no more than an acre or two, who must supplement their income by wage labor.

The disparity between urban and rural welfare is much greater in poor countries now than it was in rich countries during their early development. This huge welfare gap is demonstrably inefficient, as well as inequitable. It persists mainly because less than 20 percent of investment for development has gone to the agricultural sector, although over 65 percent of the people of Third World countries, and over 80 percent of the really poor who live on $1 a week each or less, depend for a living on agriculture.

In most Third World countries, governments have undertaken numerous measures with the unhappy side-effect of accentuating rural-urban disparities: their own allocation of public expenditure and taxation; measures raising the price of industrial products relative to farm products, thus encouraging private rural saving to flow into industrial investment because the value of industrial output has been artificially boosted; and educational facilities encouraging bright villagers to train in cities for urban jobs.

Such processes have been extremely inefficient. For instance, the impact on output of $1 of carefully selected investment is, in most countries, two to three times as high in agriculture as elsewhere, yet public policy and private market power have combined to push domestic savings and foreign aid into non-agricultural uses.

Urban bias also increases inefficiency and inequity *within* the sectors. Poor farmers have little land and much under-used family labor. Hence they tend to complement any extra developmental resources received—pumpsets, fertilizers, virgin land—with much more extra labor than do large farmers. Poor farmers thus tend to get the most output from such extra resources (as well as needing the extra income most). But rich farmers (because they sell their extra output to the cities instead of eating it themselves, and because they are likely to use much of their extra income to support urban investment) are naturally favored by urban-biased policies. It is they, not the efficient small farmers, who get the cheap loans and the fertilizer subsidies.

(continues)

Box 19.3   Continued

But am I not hammering at an open door? Certainly the persiflage of allocation has changed recently, under the impact of patently damaging deficiencies in rural output. Development plans are nowadays full of "top priority for agriculture." This is reminiscent of the pseudo-egalitarian school where, at mealtimes, Class B children get priority, while Class A children get food.

It is *not* my wish to *overstate* the case for reducing urban bias. Such a reduction is not the *only* thing necessary. But a shift of resources to the rural sector, and within it to the efficient rural poor even if they do very little for urban development is often, perhaps usually, the *overriding* developmental task.

Urban bias does not rest on a conspiracy, but on convergent interests. Industrialists, urban workers, even big farmers, *all* benefit if agriculture gets squeezed, provided its few resources are steered, heavily subsidized, to the big farmer, to produce cheap food and raw materials for the cities. Nobody conspires; all the powerful are satisfied; the labor-intensive small farmer stays efficient, poor and powerless, and had better shut up. Meanwhile, the economist, often in the blinkers of industrial determinism, congratulates all concerned on resolutely extracting an agricultural surplus to finance industrialization.

Source: Reprinted by permission of the publishers from *Why Poor People Stay Poor: Urban Bias in World Development* by Michael Lipton, Cambridge, Mass.: Harvard University Press, copyright © 1976 by Michael Lipton.

Since the mid-1980s, a substantial shift has ocurred in the emphasis of developing country policies to eliminate much of the urban bias.

In a recent article reviewing the literature on agricultural policies in developing countries, Binswanger and Deininger (1997) explore the conditions under which policy reforms are likely to be initiated. They observe that "a fiscal crisis is usually necessary for initiating reform"—the efficiency costs of the urban bias must become high enough to have an impact on the government budgeting process. They argue that the sustainability of the reform effort depends on: (1) whether people who benefit from the reform are organized into groups that can exercise some political clout; (2) whether the central bank and ministry of finance have the will and power to maintain budgetary discipline; (3) whether the reform effort is encouraged by international credit and advice; and (4) whether policy analysts can support the reforms without succumbing to political pressures.

□ 20

Policies Aimed at Lowering the Price of Food by Increasing the Supply

While the most important reasons for inadequate agricultural output are difficult to ascertain, T. W. Schultz, in the first Elmhurst Memorial Lecture to the International Association of Agricultural Economists, left no doubt as to his ranking of the causes. He stated that the level of agricultural production depends not so much on technical considerations, but in large measure, "on what governments do to agriculture."
—Bale & Lutz 1981:8

Lack of purchasing power—food prices that are high relative to income—is one of the leading causes of undernutrition. In Chapters 18 and 19, we reviewed policies aimed at lowering the consumer price of food. In this chapter we examine policies designed to lower food prices by increasing the supply of food. In developing countries, increasing the supply of locally grown food would not only bring down the local price of food but would reduce dependence on food imports, allow these countries to build up reserve stocks of food against future bad crop years, and enhance their opportunities for food exports.

Before proceeding, we will define the distinction between *increasing the supply of food* and *increasing the quantity of food supplied*. The second term refers to the farm sector's response to an increase in food price—when prices go up, farmers produce more food. Obviously, it is internally inconsistent to claim that this (an increase in food prices) will drive food prices down. The only way this could happen is if the government intervened in the market. Government programs can create a situation in which the seller receives more than the buyer pays; the government makes up the difference. These types of policies will be discussed in the first section below.

An *increase in the supply of food*—or as economists call it, an *outward shift in supply curve*—refers to a different kind of response by the

319

farm sector: that farmers are now willing to produce more food at the same price, or are willing to produce the same amount of food at a lower price. This is the type of change that would permit the quantity of food to increase while the price of food declines. What would make a farmer willing to produce more at the same price, or produce the same amount at a lower price? A reduction in the farmer's costs of production. And how can we reduce food production costs? By reducing prices farmers pay for inputs, by encouraging investment, and by developing new technologies that increase farm productivity. Policies to achieve these objectives will be considered in later sections of this chapter.

◼ SUBSIDIZING PRICES OF FARM OUTPUT

In Chapter 18, we saw how government subsidies could reduce the price paid by consumers without reducing the price received by farmers. In this section, we look at a different kind of policy—one that increases the price received by farmers without increasing the price paid by consumers. The government can institute this policy through three mechanisms: government purchases, deficiency payments, and processor-handler subsidies.

When the government purchases and resells a food commodity, it can pay farmers more than it charges consumers, and use government funds to make up the difference. This type of policy has been implemented in countries where the government was the sole buying agent for a food commodity, as described in Chapter 18. The government can also raise farm prices by setting a support price, or price floor, and buying up whatever quantity is offered at that price. Farmers will sell to the government at the support price unless and until the price offered by private buyers rises above the support price. Thus, typically, the government will buy some of the farm output, and the private sector will buy the remainder. For the quantity bought by the private sector, consumer prices will rise along with producer prices. However, the quantity purchased by the government can be sold at a loss, at lower consumer prices. Of course, for this to work, the consumers who buy from the government have to be separate from the consumers who buy from the private sector. This separation usually takes the form of a ration card that allows low-income households to buy from the government at below-market prices. (See the discussion on targeted consumer price subsidies in Chapter 18.)

Deficiency payments are the simplest form of subsidy to producers. Farmers sell their output on the private market, and receive market price. Then the farmer receives an additional amount of money from the government. This kind of program is illustrated in Figure 20.1. Because farmers are receiving a payment in addition to the market price, they increase their production; for them to sell the increased quantity to consumers, consumer prices must drop. Thus, the effect of the deficiency payment is to raise prices to farmers, reduce prices paid by consumers, and increase quantity produced.

The same results shown in Figure 20.1 can be achieved by paying a subsidy to processors or handlers of the commodity. The subsidy makes it possible for private sector businesses to pay more to farmers and to charge less to consumers. Processor subsidies have the advantage of being easier to administrate: Instead of auditing the output of thousands of farmers and making a payment to each farmer, the program deals with fewer processor-handlers. These programs tend to be less popular politically than deficiency payments because people would rather see direct government payments go to small farmers than to large processing corporations.

Subsidies paid to farmers reduce economic efficiency. As the quantity produced increases above the market quantity, the cost of producing an additional unit exceeds the value that consumers get from consuming the additional unit. The quantity of this efficiency cost is shown as triangle 1 in Figure 20.1. Subsidies also have a direct cost paid by the government. This is the amount paid per unit (producer price minus consumer price) times the number of units. This cost is shown as rectangle ABCD in Figure 20.1.

As you can see from Figure 20.1, if the supply and demand curves are very steeply sloped, it will be very costly for the government to gain a

Figure 20.1   Impact of a Deficiency Payment Program: Higher Producer Price, Lower Consumer Price, and Higher Quantity

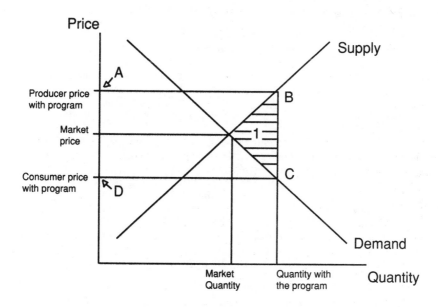

noticeable increase in quantity produced. The steepness of the supply curve is measured by the elasticity of supply (see Box 20.1).

Because both food supply and demand are inelastic, output price subsidies can become very expensive for governments. To see this, consider a hypothetical country with a supply elasticity for a basic food commodity of 0.5 and a demand elasticity for the commodity of 0.2. For the government to gain a 1 percent increase in output, farm price will have to increase by 2 percent; for the consumer to buy the increased output, consumer price will have to drop by 5 percent. Therefore, to obtain a 1

Box 20.1 Elasticity of Supply

Elasticity of supply with respect to price is the percentage change in quantity supplied to the market given a 1 percent change in price. In contrast with demand elasticities with respect to price, supply elasticities are positive; as price increases, quantity supplied increases. In Table 20.1 we see some short-run supply elasticities for several farm products in African countries. (The short run, in this case, refers to land and other fixed inputs such as tube wells not being allowed to vary in the elasticity analysis.)

Although the evidence is not conclusive, it appears that agricultural supply elasticities are somewhat higher in the developed world than in the Third World (Askari & Cummings 1976; Herdt 1970:518–519), indicating that Third World farmers are somewhat less responsive to changes in prices than are farmers in the developed world. If this is the case, it is most likely explained by three characteristics of Third World farmers: (1) They are less involved in the market economy—they sell a smaller percentage of their production and therefore are less impressed by swings in market prices; (2) they use lower quantities of purchased inputs relative to output sold and are therefore less able to adjust their production to variations in market prices; (3) they are more risk-averse than farmers in the developed world—they do not like spending large amounts on purchased inputs when a chance exists that, because of low prices, the investment may not pay off. Nevertheless, hundreds of estimates of supply response to price among Third World farmers have generally shown a positive relationship between price and production (Askari & Cummings 1976).

Similar results are obtained for long-run aggregate supply elasticities; that is, the percentage that aggregate farm output changes with a 1 percent change in real farm prices. (Aggregate supply elasticities are called long-run when all inputs, including land and major capital items, are allowed to vary with price changes. Because all inputs are allowed to vary, long-run supply elasticities are generally higher than short-run supply elasticities.) In the Third World the aggregate supply elasticity of agriculture with respect to price appears to range between 0.3 and 0.9. More-advanced Third World countries tend to have aggregate supply elasticities in the 0.6 to 0.9 range while the less-advanced countries, with poorer infrastructure, tend to fall in the range around 0.3 and 0.5 (Chhibber 1988).

Table 20.1 Short-Run Supply Elasticities, Selected Crops, African Countries

	Elasticity
Wheat	.31
Maize	.23
Sorghum	.10
Groundnuts	.24
Cotton	.23
Tobacco	.48
Cocoa	.15
Coffee	.14
Rubber	.14

Source: World Bank 1986:68; data are derived from Askari & Cummings 1976 and Scandizzo & Bruce 1980.

percent increase in output, the government will pay about 7 percent of the total amount consumers formerly spent on the food commodity.

■ SUBSIDIES FOR PURCHASED INPUTS

For the remainder of this chapter, we consider policies that are intended to shift the supply curve for food out and to the right, as illustrated in Figure 20.2. As mentioned in the introduction to this chapter, such shifts

Figure 20.2   Effect of Reduced Costs or Improved Technology on the Supply Curve

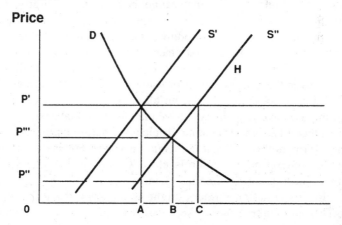

Note: When the supply curve shifts from S' to S", farmers are willing to furnish to the market: (1) an increased quantity (OC rather than OA) at the same old price (P'); (2) the same old quantity (OA) at a new prices (P"); or (3) some other combination of quantity and price—for instance, the quantity and price represented by point H on the diagram.

occur when the costs of production are reduced; therefore, the rest of the chapter will deal with policies that reduce production costs.

The most direct and obvious way to reduce production costs is to subsidize the prices farmers pay for inputs. The government can do this by compensating farmers for each unit of inputs purchased, by subsidizing the production of inputs, or by producing or distributing the inputs themselves. In this section, we will briefly explore programs that subsidize irrigation, fertilizer, and mechanization.

□ Irrigation

Publicly sponsored irrigation systems date back some 6,000 years, to when vast irrigation works were developed for the flood plain of the Tigris and Euphrates rivers in Mesopotamia. In modern times, huge dams thrown across major rivers throughout the world (the Nile, the Indus, and the Colorado, for example) have furnished low-cost irrigation water to millions of farmers. Cost-benefit analysis has shown substantial gains to society from such projects, which usually are promoted for their multiplicity of benefits—flood control, electricity generation, and irrigation water for agriculture.

In most countries, government subsidizes irrigation water. In Egypt it is free. In the Philippines, during 1980–1981, the subsidy amounted to 90 percent of the marginal cost (Bale 1985:17). We can argue that there is no need to charge the water users for the cost of the dam; without government sponsorship, the dam would not have been built. There is no efficiency gain to society in asking water recipients to pay for the dam. Once the resources are sunk into the dam, they cannot be moved, so charging users for the dam does not alter the decision on whether or not to make the investment. (This discussion does not address the question of whether the dam should have been built in the first place.)

Once the dam is built, a couple of conditions make it illogical to charge for even the marginal costs of water delivery to the farmer: (1) The water supply is so abundant that no allocation problem exists; and (2) monitoring use may be more expensive than the marginal cost of the water. In most other situations economic efficiency would be improved through charging farmers the full cost of irrigation water. For instance, in areas where the underground aquifer is close to the surface and is rapidly recharged, such as on the Ganges plain in India, tube wells give a high payoff. In this situation farmers might as well pay the full cost of the water. This will make it more likely that resources are being allocated to their highest-valued use for society.

Concerns that the introduction of irrigation and the modern technologies that go with it will lead to increased inequalities in income distribution have proved unfounded. Irrigation was found to increase substantially the income of all sectors of production, although the increases to land, fixed capital, and purchased inputs appear to be higher than those to labor and management. Just the same, poor people benefit substantially from irrigation. Gains in labor income resulting from irrigation ranged from 12 percent in the Philippines to over 400 percent in Thailand (where dry-season irrigation doubles the cropping intensity, and wet-season labor use is higher in irrigated than in nonirrigated areas) (Rosegrant 1986).

☐ **Fertilizer and Farm Chemicals**

Fertilizer subsidies are common in the Third World. During the 1980s, for example, urea sold at 56 percent below cost in Sri Lanka and at 60 percent below cost in Gambia. A long list of arguments favoring subsidies to fertilizer include encouraging learning by doing; overcoming risk aversion and credit constraints; helping poor farmers; offsetting disincentives caused by taxing or pricing policies; and maintaining soil fertility (World Bank 1986:95). Let us look briefly at each of these arguments.

- When fertilizer was a new idea, it made sense to provide it to farmers at below cost as an incentive to try it. But knowledge of fertilizer is widespread now.
- As we will discuss below, encouraging rural financial markets is the most appropriate way to deal with rural credit constraints.
- Fertilizer subsidies are an inefficient way to help poor farmers. Farmers with large operations, and those on better land, are likely to reap more benefits than the poor farmers. Examine Table 20.2 with a view to the distribution of benefits from a fertilizer subsidy among soybean farmers in Brazil.

Table 20.2 Soybean Producers and Production in Brazil, 1975

Size of Farm (Hectares)	Number of Farms	Total Production in Thousands of Metric Tons
0–10	162,859	594
10–20	149,288	1,134
20–50	127,331	1,976
50–100	26,709	1,127
100–200	10,301	1,042
200–500	6,552	1,284
500–1,000	2,286	794
1,000–10,000	1,518	650
10,000–100,000	25	16
Total	486,872	8,721

Source: Leclercq 1988:Annex 1, Table 6.

- The best way to cope with production disincentives caused by antifarm taxation or pricing policies is to eliminate urban bias. Subsidizing the price of fertilizer is an inequitable way to transfer income to the farm sector because it provides the greatest subsidy to the biggest farmers.
- Subsidizing fertilizer use to maintain soil fertility is a questionable practice, especially when making fertilizer cheap encourages farmers to substitute it for naturally occurring organic fertilizers that have better moisture-retaining properties.

Similarly, making pesticides cheap through subsidization encourages farmers to use more of the chemicals than they would if they paid the full costs. The subsidies undermine efforts to promote integrated pest management—a method of pest control that stresses biological suppression of insects and weeds and minimal use of chemical pesticides (Repetto 1985; U.S. Dept. of Agriculture 1989a).

As fertilizer use increases, scarcities often develop as the government-subsidized distribution falls behind demand. Furthermore, the cost of the fertilizer subsidy can become a major concern to government. Concern over the budgetary costs of the fertilizer subsidy in Bangladesh prompted a study of the production impact of removing the subsidy. On the one hand, it was found that eliminating the subsidy would result in an increase in the domestic price of fertilizer some 34 percent over what it would have been during 1983–1984, and that this increase in price would result in a decrease in fertilizer use. On the other hand, several factors were found to be of even greater importance than the fertilizer subsidy in stimulating fertilizer use and farm production in Bangladesh. Many of these factors were related (because of the subsidy to fertilizer) to the government's involvement in the distribution of fertilizer, with its attendant bureaucratic inefficiencies.

☐ Mechanization

Many developing countries have pursued a mix of policies that tend to accelerate mechanization beyond the pace appropriate for their labor force (Binswanger, Donovan et al. 1987:1). They do this in a variety of ways.

Governments often give preferential tariff treatment for machinery, and especially low tariffs for agricultural machinery. Farmers are sometimes given a tax shelter through deductions for farm machinery set at levels greater than the cost of the machinery. Brazil, for instance, has allowed a deduction for farm machinery of six times the value of the machine in the first year of operation. Other farm investments are treated less favorably, and labor costs enjoy no preferential tax treatment at all (World Bank 1986:97).

Countries often set the official exchange rate for their domestic currency higher than the market value. The market value for a rupee in India, for example, might be 10 (U.S.) cents, but the Indian government might declare a rupee to be worth more, say 15 cents. The upshot of this artificially inflated exchange rate is that, if you can get dollars from the government at the official rate, you can buy goods, like machinery or food, from abroad at bargain prices. When this happens, competition immediately arises for these cheap dollars, and the government has to ration them among competing uses. Commonly, agricultural machinery imports receive a substantial allocation. Cheap foreign currency and low tariffs make a substantial subsidy to imported machinery. In addition, subsidized credit (discussed below) makes capital cheaper than it otherwise would be.

The desirability of machinery subsidies has been questioned on several points. First, the benefits of machinery subsidies typically go to large farms. Thus they provide the wealthy farmers with a competitive advantage relative to their poorer neighbors. Second, mechanization does not necessarily increase yields. Binswanger (1978:73), in a careful review of the studies concerning the impact of tractorization on yields in South Asia, found that the surveys failed "to provide evidence that tractors are responsible for substantial increases in intensity, yields, timeliness, and gross returns on farms in India, Pakistan, and Nepal." It seems that, by and large, an acre of land tilled by hand or animal power does not yield less than an acre of land tilled by a tractor (Campbell 1984:47).

From the point of view of improving Third World nutrition, there can be no justification for a machinery subsidy. When machinery is profitable, farmers will buy it and society will benefit from it. If the machinery is available only in fairly large units, small farmers can benefit from using rented machinery.

Subsidizing agricultural mechanization denies funding for alternative investments that are at least as productive as the machinery and that do not reduce labor demand as much as the subsidized machinery (Binswanger, Donovan et al. 1987:1).

Stevens and Jabara (1988:272–273) list four undesirable effects from premature acceleration of agricultural mechanization resulting from subsidies: (1) reduced employment; (2) greater income disparities; (3) attempts by those with tractors and other machines to increase farm size; and (4) increased incentives to inventors and manufacturers to develop and produce even more labor-saving agricultural machinery.

■ CREDIT SUBSIDIES

□ Rationale for Subsidizing Credit

To the extent that credit can remove existing financial constraints, it can accelerate the use of capital equipment and the adoption of new technology. Third World governments commonly feel that a scarcity of credit is constraining the development of their low-income farm sector and see subsidized credit as a way of transferring income to the poor, who will then benefit by becoming more productive through the use of this cheap credit. Furthermore, as described in Chapter 19, these same governments often engage in policies that result in farm-gate prices below those the market would normally pay, and look to subsidized credit, with its below-market interest rates, as a way of compensating low-income farmers for their losses from these pricing policies (Adams et al. 1984).

Billions of dollars have been spent on subsidized credit programs in the Third World. These programs have arisen because of a number of assumptions about peasant farmers as savers and borrowers and about the credit sources that are commonly available to them. For instance, it is commonly assumed that, despite their ability to repay a loan, small farmers have difficulty obtaining loans because of a lack of collateral or the feeling among rural lenders that small farmers present too great a risk.

Dale Adams and others, having reviewed these assumptions, concluded that many of them are erroneous (see Box 20.2). To take just one example, the assumption about collateral and small farmers presenting too great a risk: The Grameen Bank—an innovative bank in Bangladesh—has had reasonable success with loans to poor families who put up no other collateral than joining and meeting regularly with a support group that promises to see to it that its members do, in fact, pay back their loans (Hossain 1988a:25–26).

As we will see below, subsidized credit is not an effective instrument for transferring income to the poor. Furthermore, subsidized credit may have harmful side effects on financial institutions and other segments of the economy, particularly the poor.

☐ Methods of Providing Cheap Credit

There are two common ways in which governments provide low-interest loans. One is directly through a government bank or quasi-government bank that loans the money to preferred borrowers at below-market interest rates. For instance, in Jamaica during the 1970s, the parastatal development bank supplied loans at less than half the commercial bank rate.

The other common way of providing low-interest loans is for the government to require commercial banks to supply a given amount of money to preferred borrowers at below-market rates. In Nigeria, for example, banks must devote 8 percent of their loans to the agricultural sector at approximately half the going commercial interest rate (Bale 1985:17).

Beginning in 1965 in Brazil, the law required commercial banks to lend at least 50 percent of their demand deposits to farmers at 17 percent interest per year. At that time the annual inflation rate was ranging from 20

Box 20.2
Common Assumptions About Lenders and Borrowers

Dale Adams and Douglas Graham

Common assumptions about saver-borrower behavior are that the rural poor cannot save and therefore will not respond to incentives or opportunities to save, that most farmers need cheap loans and supervision before they will adopt new technologies and make major farm investments, and that loans in kind are used in the form granted.

Common assumptions about lender behavior are that most informal lenders are exploitative and charge borrowers rates of interest that result in large monopoly profits, that the rural poor do not receive formal loans because formal lenders are overly risk-averse, that nationalized lenders can be forced to ignore their own profits and losses to serve risky customers and the rural poor, and that all formal lenders can be induced to follow government regulations in allocating financial services.

At a national level it is commonly assumed that cheap credit is an efficient way of offsetting production disincentives caused by low farm product prices or high farm input prices, that loan quotas established in the capital city are efficient ways of allocating loans in the countryside, that loans should be a part of a package of inputs, that only production loans should be made, and that rural financial market vitality is not related to projects and policies.

Research is showing that many of these assumptions are either unsubstantiated, weak, or incorrect.

Source: Extracted from Adams & Graham 1981.

to 40 percent per year; these loans were therefore very profitable for the borrowers. In 1971 the mandated rural interest rate was lowered to 15 percent, even though high rates of inflation continued (Sicat 1983:381).

☐ Problems Associated with Subsidized Credit

When the credit subsidy is paid for directly by government, the costs can run very high, so high that governments often use deficit financing to pay for the programs. The deficit financing, in turn, leads to inflation, which discourages saving, the basis of capital formation. The question must be asked whether the resources devoted to providing cheap credit might better be used in other government programs—more agricultural research, better rural roads, or improved educational services.

When the credit program is paid for implicitly, as happens when you force commercial credit institutions to give low-interest loans to priority borrowers, the costs of this hidden subsidy must be borne by the less preferred borrowers. They get less credit or pay higher interest rates for their loans, both of which are a constraint on development.

Sometimes governments attempt to limit the possibility that someone will make a profit (by obtaining cheap credit and then depositing the money right back in the bank at the [higher] commercial rate) by putting a ceiling on the commercial interest rate. Forcing down the interest rate in this way lessens the rewards from saving, discouraging some people from saving and motivating others to send their savings (and thus their capital) out of the country where they can get a better return.

From the point of view of income distribution, the worst aspect of subsidized credit is that it discriminates against the poor. The subsidized credit almost always goes to those in the community who are better prepared to receive it. In rural areas this means the rural elite: those well connected politically. Seldom does it go to the poorest of the poor.

The impact of a credit subsidy is thus regressive. Loans are seldom all the same size, and the size of the subsidy is directly proportional to the size of the loan. The larger farmers get larger loans and more subsidy. Medium and small farmers get proportionally smaller subsidies. The smallest farmers and landless laborers get no subsidy at all (González-Vega 1983:371).

☐ An Alternative to Subsidized Credit

Evidence shows that the availability of credit in the countryside can be greatly expanded merely by rigging the system to encourage rural financial markets to serve as intermediaries between savers and borrowers. This seems to be the appropriate alternative to subsidized credit.

Contrary to the commonly held assumption, low-income farmers do save. In a review of the available data on savings among rural households in Taiwan, Japan, South Korea, Malaysia, and India, Dale Adams found positive average propensities to save to be the norm. (The propensity to save is the percentage of income that is not spent for consumption or taxes.) Furthermore, rural households' savings are responsive to changes in the real interest rate. (The real interest rate is the difference between the nominal interest rate and the inflation rate.) In 1965 South Korea allowed the interest rate paid on time deposits and applied to loans to almost double. This resulted in real interest rates of over 8 percent per year. During the ensuing four years, total time and savings deposits in all banks increased fourteenfold. The number of savings accounts also increased sharply during this period (Adams 1983:401–405). In Korean farm households, the average propensity to save steadily increased during the 10 years following the credit reform (Table 20.3). Interestingly, the rate of

Table 20.3 **Average Propensity to Save, South Korean Farm Households, by Farm Size, 1962–1974**

Farm Size (in Cheongboa)	1962	1965	1966	1968	1970	1972	1974
0.5 or less	0.05	−0.05	0.01	0.06	0.03	0.02	0.22
0.5–1.0	0.12	0.01	0.09	0.11	0.13	0.21	0.29
1.0–1.5	0.16	0.06	0.10	0.20	0.16	0.34	0.35
1.5–2.0	0.15	0.12	0.13	0.23	0.26	0.30	0.43
2.0 or more	0.22	0.13	0.23	0.24	0.19	0.30	0.40
Average all households	0.15	0.04	0.11	0.16	0.15	0.24	0.33
Total number of households	1,163	1,172	1,180	1,181	1,180	1,182	2,515

Source: Adams 1983:404.
Note: One cheongbo equals 0.992 hectares or 2.45 acres. In this table average propensity to save was calculated as follows: (net income after taxes − consumption)/net income after taxes.

increase in propensity to save was greatest among those farm households with the smallest landholdings.

Mere convenience can be a factor in attracting rural savings. In India, when banks were encouraged to open rural branches for the primary purpose of disbursing agricultural loans, but at the same time offered a positive real interest rate on deposits, the response was so substantial that some authorities were concerned about the drain of funds from rural areas (World Bank 1986:101).

When rural people are offered convenient, secure savings institutions providing financially attractive real rates of return on savings, they seem to flock to make deposits. This increases the supply of lendable funds, eventually reducing the cost of credit through market mechanisms. Abundant credit at reasonable commercial rates eliminates the need for the capital rationing associated with subsidized credit, with its tendency to favor rural elites, and makes credit more readily available to the rural poor.

■ POLICIES TO ENCOURAGE INVESTMENT:
RURAL INFRASTRUCTURE AND PRICE STABILITY

Making credit more easily available or reducing the prices of capital goods increases farmers' *ability* to make investments that will lower production costs. In this section, we discuss some policies that can increase farmers' *desire* to make such investments. In particular, we will examine how government investments in rural infrastructure and government programs to stabilize farm prices can reassure farmers about their ability to transport their output to market and sell it.

☐ **Subsidizing Farm-to-Market Roads**

Building a new road into a region that formerly was reached only by human or animal transport can have an important impact on that region's economy. Because it dramatically reduces the cost of transporting farm products out of the region, it raises the farm-gate price of what farmers sell to country marketing agents who buy and transport food to the city. And because it simultaneously reduces the cost of transporting materials into the region, it reduces the cost of purchased farm inputs such as fertilizer. Higher farm-gate prices and lower input costs increase farm income, stimulate greater farm production, increase the demand for farm labor, and raise local wages.

In a study of the impact of new roads on 46 Philippine rural communities, Santos-Villanueva (1966) found a decrease in transportation costs of from 17 to 60 percent per kilometer and a substantial increase in the amount of agricultural products sold off the farm (see Table 20.4).

In a study of 16 villages in rural Bangladesh, it was found that villages with a good infrastructure, including good all-weather, hard-surfaced roads, used 92 percent more fertilizer per hectare than villages with poor infrastructure. They used 4 percent more labor per hectare, and they paid their agricultural laborers 12 percent more per day than did villages with poor infrastructure (Ahmed & Hossain 1990).

Higher local wage rates reduce the pressure for out-migration. In other words, good roads help keep people home! Good roads encourage private entrepreneurs to start bus services, often with very small vehicles ranging from large three-wheeled motorcycles to minibuses, and thus make it possible for rural people who live within reasonable commuting distances to work in town but continue to live at home. Good roads enable employment outside the home neighborhood.

Table 20.4   Average Increases in Volume of Sales of Selected Farm Products After the Construction of a Nearby Road from Farm to Market, Philippines

	Percentage Increase
Corn	104
Chicken	69
Swine	47
Coconuts	30
Rice	24
Bananas	12

Source: Santos-Villanueva 1966.

As roads lower the cost of transportation to and from the countryside, the annual fluctuation in the price of food is reduced. Remote communities find it cheaper to export food in good crop years and to import food in poor crop years, thus reducing price swings between the bad and the good harvests. Reducing these price swings reduces the probability that low-income families will face undernutrition during the years of bad harvest.

As a good road network reduces the cost of transporting agricultural commodities around the country, increased agricultural specialization by region can take place. For instance, perishable fruits and vegetables can be grown farther from urban markets than previously, making possible a higher-valued use of land far from market and reducing the income disparity between remote areas and the major cities.

The same sorts of advantages that accrue with new roads into a formerly remote territory apply to improvements in old roads. Putting a hard surface on a dirt road, or mending potholes on a worn-out, older, all-weather road, creates similar benefits, albeit less dramatic, as the benefits from putting in a new road.

☐ Other Aspects of Rural Infrastructure

In addition to roads, the parts of rural infrastructure that probably have the most bearing on agricultural production are the electrical system, the communications network, and the marketing system.

Rural electrification makes possible the powering of a host of time-saving and production-enhancing devices. Small irrigation pumps and power tools are efficiently driven by electricity.

Rural electrification makes communications easier in the countryside, for example by making a modern telephone switching system possible. Access to a telephone (even if there is only one per village) can save lives in a medical emergency. But efficient communications are also important in marketing farm products as well as in gaining access to purchased farm inputs.

An important function of a marketing system is to reflect back to producers the wants and preferences of consumers. As economic development brings changes in food-demand patterns, a good marketing system will efficiently transmit this information to farmers, who can then reallocate their resources to take advantage of the new production opportunities.

And as the sophistication of agricultural production increases with the adoption of new technology and improved management, a good marketing system for agricultural inputs will reflect farmers' preferences back to the farm suppliers. Bureaucratic, government-sponsored fertilizer distribution schemes usually supply only a limited choice of plant nutrient mixes. But if allowed to function in an appropriate institutional framework, a private-enterprise marketing system will make available a wide variety of fertiliz-

Box 20.3
Subsidies, Public Goods, and Public Investment

A subsidy, to quote a Merriam-Webster dictionary, is a grant or gift of money as, for instance, money granted by one state to another or a grant by a government to a private person or company to assist an enterprise deemed advantageous to the public.

Subsidies are usually granted because of a failure of the market to provide certain public goods. A small public park, a downtown sidewalk, national defense, and free public education are examples of public goods. Public goods have two critical properties: (1) It is impossible to exclude individuals from enjoying the benefits from them; and (2) it is undesirable to exclude individuals from enjoying the benefits from them, since such enjoyment does not detract from that of others (Stiglitz 1986:119).

No one wants to produce a public good because, once produced, it is available to all. The producer cannot sell it and capture his costs. Therefore government needs to give an incentive (the subsidy) to someone to provide the public good.

Because we think of investment as an expenditure that will provide production or income on into the future, the distinction between subsidy and public investment may be blurred or fuzzy. For instance, we can think of expenditure on the education of our children not only as a subsidy spent for a public good, but as investing in human capital, because educated children will be more productive later on in life than uneducated children.

Some subsidies are not available to all, but only to a particular class of people. For instance, the U.S. government has, at times, subsidized farmers by paying them to put lime on their fields, or homeowners by giving them a tax break for insulating their homes. These subsidies were available, respectively, only to farmers and homeowners. The subsidies were provided, however, because it was thought that they would improve welfare for all. The lime was to increase food production, thus lowering the price of food for all, and the home insulation was to lessen U.S. dependence on overseas sources of oil.

Because the word *subsidy* carries negative connotations for many people, we often use the phrase *public investment* when a subsidy results in increased benefits to society through time. Thus when a consortium of governments pays a public agricultural· experiment station for research to develop high-yielding varieties of rice, we may want to call it a public investment. All rice farmers can benefit from the new rice varieties, and of course the public benefits from the lower market price of rice after the higher-yielding rice varieties are put into use. We could also call the rice research and the resulting high-yielding varieties a public good. So it is with many other public expenditures for enhancing agricultural production, such as research on irrigation machinery or agricultural extension programs—they are pitched at the farm sector but they benefit the public.

The word *subsidy* is used here in a nonpejorative sense to indicate government expenditures deemed advantageous to the public, whether to another government, an institution, a company, or a person. In many cases the phrase *public investment* could be substituted for the word *subsidy.* The important thing is that you understand what happens with, what are the impacts of, the various types of expenditures governments make as they allocate their scarce resources among alternative ends in order to minimize undernutrition.

ers, allowing farmers to choose the most efficient ones for a particular situation.

Government support can supply radio stations and newspapers to pass along price information of interest to farmers. This is especially important for small farmers who, because of lack of information about market prices, might otherwise be at a disadvantage in comparison with the larger farmers who can afford to get such information on their own.

Government-sponsored terminal markets, where buyers can assemble farm products from the countryside and distribute them to retailers in the city, can increase the efficiency of the marketing system. Increasing the efficiency of the marketing system lowers prices to consumers and increases prices to producers, thus improving nutrition and stimulating increases in production. Appropriate government subsidies are important to an efficiently functioning agricultural marketing system.

☐ Price Stabilization

When farmers make decisions about whether to invest in projects that will improve their long-term productivity, they base their decisions on beliefs about future prices. Economists have found evidence that farmers are *risk-averse*—other things being equal, they would prefer a sure thing or a low-risk investment to a high-risk investment. When output prices are highly variable and unpredictable, farm investments are riskier, and farmers are less likely to make these investments. For this reason, some governments have instituted policies to stabilize prices of agricultural commodities (Newbery & Stiglitz 1981).

Governments have used four general types of policies to achieve more stable prices:

- The most direct is a policy of *administered prices,* under which the government sets prices, either by administrative fiat, or by acting as the sole buyer of the commodity. The difficulty with this type of policy is that the government frequently knows even less than farmers about likely future price levels. Therefore, the prices established by the government do not reflect underlying supply-and-demand conditions. Black markets emerge and either the programs are ineffective or they become an enormous drain on the government treasury.
- A second method is a *buffer stock* program under which the government buys the commodity when supplies are plentiful and prices are relatively low, and sells the commodity when supplies are tight and prices are relatively high. The government storage acts to even out prices over time. In theory, this program should put a ceiling and a floor on agricultural prices: When prices threaten to drop below the floor, the government buys the commodity and bids the price back up; when prices threaten to shoot through the ceiling,

the government sells the commodity and brings prices back down. In practice, governments have not been particularly adept at establishing the correct range of prices. In addition, the subsidized government storage tends to discourage storage in the private sector.

- A *buffer fund* accomplishes much the same thing as a buffer stock program, but does so without the government's actually buying and selling the commodity. Under a buffer fund, governments tax sales of the commodity in periods when prices are high (and thereby reduce the price received by farmers), and subsidize sales in periods when prices are low (effectively increasing the farm price). Buffer funds require extensive bookkeeping to verify which farmer sold what quantity at what price.
- Finally, governments can encourage the development of private market institutions, such as *forward contracting* and *futures markets,* to stabilize prices. These mechanisms allow farmers to lock in a price at the beginning of a growing season, at least for a major proportion of their crop. These types of contracts work well in theory; but farmers have been reluctant to adopt them in the United States and other developed countries.

■ POLICIES TO PROMOTE TECHNOLOGICAL IMPROVEMENT

☐ Subsidizing Agricultural Research

Technological change is one of the primary driving forces behind increasing production. Improved technology (e.g., a higher-yielding variety of rice) can increase the productivity of every item of the set of resources that a farmer uses—land, labor, management, and capital. Yet the agricultural researcher intent on developing new technology for agriculture faces an extraordinarily intricate range of scientific challenges. One recent analysis of technological change (Lele, Kinsey & Obeya 1989:42) listed these areas as important to researchers in improved crop varieties in Third World agriculture:

- Yield potential and responsiveness to available chemical fertilizers and pesticides
- Adaptation to the growing period and drought tolerance
- Disease and pest resistance
- Improvements in quality, palatability, and consumer acceptance
- Storage, transport, and other handling qualities (including processing) with available technology

- Changes in labor requirements in production and processing in relation to the available mechanical technology, in view of other requirements for household labor and incentives for labor use
- Compatibility with other social, cultural, and economic norms

Not only is the range of challenge complex, but the disciplines brought to bear on agricultural research are varied. Advancing agricultural technology involves research in biology, chemistry, and engineering, as well as in the social sciences, which are crucial to the appropriate integration of the new technology into the production system.

Despite the challenging nature of agricultural research, the payoff has been nothing short of spectacular. Agricultural research has been instrumental in dramatic increases in crop yields per acre (Box 20.4) as well as in livestock productivity. And when the costs of agricultural research are compared to the benefits to society, agricultural research turns out to be a real bargain.

In Table 20.5 (on p. 339), studies of payoffs to research done at agricultural experiment stations around the world are listed. The last column, annual internal rate of return, is of particular interest. The internal rate of return represents the average earning power of the resources used in a project

---

Box 20.4
Increases in Yield per Hectare—A Personal View

Theodore W. Schultz

Agricultural research, along with complementary inputs, has been very successful in developing substitutes for cropland (some call this land augmentation). Actual increases in yield per hectare have held and may well continue to hold the key to increases in crop production.

For example, during my first year at Iowa State College, 1931, the U.S. yield of maize was 1,500 kg/ha, a normal crop. In 1978 this yield came to 6,300 kg/ha. Although the maize area harvested in 1978 was 16 million hectares less than in 1931, total production was over 175 million metric tons, compared with 65 million tons in 1931. No wonder the estimated rates of return on maize research in the United States are exceedingly high.

The achievement with sorghum is even more dramatic. Taking 1929 as a normal year, the yield of sorghum grain rose from 870 kg/ha to 2,800 kg/ha in 1978, despite the fact that the area devoted to this crop [only] increased from 1.8 to 6.7 million hectares. Total production in 1978 was 19 million tons, which is over 15 times as much as that in 1929.

Source: Extracted from Schultz 1979.

during the project period. For an agricultural research project, this is the equivalent of the interest rate you would have to get from a savings account to receive the same return on your savings as the public got from the agricultural research project.

Consider the first item on the list in Table 20.5, returns to research on hybrid corn (maize) in the United States, calculated by the economist Griliches (1958). (The corn breeding research was carried out by many scientists.) The internal rate of return to hybrid corn research in the United States is calculated at from 35 to 40 percent. That means for every dollar the U.S. public paid for agricultural research on hybrid corn until 1955, it collected from $0.35 to $0.40 every year in benefits (mostly through lower prices for corn).

Of the 62 studies collected in Table 20.5, only four showed internal rates of return below 20 percent. Interestingly, rates of return to agricultural research run about the same for Third World countries as for developed countries. It would be hard to find another set of investments that pay off as well as agricultural research.

If agricultural research has such a spectacular payoff, why do farmers themselves not pay for it? The two reasons why it is not appropriate to ask farmers to pay are (1) most farmers have far too small an operation to sponsor and benefit from agricultural research, and (2) because the elasticity of demand for most farm products is less than one, the majority of the benefits from agricultural research goes to consumers. Farmers generally lose revenue when the new technology is widely adopted because they see their farm-gate prices fall faster than they can increase production. Long-term data from the United States, with a history of public sponsorship of agricultural research dating back to the 1870s, is illustrative:

> The decline in the real price of food has been dramatic. Available data for the period 1888 to 1891 indicate that consumers spent an average of about 40 percent of their income for food. From 1930 to 1960, the food expenditure proportion of consumer incomes ranged from 20 to 24 percent. In the seventies, the proportion of total disposable personal income spent for food dropped to a range of 1–17 percent. By the mid-eighties, that proportion for the average family had dropped to a record low of 15 percent (Lee & Taylor 1986).

Patent laws protect mechanical and chemical innovations more effectively than biological innovations. For this reason, some agroindustrial firms have been able to sponsor research in farm machinery or agricultural chemicals and capture the benefits from that research. Hybrid seeds are protectable by patents and, because they do not breed true, farmers must purchase new supplies each year. So after government-sponsored research led the way, hybrid seed companies set up their own research and are developing their own varieties. But by and large, biological innovations in agriculture have to be paid for by government. Thus, animal breeding, animal nutrition, plant breeding, plant pathology, entomology, agronomy, soil

Table 20.5   Internal Rate of Return from Agricultural Research Projects

Study	Country	Commodity	Time Period	Annual Internal Rate of Return (Percentage)
Griliches 1958	USA	Hybrid corn	1940–55	35–40
Griliches 1958	USA	Hybrid sorghum	1940–57	20
Peterson 1967	USA	Poultry	1915–60	21–25
Evenson 1969	South Africa	Sugarcane	1945–62	40
Ardito Barletta 1970	Mexico	Wheat	1943–63	90
Ardito Barletta 1970	Mexico	Maize	1943–63	35
Ayer 1970	Brazil	Cotton	1924–67	77+
Schmitz and Seckler 1970	USA	Tomato harvester	1958–69	
		With no compensation to displaced workers		37–46
		Assuming compensation of displaced workers for 50 percent of earnings lost		16–28
Ayer and Schuh 1972	Brazil	Cotton	1924–67	77–110
Hines 1972	Peru	Maize	1954–67	35–40[a] 50–55[b]
Hayami and Akino 1977	Japan	Rice	1915–50	25–27
Hayami and Akino 1977	Japan	Rice	1930–61	73–75
Hertford, Ardila, Rocha, Trujillo 1977	Colombia	Rice	1957–72	60–82
	Colombia	Soybeans	1960–71	79–96
	Colombia	Wheat	1953–73	11–12
	Colombia	Cotton	1953–72	0
Pee 1977	Malaysia	Rubber	1932–73	24
Peterson and Fitzharris 1977	USA	Aggregate	1937–42	50
			1947–52	51
			1957–62	49
			1957–72	34
Wennergren and Whitaker 1977	Bolivia	Sheep, wheat	1966–75	44.1–47.5
Pray 1978	Punjab (Br. India)	Agricultural research and extension	1906–56	34–44
	Punjab (Pakistan)	Agricultural research and extension	1948–63	23–37
Scobie and Posada 1978	Colombia	Rice	1957–74	79–96
Tang 1963	Japan	Aggregate	1880–1938	35
Griliches 1964	USA	Aggregate	1949–59	35–40
Latimer 1964	USA	Aggregate	1949–59	Not significant
Peterson 1967	USA	Poultry	1915–60	21
Evenson 1968	USA	Aggregate	1949–59	47
Evenson 1969	South Africa	Sugarcane	1945–58	40
Ardito Barletta 1970	Mexico	Crops	1943–63	45–93
Duncan 1972	Australia	Pasture improvement	1948–69	58–68
Evenson and Jha 1973	India	Aggregate	1953–71	40
Kahlon, Bal, Saxena, and Jha 1977	India	Aggregate	1960–61	63
Lu and Cline 1977	USA	Aggregate	1938–48	30.5
			1949–59	27.5
			1959–69	25.5
			1969–72	23.5

(continues)

Table 20.5   Continued

Study	Country	Commodity	Time Period	Annual Internal Rate of Return (Percentage)
Bredahl and Peterson 1976	USA	Cash grains	1969	36[c]
		Poultry	1969	37[c]
		Dairy	1969	43[c]
		Livestock	1969	47[c]
Evenson and Flores 1978	Asia (national)	Rice	1950–65	32–39
	Asia	Rice	1966–75	73–78
	(international)	Rice	1966–75	74–102
Flores, Evenson and Hayami 1978	Tropics	Rice	1966–75	46–71
	Philippines	Rice	1966–75	75
Nagy and Furton 1978	Canada	Rapeseed	1960–75	95–110
Davis 1979	USA	Aggregate	1949–59	66–110
			1964–74	37
Evenson 1979	USA	Aggregate	1868–1926	65
	USA	Technology-oriented	1927–50	95
	USA (south)	Technology-oriented	1948–71	93
	USA (north)	Technology-oriented	1948–71	95
	USA (west)	Technology-oriented	1948–71	45
	USA	Science-oriented	1927–50	110
			1948–71	45
	USA	Farm management research and agricultural extension	1948–71	110

Source: Evenson 1981:358–360. (See the source for the studies from which these data are derived.)
Notes: a. Returns to maize research only.
b. Returns to maize research, plus cultivation "package."
c. Lagged marginal product of 1969 research on output discounted for an estimated mean lag of five years for cash grains, six years for poultry and dairy, and seven years for livestock.

science, and so on are, by and large, government-sponsored (Judd, Boyce & Evenson 1987:7).

Some governments are too small to sponsor agricultural research. Their funds are best spent on adaptive agricultural research—finding out which of the innovations discovered elsewhere are most adaptable to their own situations. The Consultative Group on International Agricultural Research stations are helping to fill in the research gap felt by the smaller countries. As of 1998, 12 international agricultural research stations belonged to this group and were sponsored by a variety of sources. The group includes the International Rice Research Institute (IRRI) in the Philippines and the International Maize and Wheat Improvement Center (CIMMYT) in Mexico (both of which were mentioned in Box 11.1), as well as a number of other centers whose activities range from plant and animal breeding to food policy.

Modern-day challenges to agricultural research are legion. The techniques of recombinant DNA and cell fusion are making it possible for biotechnologists to engage in investigations with opportunities for very high rewards, developing highly productive organisms that might not ever have arisen in nature (U.S. Congress, Office of Technology Assessment 1986).

Innovative research sometimes can take unusual directions, such as the simultaneous cultivation of fish and rice in one rice paddy. Such a practice has been shown to increase the yield of rice and at the same time provide a high-protein supplement to the regular rice crop (Table 20.6). Alternatively, a tiny water fern called *azolla* can be grown with the rice. "Azolla plays host to a blue-green alga, *Anabaena azollae*, that can convert or 'fix' atmospheric nitrogen into a form that plants can use. Azolla floats on the water between the rice plants. When it dies and is incorporated into the soil, decomposition frees the nitrogen. A rice crop fertilized only with azolla can yield about 1.5 tons more per hectare than an unfertilized crop" (International Rice Research Institute 1989:1).

Low-income rural householders could benefit from research on hardy but efficient scavenging animals. High-yielding, disease-resistant breeds of chickens, ducks, goats, pigs, cattle, bees, or fish that can utilize garbage or other food that may be locally available but unfit for human consumption would be of considerable benefit to the Third World's poor.

Africa poses a particular challenge to agricultural research. Its soils are more diverse, its climate more varied, its pest and disease hazards more pronounced, and its farming systems more complex than those of monsoon Asia, where the green revolution has been such a success (Lele & Goldsmith 1989; Lipton & Longhurst 1990). African agriculture is characterized by *mixed cropping* (more than one crop at a time is grown in a

Table 20.6   Growth and Yield of Rice with and Without Fish at
Barddhaman, West Bengal, 1987 Wet Season

Characteristic	Rice Without Fish	Rice with Fish
Rice		
Plant height (cm)	133.21	120.8
Effective tillers/plant	12.0	15.2
Panicle length (cm)	26.4	26.8
Grains/panicle	158.21	178.4
Grain yield (t/ha)	4.1	4.9
Straw yield (t/ha)	5.2	6.0
Fish		
Recovery (%)	—	81.3
Increase in length (cm)	—	8.2
Increase in weight (g)	—	96.4
Fish yield (t/ha)	—	0.7

Source: Datta, Ghosh, and Bairagya 1988.

field), which occupies over 90 percent of the cropped area in most countries on the continent. Mixed cropping falls into three main categories:

1. *Intercropping:* more than one crop on a given area at one time, arranged in a geometric pattern
2. *Relay cropping:* a form of intercropping where not all the crops are planted at the same time
3. *Sequential cropping:* more than one crop (or intercrop) on a given area in the same year, the second crop being planted after the first is harvested

A special challenge for the agricultural research community working in Africa is to intensify agricultural production within this complex farm management system while maintaining its flexibility and its proven sustainability (Dommen 1988). One production innovation that holds promise for sustainability in the semiarid tropics that cover so much of Africa is *agroforestry,* a system of strip-cropping rows of trees between narrow strips of crops. The trees help conserve water, provide a ready source of organic matter, and reduce erosion.

☐ Subsidizing Technology Diffusion and Adoption

Profitable technology will spread from farmer to farmer by itself. But the rate of adoption can be accelerated by government-sponsored educational programs. Such programs are often called *extension* because they were originally conceived to extend the knowledge developed in the U.S. land-grant college system directly to the farmer. Programs that provide education and advice to farmers are now in place in most countries having a significant agricultural economy.

A classic study of Iowa's farmers illustrates the typical growth curve of knowledge that an agricultural community experiences as its farmers gradually become aware of a new technology, then try it out, and finally adopt it as part of their regular farming activities. In this case, a new chemical weed control called 2,4–D had come on the market. It took approximately 11 years between the time only a few farmers (4 percent) had even heard of it and all of them were using it. Notice in Figure 20.3 how awareness precedes trial, which precedes adoption. In 1949, for instance, about midway through the process, 74 percent of the farmers were aware of the existence of the new weedicide, but only 40 percent had adopted it. By 1955 all farmers in the area were using it. Without the vigorous extension program carried on by Iowa State University, the new technology undoubtedly would have spread, but whether it would have spread as fast is open to question. It is the charge of the extension service to accelerate the adoption of new technology, whether it be new agricultural chemicals, better plant and animal varieties, or better farm management practices.

Figure 20.3   Cumulative Percentage of Farm Operators at the Awareness, Trial,
and Adoption Stages for 2,4–D Weed Spray, by Year, Iowa, 1944–1955

Cumulative percentage

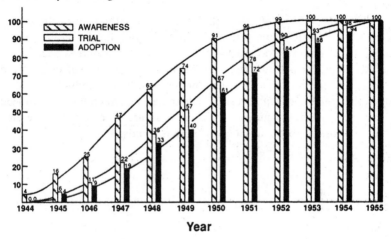

Year

Source: Adapted from Beal & Rogers 1960:8.

Accelerating the spread of technology begins with government sponsorship of agricultural training institutions—places where technicians learn the skills necessary for backstopping agriculture in the field—plant and animal sciences, and farm management and finance, for example. Not only do government-sponsored farm advisors need to know agricultural technology, but rural banks need farm appraisers, and rural tax collectors need to know about the economics of farming. Sponsoring the training of these technicians provides an important subsidy to agricultural production. The success of an agricultural extension service depends not only on the quality of training that farm advisors get at their local agricultural colleges but, perhaps more important, on the quality of the technology they have to extend. Building an array of extension agents without providing them with a set of technologies appropriate to the region where they are working does not endear them to farmers and weakens the future effectiveness of their organizations.

■ POLICIES TO PROMOTE SUSTAINABLE FARMING METHODS

Closely related to policies that promote increased productivity in the farm sector through development and adoption of new technologies are policies that promote environmentally friendly (or sustainable) farming. Here too, the government programs are directed at invention—or discovery—of environmentally appropriate practices, and extension—or teaching farmers about those methods. The kinds of policies discussed in the previous section apply here.

The importance of sustainable farming methods was discussed in Chapter 12. Agricultural production puts a strain on the natural environment. If the strain is too great—if land and water resources become sufficiently degraded—future agricultural production will suffer. Therefore, persuading farmers to adopt sustainable farming methods—methods that by definition do not entail resource degradation, which will in turn lead to future declines in production—will cause future food supply to be greater than it would be in the absence of these methods.

□ 21

Policy Concepts
and Policymaking

Governments . . . have an interest in keeping the exchange rate overvalued (one of the principal tools of depressing the incomes of small farmers) because the resulting need for rationing and allocating foreign exchange gives politically established groups extra money and power. The power of these groups is one of the strongest sources of resistance to changing exchange rates in many countries. Rents caused by economically inefficient interventions present political resources which can be used to organize political support.

Farming interests are opposed by urban workers who want low-priced food; urban industrialists, who want low wages and low prices for raw materials; bureaucrats and white collar workers who want higher salaries and lower food prices; and politicians who run governments which need taxes and which are major employers and industrialists in their own right.

—Streeten 1987:77

Part 3 of this book is about policy approaches to undernutrition. We have examined and evaluated a number of policy alternatives that have been proposed for the alleviation of Third World hunger. In this chapter we look formally at policy concepts, policy conflicts, the types of policy instruments available, the modes of policy formulation, and finally, at an action framework for policy reform.

■ POLICY OBJECTIVES
AND POLICY INSTRUMENTS

A public policy can be defined as course or direction taken by government, selected from among various alternatives in light of given conditions and designed to guide and determine present and future decisions.

Public policies almost always motivate a particular type of behavior or affect distribution of income, wealth, education, health care, and so on. You can usually break a public policy into one or more policy objectives and one or more policy instruments. The policy objective is the desired result. The policy instrument is the specific technique used to motivate the desired behavior or to affect distribution.

Some examples will help to make this clear. Let us start with simple automobile traffic policies:

Policy objective: Improve efficiency of traffic flow at major intersections
Policy instrument: Install traffic lights

Policy objective: Reduce traffic deaths caused by excessive speed
Policy instrument: Establish and enforce low speed limits

Tax policy takes a multitude of forms. Here is one designed to affect distribution:

Policy objective: Have rich people pay more tax per dollar earned
Policy instrument: Institute a progressive income tax structure

Taxes are often used to promote certain types of human behavior; for example:

Policy objective: Promote human fertility
Policy instrument: Provide a tax break for each dependent child in the family

There are public health policies:

Policy objective: Promote better health through a reduction of cigarette smoking
Policy instrument: Publish a health warning on the side of each cigarette package

Policy objective: Promote better health through reduction in marijuana smoking
Policy instrument: Make possession of marijuana illegal

One U.S. agricultural policy began with a law signed by Abraham Lincoln in 1862:

Policy objective: Promote the production of food
Policy instrument: In every state set up a college that teaches and conducts research and extension in agriculture and the mechanical arts (the land-grant college system)

U.S. policy toward the Third World can be defined in the same terms; for example:

Policy objective: Promote economic development in the Third World
Policy instrument: Pay for projects in economic development administered through the Agency for International Development (AID)—the U.S. foreign assistance agency

■ TYPES OF PUBLIC POLICY INSTRUMENTS

Government has available to it six broad categories of policy instruments: (1) moral suasion, (2) the tort system, (3) regulations, (4) charges, (5) subsidies, and (6) markets in rights. We will examine briefly each of these categories and, when possible, mention examples of specific nutrition policy instruments advocated under each category.

☐ Moral Suasion

When governments engage in admonitions, advertising, or education as a means to persuade people to behave in certain ways, they are using moral suasion. The health warning on a cigarette package is an example. For nutrition, campaigns to promote breast-feeding or oral rehydration therapy fit this category, as do campaigns to persuade people to eat less fat or less salt or to have smaller families.

☐ The Tort System

An old principle from Roman law states that you should, at all times, conduct yourself in a way that will not damage someone else, and that if you do damage them, you must compensate them for it. This is the principle that allows people to sue for damages. Lawyers call the entire process the *tort system.* It is a cumbersome way to motivate people to behave properly, because it involves time and money in court. But it does influence people's behavior. One reason you drive carefully is to avoid having to pay for the damage to someone else's car should you be at fault in an accident.

The tort system is seldom used to promote better nutrition. However, it was used recently in one well-publicized case in the United States in an effort to improve infant nutrition. In a New York State court the Beech-Nut company was found guilty of cutting costs by reducing or removing apples from its apple juice. It had sold millions of bottles of baby food labeled "apple juice" that contained little or no apple juice at all—only sugar, water, flavoring, and coloring. As a result of the lawsuit, Beech-Nut paid a $250,000 fine to the State of New York and a $2 million fine to the U.S. government. Two Beech-Nut executives each paid $100,000 fines and were sentenced to prison terms of a year and a day (Traub 1988).

☐ Regulations

Regulations backed by police power are the most commonly thought-of method for changing behavior. A host of regulations have been advocated and tried out in attempts to reduce Third World undernutrition. They include raising the legal marriage age, land reform (which commonly places a ceiling on the amount of land an individual may own), minimum-wage laws, food rationing, low administered prices for food, overvalued domestic currency, and limits on cash cropping. The last three regulations mentioned are examples of regulations that result in an implicit tax on agriculture. No money is collected directly by government, as is done in explicit taxation, which is next on our list.

☐ Charges

Fees, taxes, and other charges are not only a way for government to gain purchasing power; they also direct people to behave in particular ways. The high tax on gasoline in Europe has persuaded most Europeans to purchase small, fuel-efficient cars.

Third World tax policy commonly results in disincentives to agricultural production. For instance, noncompetitive procurement of food from farmers acts like a commodity tax levied at the farm gate and discourages farm production. In a rice-exporting country an export tax on rice lowers the price to the producer and acts as a disincentive to production.

Tax policy can also be used to modify distribution. Progressive taxation is a policy instrument designed to redistribute income and wealth from the rich to the poor.

☐ Subsidies

Subsidies that pay people or institutions for behaving in a particular way can be very expensive. They can also result in paying people for behavior they would have engaged in anyway. For instance, it has been advocated that we pay high school students who have dropped out of school a bonus for going back and finishing. If such a policy were instituted, students would drop out and reenter whether or not they would have even considered it in the absence of the subsidy.

Sometimes subsidies and tax policies overlap. Providing a tax break to couples who have children or a tax write-off of more than 100 percent for purchasing a tractor are examples of tax policies that result in subsidies. In the name of better nutrition, subsidies have been advocated and tried out for farm mechanization, farm credit, and direct distribution of food to the needy, to name a few. From the point of view of improving nutrition of the poor in the Third World, some of the most beneficial subsidies that government can engage in are those to education, agricultural research, mother-and-child health centers, family-planning services, and sanitary water and sewage facilities.

☐ Markets in Rights

Governments can establish a market in rights to behave in a certain way or to engage in a particular activity. You might, for instance, bid for the right to pasture your livestock on public rangeland, or for the right to add a certain amount of pollutant to a stream.

The concept of markets in rights is relatively new on the public policy scene, but proposals abound. Few have to do with improving nutrition, but one proposal, advanced by economist Kenneth Boulding (1964:135–136), albeit humorously, was to establish markets in rights to have babies. Marketable rights for babies, claimed Boulding, would combine the efficiency of the marketplace with controls necessary to slow or halt population growth.

> Each girl on approaching maturity would be presented with a certificate which will entitle its owner to have, say 2.2 children, or whatever number would ensure a reproductive rate of one. The unit of these certificates might be the "deci-child" and accumulation of ten of these units by purchase, inheritance, or gift would permit a woman in maturity to have one legal child. We would then set up a market in these units in which the rich and the philoprogenitive would purchase them from the poor, the nuns, the maiden aunts, and so on. The men perhaps could be left out of these arrangements, as it is only the fertility of women which is strictly relevant to population control.

Boulding points out that his plan would have the

> advantage of developing a long-run tendency toward equality in income, for the rich would have many children and become poor and the poor would have few children and become rich. The price of the certificate would of course reflect the general desire in a society to have children. Where the desire is very high the price would be bid up; where it was low the price would also be low. Perhaps the ideal situation would be found when the price was naturally zero, in which case those who wanted children would have them without extra cost.

If, sometime in the future, you are trying to create a new public policy, you may want to refer back to the above checklist of alternative policy instruments. By and large, the last four in the above set have been found stronger and more efficient than the first two.

■ POLICY CONFLICTS AND POLICY DILEMMAS

Whether in a dictatorship or a democracy, public policy is made and revised in the hot crucible of competing and conflicting interests. As Streeten (1987) pointed out, Third World farm and nonfarm interests are frequent competitors. Urban bias is commonplace in the Third World and repeatedly leads to policies that have an adverse impact on the poor, such as industrial protectionist policies (import substitution) instead of export-led growth policies.

But even in the absence of urban bias, nutrition policy planners continually grapple with the dilemma of, on the one hand, low administered food prices making it easier for the poor to purchase food and, on the other hand, discouraging food production and creating other social costs, such as increased unemployment, which adversely affect the poor.

A common policy conflict affecting Third World nutrition is that between food self-sufficiency and economic efficiency. Food self-sufficiency is a politically attractive slogan and conjures up images of independence, Henry David Thoreau, Robinson Crusoe, and all that. But food self-sufficiency requires policies that raise the domestic price of food, as when more-expensive, domestically produced food must be substituted for cheaper, foreign-produced food. This may be one of the consequences of policies that limit the production of export crops in favor of the production of food crops. The poor suffer from a food self-sufficiency policy as the prices of their food rise.

Whether to promote more vigorously increased grain or livestock production is a thorny problem frequently faced by Third World planners. Because of the lower demand elasticities for grain, promoting grain production benefits farmers less and lower-income consumers more than does promoting livestock production. Promoting livestock production increases the demand for grain and raises its price as livestock consume increasing amounts of grain; this may adversely affect the nutrition of the poor while lowering the price of livestock products, which are consumed largely by the already overfed rich. On the other hand, livestock production is more labor-intensive than grain production, and promoting livestock production does increase demand for rural labor.

Just the same, if we are to improve the nutritional status of the Third World's poor, decisions on policy reform must be made. As John Mellor (1985b) put it: "In allocating a government's resources, it is not enough to inventory the things that must be done to facilitate agricultural development: the next step of dividing the tasks between the private and the public sectors and setting priorities must also be taken." In this context the importance of increasing agricultural production should not be overlooked. Again, John Mellor (1986a): "In developing countries, rising incomes of low-income people, derived from employment growth, are converted by remarkably high demand elasticities to increased effective demand for food: 60 to 80 percent of incremental income is so spent. Thus in developing countries, increased food supplies and increased employment are two sides of the same coin; one cannot proceed long without the other."

■ MODES OF POLICY FORMULATION

Policy formulation always involves choice among alternatives. We would like to think that all choices of decisionmakers in government are rational. Unfortunately, such is not the case. Sometimes, choice making in policy formulation is far from rational, but let us begin this discussion with the assumption that governmental decisionmaking regarding policy alternatives is rational. In this case, how does it go?

□ Rational Choice Using the Alternatives-Consequences Model

Let us take an idealized situation. Government policymakers identify a problem of strategic importance—say 27 percent of the preschoolers in the country classify as moderately to severely undernourished (the rate quoted for the Philippines in Chapter 4). The next step is to identify objectives relative to the problem. Say the policymaking group decides to cut the rate of moderately to severely undernourished preschoolers by 50 percent during the next 10 years.

Once the goal has been agreed upon, the policy options must be considered. A set of programs and policies that influence preschool nutrition are already in place, so examination of policy options is largely a matter of considering changes in the present policy structure. The range of policy objectives and policy instruments relative to the above goal must be laid out. These can be called the *public policy alternatives*. Each alternative will generate a set of consequences. Examination of the consequences of each proposed policy alternative will, in turn, lead the policymakers back to the most appropriate set of policy alternatives for achieving their policy goal. In Figure 21.1, the alternatives-consequences model is diagrammed.

In this system the quality of policy analysis is crucial. Bad analysis of the consequences of policy alternatives will lead to bad policy. Good analysis, combined with rational choice makers, will result in good policy.

□ Applying the Alternatives-Consequences Model

We have attempted to furnish a framework for the application of the rational alternatives-consequences model in choosing policy objectives and policy instruments for alleviating Third World undernutrition. The thesis

Figure 21.1   **The Rational Alternatives-Consequences Model in Policy Decisionmaking**

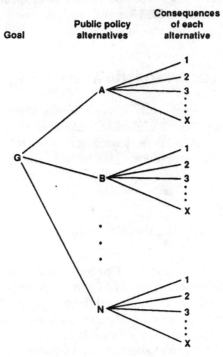

of this book postulates that particular economic, demographic, and health variables deliver undernutrition to millions of people in the Third World. A corollary of this thesis preposes that alleviation of hunger requires changes in policies to adjust these variables. Because these variables deliver undernutrition, we have called them *nutrition impact vehicles.*

We have examined policy instruments, grouped by policy objectives, designed to adjust these variables to reduce undernutrition by improving health, lowering high population growth rates, reducing income and wealth inequalities and raising income of the poor, lowering the price of food through explicit subsidized consumption, lowering the price of food through implicit subsidized consumption, and lowering the price of food through subsidized production. Our policy objectives, plus sample policy instruments commonly proposed in association with these objectives, are listed and organized in Table 21.1.

In choosing policies to alleviate undernutrition, we must deal with the real-world complexity that a policy instrument proposed to improve nutrition through adjusting one nutrition impact vehicle often affects one or more of the other nutrition impact vehicles. Improving health, for instance, may be supposed to have a positive impact on nutrition and yet it can

Table 21.1 Commonly Proposed Policy Alternatives for Reducing Third World Undernutrition

Policy Objective	Generalized Policy Instrument	Specific Policy Instrument
Improve health	Food fortification	Iodized salt Iron, vitamins in grain
	Mother and child health centers	Immunization Oral rehydration therapy education Vitamin A distribution Promotion of breast-feeding Family planning
	Interrupt transmission of diarrhea	Improved sewage handling Hygiene education Sanitary water supply
Reduce high population growth rates	Eliminate pronatalist policies	
	Upgrade the status of women	Equal educational opportunities for both sexes Equal employment opportunities for both sexes
	Adopt antinatalist policies	Contraceptive research Economic incentives for small families Economic disincentives for large families Moral suasion Raise legal marriage age Legal regulation of fertility Subsidize family-planning services
Reduce income and wealth inequalities and raise income of the poor	Land reform Progressive taxation Encourage rural financial markets Minimum-wage laws Employment creation	
	Human capital-intensive programs for reducing inequality	Provide public education, especially primary and secondary Reduce human fertility Improve health care Famine, disaster relief Marketwide explicit food subsidies
Lower the price of food	Explicit subsidized consumption	Famine, disaster relief Marketwide explicit food subsidies Subsidies targeted to the needy: Self-targeting Direct distribution Rationing Food stamps Food-for-work

(continued)

Table 21.1   Commonly Proposed Policy Alternatives for Reducing Third World Undernutrition

Policy Objective	Generalized Policy Instrument	Specific Policy Instrument
	Implicit subsidized consumption	Noncompetitive procurement Administered prices Export taxes Overvalued domestic currency Limits on cash cropping
	Subsidized production	Subsidize: Credit Mechanization Technology creation Technology diffusion and adoption Purchased inputs: Irrigation water Fertilizer Pesticides Rural infrastructure: Electrification Communication Marketing system Roads Tax shelter Preferential tariffs on machine imports

Note: The distinction between policy goals (objectives) and instruments is not always clear-cut. For instance, improved health is the first policy goal listed, yet improved health care is listed as a specific policy instrument for reducing income and wealth inequalities and raising income of the poor.

simultaneously lead to negative nutrition impacts if it leads to increased population growth rates. Solving the world food problem will require the use of a multiplicity of policy instruments. There is no "single-bullet" solution to this complex problem.

As we evaluate alternative policy instruments proposed to reduce undernutrition, we must, therefore, examine the impact of each proposed instrument on each nutrition impact vehicle, at least to the extent that it affects it significantly. We attempted to do this in Part 3; the discussion in these chapters is capsulized in Table 21.2, where policy instruments, grouped by policy objectives, are listed in the left-hand column. Across the top are listed the nutrition impact vehicles. Because production incentives in agriculture are so important to agricultural production, which, in turn, influences both employment and the price of food, production incentive to agriculture is included as a nutrition impact vehicle in column 6.

On occasion in Chapters 15 through 20, the question of the impact of a particular policy instrument on overall economic efficiency was discussed.

Table 21.2 Direction of Probable Effect of Selected Policy Instruments on Nutrition Impact Vehicles

Policy Objective (Related Chapter) or Policy Instrument	Nutrition Impact Vehicle						
	1	2	3	4	5	6	7
	Improve health of the poor	Decrease population growth rate	Increase equality of income and wealth	Increase income and/or employment of the poor	Lower price of food for the poor	Production incentive to Third World agriculture	Improve overall economic efficiency
Improve Health (15)							
Food fortification	+						
Immunization	+	−					
Oral rehydration therapy education	+	−					
Vitamin A distribution	+	−					
Promotion of breast-feeding	+	+	+	+	+		
Improved sewage handling	+	−					
Hygiene cducation	+	−					
Sanitary water supply	+	−					
Lower high population growth rates (16)							
Elimination of pronatalist policies		+	+	+	+		
Equal educational opportunities for both sexes		+	+	+	+		
Equal employment opportunities for both sexes		+	+	+	+		
Contraceptive research		+	+	+	+		
Economic incentives for small families		+	+	+	+		
Economic disincentives for large families		+	+	+	+		
Moral suasion		+	+	+	+		
Raising legal marriage age		+	+	+	+		
Legal regulation of fertility		+	+	+	+		
Subsidizing family planning services		+	+	+	+		
Reduce wealth inequalities and raise income of the poor (17)							
Land reform			+/−		−	−	
Progressive taxation			+				

(continues)

Table 21.2 Continued

Policy Objective (Related Chapter) or Policy Instrument	1 Improve health of the poor	2 Decrease population growth rate	3 Increase equality of income and wealth	4 Increase income and/or employment of the poor	5 Lower price of food for the poor	6 Production incentive to Third World agriculture	7 Improve overall economic efficiency
							Nutrition Impact Vehicle
Encouraging rural financial markets			+	+		+	+
Roads			+	+	+	+	+
Minimum-wage laws			−	−		−	−
Employment creation			+	+		+	+
Providing public education, especially primary and secondary	+	+	+	+	+	+	+
Reducing human fertility	+	+	+	+	+		
Improving health care	+	−	+	+			
Lower the price of food through explicit subsidization consumption (19)							
Famine, disaster relief	+	−	+		+	−	
Marketwide explicit food subsidies	+	−	−		+	−	
Subsidies targeted to the needy							
Self-targeting	+	−	+		+	−	
Direct distribution	+	−	+		+	−	
Rationing	+	−	+		+	−	
Food stamps	+	−	+		+	−	
Food-for-work	+	−			+	−	
Lower the price of food through implicit subsidization consumption (18)							
Noncompetitive procurement	−		−		+	−	−
Low administered prices	−		−		+	−	−
Export taxes on farm products	−		−		+	−	
Overvalued domestic currency	−		−		+	−	
Limits on cash cropping	−		−		+	−	
Lower the price of food through subsidized production (20)							
Subsidization of							
Credit			−	−			
Mechanization			−	−		+	
Technology creation			+		+	+	+
Technology diffusion and adoption:							

(continued)

Table 21.2   Continued

Policy Objective (Related Chapter) or Policy Instrument	\multicolumn{7}{c}{Nutrition Impact Vehicle}						
	1	2	3	4	5	6	7
	Improve health of the poor	Decrease population growth rate	Increase equality of income and wealth	Increase income and/or employment of the poor	Lower price of food for the poor	Production incentive to Third World agriculture	Improve overall economic efficiency
High-yielding grains			+	+		+	+
Grain-fed livestock			+	−		+	+
Purchased inputs							
Irrigation water			+	+		+	
Fertilizer	−		+	+		+	−
Pesticides	−		+	+		+	−
Rural infrastructure							
Electrification	+		+	+		+	+
Communication	+		+	+		+	+
Marketing system	+		+	+		+	+
Roads	+		+	+		+	+

This is because policies that lessen overall economic efficiency reduce total income available for taxation and thus reduce the resources available for programs to alleviate undernutrition. Policies that lessen overall economic efficiency also reduce employment opportunities, overall economic growth, and so on, which, in turn, affect nutrition. Because of its importance, the improvement of overall economic efficiency is also listed as a nutrition impact vehicle (column 7).

We have the opportunity in Table 21.2 to examine and compare the impact of various nutrition policy instruments on the various nutrition impact vehicles as an aid in selecting an appropriate set of policy instruments for solving the hunger problem. Pluses and minuses have been assigned where data or logic seem to lend strong support to such a relationship. The table is constructed in such a way that a plus indicates a relationship that will result in an improvement in nutritional status; a minus indicates a relationship that will result in a worsening of nutritional status. Where the relationship is virtually nonexistent, weak, or highly debatable, the cells in the table have been left blank.

For instance, vitamin A distribution is expected to improve health through a reduction in xerophthalmia and at the same time reduce deaths from diarrhea, thus increasing the population growth rate. The impact of vitamin A distribution on the variables listed in columns 3 through 7 was not deemed clear enough or strong enough to categorize.

Successful promotion of breast-feeding will improve infant health (a plus in column 1), but the reduction in births attributable to the contraceptive effects may be great enough to reduce the birth rate more than the death rate is reduced by the positive health effects. The plus in column 2 is therefore plausible, but debatable.

A reduction in high population growth rates will probably improve mother and child health, decrease population growth, increase equality of income and wealth (review Table 9.7), reduce unemployment, and decrease the demand for food, therefore helping lower its price. Thus, programs that successfully reduce the birth rate get a plus in columns 2 to 5.

Land reform has positive or negative impacts on distribution, depending on the situation. It gets both a plus and a minus in column 3 to suggest this. Conversely, because such programs seldom increase the level of food productivity and frequently reduce it, it gets a minus in column 5. And because the threat of land reform may reduce investment in agriculture, it ranks a minus in column 6.

In some cases the direction of influence will depend on the assumptions we make. For instance, in Table 21.2 it is assumed that explicit subsidized consumption will be supported in greater measure by donor countries than by Third World countries, and that the price effect on food bought at discount prices will act as a production incentive in the donor countries, but that the price effect of the sale of surpluses from overseas will act as a production disincentive to agriculture in the recipient country. Therefore, explicit food subsidies rate a minus in column 6.

Look through the table and see if the assignment of pluses and minuses makes sense to you. In cases where it does not, go back to the chapter in which the relationship is discussed and review the data or the reasoning process (the numbers of the related chapters are given in parentheses after each major subhead in the table).

After you have worked through the consequences of the various proposed policy instruments, you will not necessarily be a nutrition policy expert, but you will have a better feel for the types of policy adjustments that will have to be made in order to reduce Third World undernutrition.

☐ **Nonrational Policymaking**

So far in this section we have examined policy formulation in the rational decisionmaking framework. But government policymaking is not always rational.

Graham Allison (1971), a perspicacious observer of government decisionmaking, postulates three modes of policy formulation. The first is the mode of the *rational actor,* working with the alternatives-consequences model, which we assumed above. The second mode he calls the *organizational process.* The third he calls *governmental politics.* Because the last two modes are important in the policymaking process, let us look at them briefly.

Organizational process. In Allison's view, "government consists of a conglomerate of semi-feudal, loosely allied organizations, each with a substantial life of its own" (p. 67). These individual organizations carry weighty names such as Ministry of Agriculture, or Ministry of Defense, or Ministry of Health. In the United States they are called *departments*. These organizations develop their own bureaucracies, each with its own institutionalized way of doing things—the standard operating procedures.

In the short run, decisionmaking within the organization is limited by the standard operating procedures. (That is why we often find bureaucracies so frustrating to deal with.) In the long run, decision outputs can be influenced by gradually changing organizational goals, still modified by the entrenched standard operating procedures. Top government leaders can influence the bureaucracies, but only with some difficulty and much effort.

Governmental politics. Top government leaders are, of course, not always paragons of virtue, with no interests at heart except the welfare of the population. They reached the top in a competitive struggle, and each one has an agenda, strategic objectives, and personal goals. As Allison puts it, "the name of the game is politics: bargaining along regularized circuits among players positioned hierarchically within the government" (p. 144).

Sometimes one individual or group will succeed in putting its pet policy in place unscathed by the bargaining process. More likely, in this mode, policy choices are the result of bargains and compromises representing a mixture of conflicting preferences and the unequal power of various groups and individuals holding diverse stakes and stands. In this mode, what finally motivates the policy choice is not rational decisionmaking, not the routines of government organizations, but "the power and skill of proponents and opponents of the action in question" (p. 145).

■ AN ACTION FRAMEWORK FOR POLICY REFORM

If you want to do something significant about the problem of Third World hunger, you will, ultimately, have to exert some influence in the adjustment of the nutrition impact vehicles so that less undernutrition is delivered to the Third World's poor. This will involve not only supporting careful policy analysis for the use of rational decisionmakers, but coping with the less-than-rational modes of the policymaking process, described above. You will have to become involved in power struggles, such as the one alluded to by Streeten (1987). This is the stuff of which policy reform is made.

Achieving changes in policies is a process of social action. Two sociologists at Iowa State University (Beal & Hobbs 1969) studied this process and described a model for successfully, and nonviolently, achieving social change. The essence of their model is presented below.

Establish convergence of interest. If you play an active role in achieving nutrition policies, and if you help instigate the changed policies yourself, you are a *change agent*. A change agent must realize that all social action takes place within the context of social systems. And any social action must begin with a convergence of interest, a common definition of need, on the part of two or more people. In other words, to motivate social change, you have to work with groups, and you have to find or create allies who will work with you.

Analyze the social system. After you have found some allies in your cause, take a careful look at the social system you must deal with. All kinds of groups make up the social system. Try to figure out which of these *subsystems,* as these groups are called, are relevant to your cause. That is, determine which ones are likely to give you support, and also which ones may give you opposition.

Establish initiating sets. Your original small group should now undertake to contact key leaders in the organizations and groups. You will be seeking support from some groups and trying to find ways to neutralize the potential opposition from others.

Legitimize. The more people you can get to support your cause the better. But it is especially important to seek out and try to gain the support of people of status who have the power to make or break your action program— the *legitimizers.* Legitimizers may be formal; for example, the official heads of the relevant groups. Or legitimizers may be informal, in which case they may not be so easy to identify. In either case they are important. A relevant legitimizer may not lift a finger to help your cause. But if you fail to contact her or if you somehow antagonize her somewhere along the line, her opposition could spell delay or even disaster for your cause.

Find and use diffusion sets. If everything is going well so far in your campaign and if the legitimizers are on your side, support for your cause should be growing. Then it is time to broadcast your ideas more widely. Here you need people who can be instrumental in diffusing information throughout the community, region, or nation, whatever is the eventual target of your social action program. Newspaper editors can help here, as well as others associated with the mass media. So can other communicators, such as teachers, school administrators, farm advisors, or religious leaders.

Generalize the movement. Now your objective is to influence the general population, or at least a majority of the decisionmakers, to favor your stand. As the information diffuses through the mass media, you can assist in developing a general "felt need" for your program by promoting discussions, carrying out surveys, doing anything you can to make your cause a "people's problem."

Use personal contact. Observers of social change feel that people are made aware by impersonal methods of communication (newspapers, postcards, and so on), but they are only persuaded or convinced by face-to-face contact. Of course, you or your original allies cannot possibly make all the necessary personal contacts at this time. That is why you must bring together as many groups as possible in the service of your cause. Keep in mind throughout your entire effort that social action happens within the context of social systems. You must work with groups.

Move toward action. After the relevant groups agree that the problem really exists, and after a general feeling of support for your cause has been built up, you now move toward a specific action program. Perhaps the original goals that your initial allies had in mind will turn out to be too vague for this stage of the game. More-specific goals may have to be set. So the process of looking at alternative public policies and their consequences must begin again, this time with rather more specific policy alternatives in mind.

With lots of hard work, and probably after a long time, you and the others who began work on the program together may well be able to participate in the final stages of the social action process, setting up the plan of work and carrying out the action program. Perhaps this will be worked out in some government agency, maybe in the legislature. The important thing, of course, is that your efforts ultimately yield a change in public policy in the right direction.

Evaluate throughout. Throughout the social action process, you must continually evaluate progress so far, decide whether progress is satisfactory, and plan for the next step. Continual evaluation will help you avoid the mistake of moving too fast or too far and thus jeopardizing the chances of your next step's being a success.

□ **22**

World Food Supply and Demand for the Next Half Century: Some Alternative Scenarios

And I beheld a black horse; and he that sat on him had a pair of balances in his hand. And I heard a voice . . . say, A measure of wheat for a penny, and three measures of barley for a penny. . . . And power was given unto them over the fourth part of the earth, to kill with the sword, and with hunger, and with death, and with the beast of the earth.

Revelation 6:5–8

Famine is one of the Four Horsemen of the Apocalypse. And when our visions of the future take an apocalyptic turn, the spectre of widespread hunger is likely to appear. What does the future hold? Will the progress of the last 30 years continue? Or are we on the brink of a slide into catastrophe? Having boldly asked these questions, we less boldly reply, "It all depends . . . " This chapter will briefly review schools of thought about the future of the world food problem and will present a framework for building scenarios about the future.

There are several points on which there is universal agreement. Of course, any prediction is likely to be wrong in certain fundamental ways. But the four Ps identified in Chapter 1—population, prosperity, productivity, and pollution—are almost certain to be the major factors shaping the future. Growth in population and in per capita income will determine, to a considerable extent, demand for food. Growth in yields per hectare and limitations imposed by environmental quality will determine, to a considerable extent, supply of food. The interplay of these factors will ultimately be reflected in the fifth P—the price of food. If demand grows more rapidly than supply, food prices will increase and hunger may become more widespread. If supply grows more rapidly than demand, food prices will drop. The sixth P—policy—is the means by which humankind can hope to influence the future.

■ TWO VIEWS OF THE FUTURE

It is tempting to characterize people's views about the future of world food supply and demand as "optimistic" or "pessimistic." (In fact, at several points in this book, such characterizations are made.) But a more accurate division might be between the *establishment* view and the *anti-establishment* view. The establishment view is reflected in recent reports by the FAO (Alexandratos 1995), the World Bank (Mitchell et al. 1997), the International Food Price Research Institute (Pinstrup-Andersen et al. 1998, and other IFPRI 2020 reports), and the U.S. Department of Agriculture (1998). These reports embrace a common vision of the future in which world agricultural production continues to grow (with slight growth in agricultural area and yield growth in the 1 to 1.5 percent per year range), world population continues to grow but ever more slowly than the current 1.4 percent rate, and income per capita continues to grow. Implicit in their vision is an assumption that there will be no catastrophic changes in environmental conditions.

The anti-establishment view is reflected in the work cited in Chapters 11 and 12 by David Pimentel of Cornell and by Lester Brown and his colleagues at the WorldWatch Institute. This view puts a much greater emphasis on the possibility of environmental catastrophe. The types of catastrophe that could occur include losses of agricultural land due to erosion or degradation, reductions in availability of usable water for agriculture, due to overirrigation, and global warming that could (in the worst cases projected by scientists) cause significant loss of land to rising sea levels, and significant yield reductions from changing climate patterns. The anti-establishment view is also notably less confident about the possibility of a "technological fix" for these future catastrophes if they do occur. As described in Chapter 11, this lack of confidence is based on the slowing of yield growth, and the belief that we are unlikely to see any significant breakthroughs in basic science that would provide a foundation for a new spurt of growth in yields.

Past predictions of global food shortages have been wrong in large part because they underestimated the ability of technological progress to increase food output. The establishment view has confidence that the institutions and processes that generated yield growth in the past will continue to generate yield growth in the future. The anti-establishment view sees the yield growth of the past 50 years as a one-time stroke of good fortune that is unlikely to be repeated.

Both the establishment and anti-establishment views accept the premise that human actions—especially government policies—can influence the future state of the world. The establishment view is more sympathetic to incrementalism—small changes in policies to ensure the world continues to make progress. The anti-establishment view is that major sweeping changes—especially in environmental and population policies—must be made to accommodate and ameliorate future problems.

The anti-establishment view tends to see current prosperity—and the fact that "only" 20 percent of the world's population is currently undernourished—as coming at the expense of future generations. In effect, they argue, we are "eating the seed"—satisfying our current hunger by guaranteeing even more severe and widespread problems in the future. The appropriate response, therefore, is a radical reduction in current levels of consumption of food and nonfood alike. At the extreme, it is argued, accomplishing this radical reduction may require radical restructuring of economic and political systems. The establishment view does not accept the vision of inherent conflict between present and future generations: Current prosperity will not cause future poverty; future generations will be on average at least as prosperous as we are today. This attitude leads to a broad endorsement of existing institutions. This is not quite the same thing as saying the establishment view endorses a "business as usual" policy. Rather, the kinds of policies endorsed by the establishment view—market-oriented pricing, increased government funding of research and development, appropriate macroeconomic policies to promote general economic growth, for example—tend to be policies that can be pursued within the existing institutional framework.

■ PREDICTING THE FUTURE: PRINCIPLES FOR SCENARIO BUILDING

Looking at different scenarios for the future allows us to see how intelligent, well-informed people can arrive at such different views about the future. In this section, we present a few alternative scenarios. The main purpose is not to prove that one or the other of these scenarios is "correct," but rather to provide a template from which readers can construct their own scenarios.

These scenarios make projections 50 years into the future. This is further than most projections; but most projections are intended for policymakers, who recognize that today's projections will be replaced by a new set within a few years. The 50-year period was chosen to give readers a view of world food supply and demand during their lifetimes.

All scenarios are based on assumptions about annual rates of growth: growth in population, growth in per capita income, growth in area harvested, and growth in yields per hectare. The rates of growth assumed are *average* rates for the entire 50-year period. Growth may be higher than average for some years, and lower than average for others. As laid out at the end of Chapter 10, projections about world food demand are based on assumptions about growth in population and growth in income per capita. As suggested at the beginning of Chapter 11, projections about world food supply are based on assumptions about growth in agricultural land area and growth in yields.

In developing scenarios, we use a set of assumptions that is internally consistent. The complexity of interconnections among the factors has been illustrated throughout the book. Agricultural productivity, and the concomitant prosperity in the farm sector, contributes to economy-wide prosperity and growth in per capita income. Higher per capita income is associated with better health care and sanitation, and therefore lower infant mortality; this in turn leads to reduced fertility and ultimately lower population growth rates. Environmental catastrophes, should they occur, are likely to be associated with lower per capita incomes, and increased mortality—therefore possibly lower population growth.

☐ An "Establishment View" Scenario

At the end of Chapter 10, we presented some sample scenarios for growth in total food demand. There we saw a number of different assumptions that were consistent with a doubling of demand for food over the next 50 years. Here, we revisit that, and expand it to include the supply side. The assumptions and conclusions are summarized as scenario A in Table 22.1.

Population. Chapter 7 showed us that both the U.S. Census Bureau and the UN medium variant projected average population growth of slightly less than 1 percent per year. Here we use an average growth rate of 0.95 percent per year. At the end of 50 years, population will be 60 percent higher than the current population.

Income and calories per capita. Chapter 9 showed that over the last 10 years, growth rates in the income per capita worldwide have been about 1 percent per year. Nevertheless, the "establishment view" studies cited above typically project average growth in the 2 to 3 percent per year range. However, the studies are for shorter periods than the 50 years here. For our establishment view projection, we assume an average worldwide income growth of 1.5 percent per year. This means that by the end of the 50-year period, the average income will be more than twice as high as the current level (210 percent of the current level). As described in Chapter 8, assuming an income elasticity for food of 0.14, this means that calories per capita will increase by about 15 percent over the 50-year period. In addition, we assume an increase in calories from animal sources will increase the effective demand per person by an additional 13 percent. The cumulative effect is to increase (plant-equivalent) calories per capita by 30 percent.

Total shift in demand. The above allows us to project that at the end of 50 years, food demand (at constant prices) would be (1.60 x 1.30 =) 208

Table 22.1   Assumptions and Outcomes of Different Scenarios for the Food Supply and Demand Situation: Comparison of the Situation as Projected 50 Years in the Future to the Current Situation

Scenario	Population	Income per Capita	Plant-Equivalent Calories per Capita	Agricultural Land	Yields per Acre	Total Demand for Food	Total Supply of Food	Price of Food	Calories per Capita per Day After 50 Years[a]
A	+60%	+110%	+30%	+13%	+86%	+108%	+110%	-3%	3518
A-1	+32%	+110%	+30%	+13%	+86%	+72%	+110%	-54%	3743
A-2	+60%	+110%	+30%	+13%	+49%	+108%	+68%	+57%	3316
B	+60%	+28%	+6%	-15%	+10%	+70%	-7%	+110%	2505
B-1	+120%	+0%	0%	-15%	+10%	+120%	-7%	+181%	2258
B-2	+60%	+28%	+6%	-15%	+49%	+70%	+27%	+61%	2658

Notes: A number such as "+60%" means that the scenario projects that, after 50 years, the level of the variable will be 60% higher than the current levels. The details of the scenarios are described in the text.

a. For purposes of comparison, average calories per capita per day are about 2700 in 1998.

percent of its current level—slightly more than twice current demand. Can supply keep pace?

Increase in agricultural land. Chapter 11 discusses the potential for increasing agricultural land. Here we assume that land in agriculture increases by 2.5 percent per decade (not per year), or 13 percent over the 50-year period.

Increases in agricultural yields. As mentioned above, the establishment view projects increases of from 1.0 to 1.5 percent per year in yields. The graphs in Chapter 11 show that this range is consistent with historical trends and experience. Here we take the midpoint of that range (1.25 percent per year) as our assumption. Under this assumption, yields grow to 186 percent of current levels over the next 50 years.

Total increase in supply. Under these assumptions, total food supply (at constant prices) would increase to (1.13 x 1.86 =) 210 percent of current levels.

Effect on price. If food demand grows to 208 percent of current levels while supply grows to 210 percent of current levels, we see a slight downward pressure on prices. Assuming a demand elasticity of 0.2 and a supply elasticity of 0.5, food price would decline by about 3 percent from current levels.

Extent of undernutrition. Of course, we cannot estimate what happens to the extent of undernutrition with any precision by using only these worldwide aggregate numbers. But ample evidence shows that the extent of undernutrition will decline substantially under this scenario. The projected calories per capita per day increase from the current 2,700 to 3,500 (about the level in the United States during the mid-1980s). In addition, notice that while the price of food (in this scenario) is essentially unchanged at the end of 50 years, average income per capita has doubled. This should lead to a substantial reduction in the extent of undernutrition. In fact, this is the prediction of the establishment view. For example, the FAO projects that the number of food-insecure people should drop from 840 million (about 20 percent of the developing world's population) in the early 1990s to 680 million in 2010 (about 12 percent of the population). The International Food Policy Research Institute projects that by 2020, the number of malnourished children will have dropped 20 percent from 1993 levels; during the same period, total population will increase by more than 30 percent.

□ **"Sensitivity Analysis":**
What Happens If We Change Assumptions?

The base scenario permits us to modify assumptions one at a time and see how sensitive the results are to changes in the assumptions.

Scenario A-1: lower population growth. If population grows at the UN low-variant, or about 0.55 percent per year, population at the end of 50 years is higher by only 32 percent. If we hold all other assumptions constant, this would mean supply growing much faster than demand, and huge price decreases (54 percent declines). Although the supply curve shifts out by 110 percent, the price decline causes a movement along the supply curve of 27 percent (based on a 0.5 supply elasticity). Thus, the total increase in quantity of food supplied is 83 percent.

Scenario A-2: lower yield growth. If average yield growth is 0.8 percent per year, rather than 1.25 percent in the base scenario, yields at the end of 50 years will have increased by 49 percent above current levels. Total supply of food increases slightly more rapidly than population; so here again food availability per capita increases. However, food supply increases less rapidly than food demand; therefore prices rise substantially, although less rapidly than the increase in incomes. A scenario of higher population growth (at the UN high-variant of 1.3 percent annual growth) yields results that are qualitatively similar: Demand grows faster than supply; supply per capita increases slightly; food prices increase but less than the increase in average incomes.

The reader is invited to create other alternative scenarios. Again, let us stress the importance of consistency. For example, if we construct a high-income-growth scenario, but maintain our initial assumption about yield growth, we will conclude that demand growth outstrips supply growth and prices rise. But economy-wide prosperity is likely to be linked to increased agricultural productivity: If the economy is prosperous, more money can be invested in agricultural productivity; in developing countries where agriculture is a large sector of the economy, agricultural productivity is a prerequisite for high rates of economic growth.

☐ An "Anti-establishment View" Scenario

A scenario (scenario B in Table 22.1) that is consistent with the anti-establishment view is likely to reflect the following assumptions.

Population. The anti-establishment view does not take a strong stand on population projections. At least at the outset, population growth is assumed to be the same as in the establishment-view scenario—average annual growth of 0.95 percent per year. If the base-case scenario (with the UN medium-variant and U.S. Census population growth) appears to entail widespread undernutrition, we can revisit the scenario with lower population growth.

Income and calories per capita. The anti-establishment view is similarly silent on explicit projections about growth in income per capita.

However, the view does predict a considerable degree of stagnation or depression in the agricultural economy. Therefore, to be consistent with the anti-establishment view, we will assume that income per capita grows much more slowly—at a rate of 0.5 percent per year. This translates into an increase in income of 28 percent over the 50-year period, and an increase in calories demanded per capita of about 4 percent. We will assume that the impact of dietary diversification is an additional 2 percent. The cumulative effect is to increase plant-equivalent demand per capita by 6 percent. (It is important to note here that this is an increase in demand—holding prices constant. If prices increase—as is likely under the anti-establishment scenario—actual food intake per capita may decline.)

Total shift in demand. Given the above assumptions, total demand for food will be higher by a factor of (1.60 x 1.06 =) 170 percent—70 percent higher than current demand.

Increase in agricultural land. As noted in Chapter 11, the anti-establishment view believes there may be declines in agricultural land due to degradation and a rise in sea level from global warming. In this scenario, we assume that agricultural area decreases by 15 percent over the 50-year period.

Increases in agricultural yields. The anti-establishment view is doubtful that historical rates of growth can be continued. It may be reasonable (from the standpoint of this view) to assume that yields do not increase at all, or even that they decline as irrigation and land quality decline. Here we assume that yields do continue to grow, but at only a 0.2 percent rate for the next 50 years. Under this assumption, yields grow by 10 percent over the next 50 years.

Total increase in supply. Under these assumptions, total food supply (at constant prices) would decrease to (0.85 x 1.10 =) 93.5 percent of current levels.

Effect on price. If demand grows by 70 percent and supply declines by 7 percent, price must increase. Using the 0.2 demand elasticity and 0.5 supply elasticity, this 77 percent difference between quantity demanded and quantity supplied at current prices means that the price must rise by 110 percent to return supply and demand to equilibrium.

Extent of undernutrition. The anti-establishment conclusion is that the extent of undernutrition increases substantially. The decline in average purchasing power supports this conclusion—average incomes increase by 28 percent while prices increase by 110 percent. Additional evidence of food shortage is found in food available per capita. In terms of calories per capita per day, with the current level being 2,700, this scenario implies that at the end of 50 years, there would be available about 2,500 calories per capita per day. (Although the supply curve declines under this scenario, we see an increase in quantity supplied in response to the much higher prices. See appendix for details.)

Under this scenario, worldwide calories per capita per day have fallen to levels seen in the mid-1960s. During this period, population was growing at a faster rate than currently and incomes were lower than they are currently. So we might want to investigate what happens under this scenario when population grows more rapidly and income is stagnant. This is shown in scenario B-1. Here, we assume that the population at the end of 50 years has more than doubled—growing by 120 percent. (This rate of population growth is even higher than the UN high-growth variant, but is not as high as growth rates experienced during the 1960s.) Income growth, and growth in demand per capita, is assumed to be zero. The outcome of this scenario is catastrophic: Food prices increase by 181 percent and worldwide calories per capita per day decline to 2,258. This is less than the current level of food availability in Africa. At this level, there would undoubtedly be much more widespread undernutrition and large increases in infant and child mortality. The large population results from high fertility and includes therefore many children who die before the age of five.

Scenario B-2 shows that if yields grow a little more strongly (0.8 percent per year rather than 0.2 percent per year as in scenarios B and B-1) major catastrophe is avoided. Maintaining the other assumptions of scenario B, we see that demand grows by 70 percent while supply grows by 27 percent. This leads to a food price increase of 16 percent. The scenario also predicts a slight decline in average food availability per capita from the current 2,700 calories per capita per day to 2,658.

☐ Policies

Scenarios such as those presented here may be useful in evaluating the likely impacts of various policies. Policy action or inaction will influence the future course of events and the severity of the worldwide hunger problem. Experts do not agree on all details about what comprises a "best policy," nor do they agree on the likely impacts of any policy option. However, there is widespread agreement that policy initiatives should focus on the following objectives:

Reduce the rate of population growth. In addition to economic incentives to promote small families, general economic prosperity and improved health and education systems can be an important part of these policies.

Invest in improved agricultural productivity. Direct government investment in agricultural research and extension, and improved access to rural credit and markets will play an important role here.

Protect soil and water resources. Agricultural research can assist in this. In addition, clearly assigned and enforceable property rights will give resource owners a personal stake in environmental protection.

Encourage economic growth among the poorest. Appropriate macroeconomic policies, reliance on competitive markets, and investment in human capital are likely to be important elements of this policy.

> *It is for us, the living, to be dedicated to the unfinished task.*
> —Abraham Lincoln, The Gettysburg Address

■ APPENDIX:
MATHEMATICS USED IN MAKING PROJECTIONS

□ Using Growth Rates to Project the Future

To understand the calculations behind the scenarios presented in Chapter 22, it is necessary to know some elementary mathematics of growth. A simple example explains the basic point. Suppose a city starts the year with a population of 100,000, and suppose the population grows by 10 percent during the year. At the end of the year (year 1), the city's population will be 110,000. We get this by multiplying the population at the beginning of the year (100,000) by 1 plus the annual growth rate (10 percent or 0.10):

$$110,000 = 100,000 \times (1 + 0.10)$$

end of year value = beginning of year value times 1 plus growth rate

To conserve verbiage, we assign symbols to these words with V_1 being the value at the end of year 1, V_0 being the value at the beginning of year 1 (or at the end of year zero), and r being the growth rate.

$$V_1 = V_0 (1 + r) \tag{1}$$

Now suppose the population grows by 10 percent for the second year. We can use equation (1) to calculate the population at the end of year two. The population at the end of year 2 will be

$$110,000 \times (1 + 0.10) = 121,000$$

Notice that we can also write this as:

$$(100,000 \times [1 + 0.10]) \times (1 + 0.10) = 121,000$$

Similarly, at the end of year 3 (if growth continues at 10 percent) the population would be

([100,000 x (1 + 0.10)] x (1 + 0.10)) x (1 + 0.10) = 121,000 x (1 + 0.10) = 133,100

The last two calculations show us a pattern:

$$V_1 = V_0 (1 + r)^1$$
$$V_2 = V_0 (1 + r)^2$$
$$V_3 = V_0 (1 + r)^3$$

The general rule used to calculate values at the end of T periods is

$$V_T = V_0 (1 + r)^T \qquad (2)$$

To return to Chapter 22, and see how equation (2) is applied, look at the assumption about population growth in scenario A. Population is assumed to grow at an average rate of 0.95 percent (or 0.0095) over the 50-year period. Applying equation (2) gives us

$$V_{50} = V_0 (1+.0095)^{50} = V_0 \times 1.6044$$

This means that population at the end of 50 years is "160 percent of current levels" or "60.44 percent higher than population at the beginning of the 50-year period." This information is entered in Table 22.1 as "+60 percent" in the population column of scenario A. Similarly, yield growth of 1.25 percent (0.0125) per year for 50 years gives us a yield at the end of the period that is $(1.0125)^{50}$ or 1.86 times the level at the beginning of the 50 years. This information is entered in Table 22.1 as "+86 percent" in the yield column of scenario A.

☐ **Calculating the Total Impact**
When Two Multiplicative Factors Are Growing

Total Demand is demand per capita times the number of people. In our scenarios, both of these factors (demand per capita and population) grow. As explained in Chapter 10, when this happens, growth rate for total demand is calculated as follows. Following scenario A for an example, if population grows by 60 percent over the 50-year period, and if (plant-equivalent) calories per capita grows by 30 percent over the period, growth in total demand is calculated as follows:

$$(1 + .60) \times (1 + .30) = 2.08$$

Total demand at the end of the 50-year period is 2.08 times (or 208 percent of) demand at the beginning of the period; or demand has increased by 108 percent. Likewise, total supply is number of hectares (area) times yield per hectare; so growth in total supply is calculated in a similar fashion.

☐ Calculating the Price Change

The changes in demand and supply in our scenarios assume constant prices—we are projecting the degree to which demand and supply curves shift in the future. (Those with more training in economics will notice that our demand factors—population and income—are traditional demand shifters in economic theory; however, our supply factors—area and yield—are not consistent with theoretical economics of supply. We analyze growth in supply using these supply factors because they make the supply side of the equation easier to understand. It is also interesting to note that historical trends in these variables are observed for a period in which real agricultural prices were declining slightly—see Chapter 5.) If demand grows faster than supply, equilibrium price will increase from current levels. If supply grows faster than demand, equilibrium price will decrease.

How do we calculate the size of the price change? Scenario A illustrates the calculation. In scenario A, supply is projected to grow by 110 percent and demand is projected to grow by 108 percent. Thus, at constant prices, quantity supplied would exceed quantity demanded by 2 percent. We expect the price to fall. If the price fell by 1 percent, quantity supplied would drop by 0.5 percent (the elasticity of supply is assumed to be 0.5) and the quantity demanded would increase by 0.2 percent (the elasticity of demand is assumed to be 0.2). To erase the 2 percent difference in supply and demand, the price would need to drop by 2.86 percent. This would create a drop in quantity supplied of 1.43 percent, and an increase in quantity demanded of 0.57 percent.

The general calculation uses the following:

$$\text{Price Increase} = \frac{\% \text{ growth in demand} - \% \text{ growth in supply}}{\text{elasticity of supply} + \text{elasticity of demand}}$$

(where elasticities are expressed as absolute values). If growth in demand is less than growth in supply, the "price increase" is negative—that is, the price declines. Given the assumptions about elasticities, this becomes

$$\text{Price Increase} = \frac{\% \text{ growth in demand} - \% \text{ growth in supply}}{0.7}$$

☐ Calculating the Calories per Capita per Day

To calculate the total quantity supplied, we adjust the growth in supply by movement along the supply curve implied by the projected price change. So the total quantity supplied increases by supply growth plus 0.5 times the price change. If population remained constant, calories per capita per day would increase from the current level of about 2,700 by this amount.

But population does not remain constant in our scenarios. Therefore, we divide the growth in quantity supplied by the growth in population and multiply this by the current level (2,700 calories per capita per day) to calculate future food intake.

Calories per
capita per day $=$ $\dfrac{2700 \times ([1 + \text{growth in supply}] + [0.5 \times \text{price increase}])}{1 + \text{growth in population}}$
in 50 years

□ References

Adams, Dale W. 1983. Mobilizing household savings through rural financial markets. In *Rural financial markets in developing countries, Their use and abuse,* ed. J. D. Von Pischke, et al., 399–407. Baltimore: Johns Hopkins Press.

Adams, Dale W., and Douglas H. Graham. 1981. A critique of traditional agricultural credit projects and policies. *Journal of Development Economics* 8:347–366.

Adams, Dale W., et al., ed. 1984. *Undermining rural development with cheap credit.* Boulder: Westview Press.

Adelman, I., and C. T. Morris. 1973. *Economic growth and social equity in developing countries.* Stanford: Stanford University Press.

Ahluwalia, Montek S. 1976a. Income distribution and development: Some sytlized facts. *American Economic Review* 66 (May):128–135.

———. 1976b. Inequality, poverty and development. *Journal of Development Economics* 3 (September):307–342.

Ahluwalia, Montek S., N. Carter, and H. Chenery. 1979. Growth and poverty in developing countries. Chapter 11 in *Structural change and development policy,* ed. H. Chenery. Oxford: Oxford University Press. Also available in *Journal of Development Economics* 6 (September):299–341.

Ahmed, Raisuddin. 1988. Structure, costs, and benefits of food subsidies in Bangladesh. In *Food subsidies in developing countries,* ed. Per Pinstrup-Andersen, 219–228. Baltimore: Johns Hopkins University Press.

———. 1989. Making rural infrastructure a priority. Washington, D.C.: International Food Policy Research Institute. *IFPRI Report.* Vol. 11, No. 1, pp. 1, 4.

Ahmed, Raisuddin, and Mahabub Hossain. 1990. *Developmental impact of rural infrastructures: Bangladesh.* Washington, D.C.: International Food Policy Research Institute. IFPRI Research Report 83.

Alberts, Tom. 1983. *Agrarian reform and rural poverty: A case study of Peru.* Boulder: Westview Press.

Alderman, Harold. 1986. *The effect of food price and income changes on the acquisition of food by low-income households.* Washington, D.C.: International Food Policy Research Institute.

Alderman, Harold, and Joachim von Braun. 1984. *The effects of the Egyptian food ration and subsidy system on income distribution and consumption.* Washington,

378   *References*

D.C.: International Food Policy Research Institute. IFPRI Research Report 45.

Alexandratos, N., ed. 1995. *World agriculture: Towards 2010, an FAO study.* London: John Wiley.

Allison, Graham T. 1971. *Essence of decision: Explaining the Cuban missile crisis.* Boston: Little, Brown and Company.

Alston, Philip. 1997. Recognition of the right to food. *UN/FAO world food summit fact sheet.* Rome: UN/FAO. Available at http://www.fao.org./wfs/fs/e/img/right-e.pdf

Anderson, J. R., and J. A. Roumasset. 1985. Microeconomics of food insecurity: The stochastic side of poverty. Unpublished paper available through the Department of Economics, U. of Hawaii, Manoa.

Anderson, Jock, et al. 1985. *International agricultural research centers: A study of achievements and potential; Summary.* Washington, D.C.: World Bank, Consultative Group on International Agricultural Research.

Anderson, Mary Ann, et al. 1981. *Nutrition intervention in developing countries, study I: Supplementary feeding.* Cambridge, Mass.: Oelgeschlager, Gunn and Hain.

Angé, A. L. 1993. *Trends of plant nutrient management in developing countries.* Rome: FAO.

Angel, J. Lawrence. 1984. Health as a crucial factor in the changes from hunting to developed farming in the Eastern Mediterranean. In *Paleopathology at the origins of agriculture,* ed. M. N. Cohen and G. J. Armelagos, 51–73. New York: Academic Press.

Anonymous. 1974. How hunger kills. *Time,* 11 November, 68.

Anonymous. 1988. Women and development: Education and fertility. *Finance and Development* (September) 43.

Arnold, Jesse C., R. W. Engel, D. B. Aguillon, and M. Caedo. 1981. Utilization of family characteristics in nutritional classification of preschool children. *American Journal of Clinical Nutrition* 34 (November):2546–2550.

Aron, Robert, et al. 1962. *Les origines de la guerre d'Algerie.* Paris: Fayard.

Askari, Hossein, and John T. Cummings. 1976. *Agricultural supply response: A survey of the econometric evidence.* New York: Praeger.

Astawa, I. B. 1979. Using the local community: Bali, Indonesia. In *Birth control: An international assessment,* ed. M. Potts and P. Bhiwandiwala, 55–70. Baltimore: University Park Press.

Bale, Malcolm D. 1984. Opening of the discussion on plenary paper 5. In *Proceedings of the fourth congress of the E.A.A.E., agricultural markets and prices.* In *European Review of Agricultural Economics* 12:82–83.

———. 1985. *Agricultural trade and food policy: The experience of five developing countries.* Washington, D.C.: World Bank Staff Working Paper No. 724.

Bale, Malcolm D., and Ernst Lutz. 1981. Price distortions in agriculture and their effects: An international comparison. *American Journal of Agricultural Economics* 63 (February):8–22.

Bautista, Romeo M. 1987. *Production incentives in Philippine agriculture: Effects of trade and exchange rate policies* Washington, D.C.: International Food Policy Research Institute. IFPRI Research Report 59.

Baylor, K. 1996. *Biochemical studies on the toxicity of isocyanates: Abstract from a PhD thesis submitted to University College Cork (Ireland), May 1996.* http://www.connect.net/dreggie/Methyl%20I.htm

Beal, George M., and D. J. Hobbs. 1969. *Social action: The process in community and area development.* Ames, Iowa: Iowa State University Cooperative Extension Service, Soc-16. August.

Beal, George M., and Everett M. Rogers. 1960. *The adoption of two farm practices in a central Iowa community.* Ames, Iowa: Iowa State University Agricultural and Home Economics Experiment Station Special Report No. 26.

Beaton, George H., and Hossein Ghassemi. 1982. Supplementary feeding programs for young children in developing countries. *American Journal of Clinical Nutrition* 35 (April):864–916.

Becker, Gary. 1975. *Human capital.* New York: Columbia University Press.

Becker, K., Chief, Basic Data Unit, Statistics Division, FAO, Rome. 1989. Letter to author. January 16.

Belmont, Lillian, and Francis A. Marolla. 1973. Birth order, family size, and intelligence—A study of a total population of 19-year-old men born in the Netherlands. *Science* Vol. 182, No. 4117 (December):1096–1101.

Bengoa, J. M. 1972. Nutritional significance of mortality statistics. In *Proceedings of the Third Western Hemisphere Nutrition Congress.* New York: Futura.

Berg, Alan. 1973. *The nutrition factor—Its role in national development.* Washington, D.C.: Brookings.

———. 1987. *Malnutrition—What Can Be Done?* Baltimore: Johns Hopkins Press.

Berry, A. R., and W. R. Cline. 1979. *Agrarian structure and productivity in developing countires.* Baltimore: Johns Hopkins University Press.

Bettany, G. T. 1890. Introduction. An essay published with the 1890 Ward edition of the *Essay on population,* by T. R. Malthus.

Bezuneh, Mesfin, Brady J. Deaton, and George W. Norton. 1988. Food aid impacts in rural Kenya. *American Journal of Agricultural Economics* 70 (February):181–191.

Bhargava, Alok. 1996. Econometric analysis of psychometric data: A model for Kenyan schools. Washington, D.C.: World Bank, Policy Research.

Binswanger, Hans. 1978. *The economics of tractors in South Asia: An analytical review.* New York: Agricultural Development Council; and Hyderabad, India: International Crops Research Institute for the Semi-Arid Tropics.

Binswanger, Hans, and Klaus Deininger. 1997. Explaining Agricultural and Agrarian Policies in Developing Countries. *Journal of Economic Literature* 35 (December):1958–2005.

Binswanger, Hans, Graeme Donovan, et al. 1987. *Agricultural mechanization, issues and options.* Washington, D.C.: World Bank Policy Study.

Birdsall, Nancy. 1984. Population growth, its magnitude and implications for development. *Finance and Development* 21 (September):10–13.

Blake, Judith. 1989. *Family size and achievement.* Berkeley: U. of California Press.

Bleichrodt, Nico, and Marise PH. Born. 1994. A metaanalysis of reseearch on iodine and its relationship to cognitive development. In Stanbury 1994.

Bliss, C. J., and N. Y. Stern. 1982. *Palanpur: The economy of an Indian village.* Oxford: Clarendon Press.

Boediono. 1978. Elastisitas permintaan untuk berbagai barang di Indonesia; Penerapan metode Frisch. *Ekonomi dan Keuangan Indonesia* 26 (September): 362.

Bongaarts, John. 1982. The fertility-inhibiting effects of the intermediate fertility variables. *Studies in Family Planning* 13:179–189.

Boserup, Ester. 1981. *Population and technological change: A study of long-term trends.* Chicago: University of Chicago Press.

Bouis, Howarth E. 1991. The changing focus of economic research on nutrition. Washington, D.C.: International Food Policy Research Institute, *IFPRI Report* Vol. 13, No. 2, pp. 1, 4.

Bouis, Howarth E., and Lawrence Haddad. 1990. *The effects of agricultural commercialization on land tenure, household resource allocation, and nutrition in the Philippines.* Washington, D.C.: International Food Policy Research Institute, IFPRI Research Report 79.

———. 1992. Are estimates of colorie-income elasticities too high? *Journal of Development Economics* 39:333–364.

Boulding, Kenneth. 1964. *The meaning of the 20th Century.* New York: Harper and Row.

Bread for the World. 1997. *Hunger in the global economy: Hunger 1998.* Silver Spring, Md.: Bread for the World Institute.

Briscoe, J. 1979. The qualitative effect of infection of the use of food by young children in poor countries. *American Journal of Clinical Nutrition* 32 (March):648–676.

Bromley, Daniel. 1981. The role of land reform in economic development, policies and politics: Discussion. *American Journal of Agricultural Economics* 63 (May):399–400.

Brown, Lester R. 1970. *Seeds of change: The green revolution and development in the 1970's.* New York: Praegar.

———. 1974. *In the human interest—A strategy to stabilize world population.* New York: Norton.

———. 1983. *Population policies for a new economic era.* Washington, D.C.: Worldwatch Paper 53.

———. 1988. *The changing world food prospect: The nineties and beyond.* Washington, D.C.: Worldwatch Paper 85.

Brown, Lester, and Hal Kane. 1994. *Full house: Reassessing the earth's population carrying capacity.* Washington, D.C.: Worldwatch Institute.

Brown, Lynn. 1997. The potential impact of AIDS on population and economic growth rates. *2020 Brief* 43 (June). Washington D.C.: IFPRI. Available at http://www.cgiar.org/ifpri/2020/briefs/2br43.htm

Bulatao, Rodolfo A. 1984a. Fertility control at the community level: A review of research and community programs. In *Rural Development and Human Fertility*, ed. W. Schutjer, and C. Stokes, 269–290. New York: MacMillan.

———. 1984b. *Reducing fertility in developing countries: A review of determinants and policy servers.* Washington, D.C.: World Bank Staff Working Paper No. 680, Population and Development Series No. 5.

Bumb, Balu L., and Carlos A. Baanante. 1996. World trends in fertilizer use and projections to 2020. *2020 Brief* 38 (October) Washington D.C.: IFPRI.

Burki S., and Robert Ayres. 1986. A fresh sook at development aid. *Finance and Development* 23 (March):6.

Caldwell, John C. 1983. Direct economic costs and benefits of children. In *Determinants of fertility in developing countries, Vol. 1, Supply and demand for children.* ed. Rudolfo A. Bulatao et al., 458–493. New York: Academic Press.

Calegar, Geraldo M., and G. Edward Schuh. 1988. *The Brazilian wheat policy: Its costs, benefits, and effects on food consumption.* Washington, D.C.: International Food Policy Research Institute. IFPRI Research Report 66.

Campbell, Joseph K. 1984. Machines and food production. In *World food issues*, ed. Matthew Drosdoff, 47–50. Ithaca: Cornell University College of Agriculture.

Carner, George. 1984. Survival, interdependence, and competition among the Philippine rural poor. In *People-centered development.* ed. David Korten and Rudi Klauss, 133–145. West Hartford, Conn.: Kumarian Press.

Carson, Rachel. 1962. *Silent spring.* Greenwich, Conn.: Fawcett.

Carter, Michael. 1989. *U.S. farm exports and third world agricultural development.* Madison: Department of Agricultural Economics, U. of Wisc. Economic Issues, No. 111.

Cassidy, Claire. 1980. Benign neglect and toddler malnutrition. In *Social and biological predictors of nutritional status, physical growth, and neurological development,* ed. Lawrence S. Greene, 109–139. New York: Academic Press.

———. 1987. World-view conflict and toddler malnutrition: Change agent dilemmas. In *Child survival: Anthropological perspectives on the treatment and maltreatment of children,* ed. Nancy Scheper-Hughes, 293–324. Norwell, Mass.: Reidel.

Cavallo, Domingo, and Yair Mundlak. 1982. *Agriculture and economic growth in an open economy: The case of Argentina.* Washington, D.C.: International Food Policy Research Institute. IFPRI Research Report 36.

CGIAR (Consultative Group on International Agricultural Research). 1995. Wheat is doing well in Syria. *CGIAR Newsletter* (October). Washington, D.C.: World Bank. Available at http://www.worldbank.org/html/cgiar/newsletter/Oct95/3syria.htm

———. 1997. *25 years of food and agriculture improvement in developing countries.* Washington D.C.: World Bank. Available at http://www.worldbank.org/html/cgiar/25years/25cover.html

Chambers, Robert, Richard Longhurst, David Bradley, and Richard Feacham. 1979. *Seasonal dimensions to rural poverty: Analysis and practical implications.* Brighton, England: University of Sussex, Institute of Development Studies. Discussion Paper 142.

Champakam, S., S. C. Srikantia, and C. Gopalan. 1968. Kwashiorkor and mental development. *American Journal of Clinical Nutrition* 21 (August):844–852.

Chandra, Ranjit K. 1980. Immunocompetence in undernutrition and overnutrition. *Nutrition Review* 39:225–231.

———. 1988. Nutritional regulation of immunity: An introduction. In *Nutrition and immunology,* ed. Ranjit Chandra, 1–7. New York: Alan R. Liss.

Chavez, Adolfo, and Celia Martinez. 1982. Growing up in a developing community—A bio-ecological study of the development of children from poor peasant families in Mexico. Mexico: Instituto Nacional de la Nutricion. (Translated from the Spanish.)

Chen, P. C. 1981. China's birth planning program. In *National research council committee on population and demography: Research on the population in China, proceedings of a workshop,* 78–90. Washington, D.C.: National Academy Press.

Chen, P. C., and A. Kols. 1982. Population and birth planning in the People's Republic of China. *Population Reports,* Series J, Number 25, January-February, Volume X, Number 1:577–618.

Chenery, Hollis B. 1971. Growth and structural change. *Finance and Development Quarterly* 3:16–27.

Chen, R. S. 1990. Global agriculture, environment, and hunger: Past, present, and future links. *Environmental Impact Assesment Review* 10 (4):335–358.

Chenery, Hollis, Sherman Robinson, and Moshe Syrquin. 1986. *Industrialization and growth: A comparative study.* New York: Oxford University Press.

Chevalier, P. 1995. Zinc and duration of treatment of severe malnutrition [letter; comment]. *Lancet* 345, no. 8956 (April 22):1046–1047.

Chhibber, Ajay. 1988. Raising agricultural output: Price and nonprice factors. *Finance and Development* (June):44–47.

Chidambaram, G. 1989. *Tamil Nadu integrated nutrition project: Terminal evaluation.* Madras, India: State Planning Commission.

References

Chisholm, Anthony H., and Rodney Tyers, eds. 1982. *Food security: Theory, policy, and perspectives from Asia and the Pacific rim.* Lexington, Mass.: Lexington Books.

Chu, Yung-Peng. 1982. Growth and distribution in a small, open economy. Ph.D. diss., University of Maryland.

Clark, Colin G. 1973. More people, more dynamism. *CERES* Rome: FAO (Nov.-Dec).

Clarendon Press. 1959. *The shorter Oxford economic atlas of the world.* Second edition. Oxford: Oxford University Press, 1959.

Clay, Jason W., and Bonnie K. Holcomb. 1986. *Politics and the Ethiopian famine 1984–1985.* Cambridge, Mass.: Cultural Survival.

Cleaver, Kevin M. 1985. *The impact of price and exchange rate policies on agriculture in sub-Saharan Africa.* Washington, D.C.: World Bank. Staff Working Paper No. 728.

Coale, Ansley J., and Edgar M. Hoover. 1958. *Population growth and economic development in low-income countries: A case study of India's prospects.* Princeton: Princeton University Press.

Cohen, Joel. 1996a. *How many can the earth support?* New York: Norton.

———. 1996b. Maximum occupancy. *American Demographics* (February).

Cohen, Mark N. 1984. An introduction to the symposium. In *Paleopathology at the origins of agriculture,* ed. Mark Cohen and George Armelagos, 1–11. New York: Academic Press.

Cohen, Mark N. and George Armelagos, eds. 1984. *Paleopathology at the origins of agriculture.* New York: Academic Press.

Cook, Robert C., 1962. How many people have ever lived on earth? *Population Bulletin,* Vol. 18 (February).

Cowell, F. A. 1977. *Measuring inequality: Techniques for the social sciences.* New York: John Wiley.

Crosson, Pierre. 1996a. Who will feed China? *Perspectives on the Long-Term Global Food Situation* 2 (spring). Available at http://www.fas.org/food/issue2.html

———. 1996b. Resource degradation? *Perspectives on the Long-Term Global Food Situation* (summer). Available at http://www.fas.org/food/issue2.html

Cunningham, A. S., D. B. Jelliffe, and E. F. P. Jelliffe. 1991. Breastfeeding and health in the 1980s: A global epidemiological review. *Journal of Pediatrics* 15:659–668.

Dagum, Camilo. 1987. Gini ratio. In *The new Palgrave: A dictionary of economics,* Vol. 2, ed. John Eatwell et al., 529–532. New York, Stockton Press.

Dalrymple, Dana G. 1964. The Soviet famine of 1932–1934. *Soviet Studies* 15 (January):250–284.

———. 1979. The adoption of high-yielding grain varieties in developing countries. *Agricultural History* 53 (October):704–726.

———. 1985. The development and adoption of high-yielding varieties of wheat and rice in developing countries. *American Journal of Agricultural Economics* 67 (December):1067–1073.

———. 1986a. See U.S. Department of State 1986a.

———. 1986b. See U.S. Department of State 1986b.

Dam, Marjory. 1989. *Report of world health.* Geneva: WHO (September).

Das Gupta, Monica. 1988. Selective discrimination against female children in rural Punjab, India. *Population and Development Review* 13:77–100.

Datta, S. K., S. H. Ghosh, and C. N. Bairagya. 1988. Growth and yield of wet season rice with tilapia fish. *International Rice Research Newsletter* 13 (August): 46.

Deininger, Klaus, and Lyn Squire. 1997. Economic growth and income inequality: Reexamining the links. *Finance and Development* (March):38–41.

De Janvry, Alain. 1981. The role of land reform in economic development: Policies and politics. *American Journal of Agricultural Economics* 63:384–392.

DeLong, G.R., et al. 1996. Effect of iodination of irrigation water on crop and animal production in Long Ru, Hotien County, Xinjiang. *Mineral problems in sheep in northern China and other regions of Asia: Proceedings of a work-shop held in Beijing, People's Republic of China, 25–30 September 1995*. Canberra: Australian Centre for International Agricultural Research, 49–51.

De Zoysa, Isabelle, et al., 1985. *Focus on Diarrhoea*. London: Ross Institute, London School of Hygiene and Tropical Medicine, Keppel St., WC1E 7HT. For The Save the Children Fund (U.K.).

Deaton, Angus, and John Muellbauer. 1980. *Economics and consumer behavior*. Cambridge: Cambridge University Press.

Dever, James R. 1983. Determinants of nutritional status in a North Indian village: An economic analysis. Master's thesis, University of Maryland.

Diamond, Jared. 1987. The worst mistake in the history of the human race. *Discover* (May):64–66.

Dickens, Charles. 1958. *A tale of two cities*. London: Oxford U. Press.

Diro Pusat Statik. 1981. Statistik harga yan diterima dan yan dibayar pentani untuk biaya produksi pertanian dan Kebutuhan Rumah Tangga Tani. Jawa: Madura dan beberapa Propinsi Luar Jawa. Jakarta, Indonesia (December).

Dixon, John A. 1982. *Food consumption patterns and related demand parameters in Indonesia: A review of available evidence*. Washington D.C.: International Food Policy Research Institute, International Fertilizer Development Center, and the International Rice Research Institute. Working Paper No. 6.

Dommen, Arthur J. 1988. *Innovation in African agriculture*. Boulder: Westview Press.

Dover, Michael, and Lee M. Talbot. 1987. *To feed the earth: Agro-ecology for sustainable development*. Washington, D.C.: World Resources Institute.

Dreze, Jean, and Amartya Sen. 1989. *Hunger and public action*. Oxford: Oxford University Press.

————, eds. 1990. *The political economy of hunger*, 3 vols. Oxford: Oxford University Press.

Duke, Lynne. 1998. Land reform plan divides Zimbabweans. *Washington Post*, Sunday, February 15, 1998, A27.

Durand, C. H., and J. P. Pigney. 1963. Revue de 410 cas de diarrhees aqueuses infectieuses chez le nourisson et l'enfant de moins de deux ans, traites pendant quatre ans dan les meme service hospitalier. *Ann. Pediat.* 39:1386.

Edirisinghe, Neville. 1987. *The food stamp scheme in Sri Lanka: Costs, benefits, and options for modification*. Washington, D.C.: International Food Policy Research Institute.

Edirisinghe, Neville, and Thomas T. Poleman. 1983. *Behavioral thresholds as indicators of perceived dietary adequacy or inadequacy*. Ithaca, N.Y.: Cornell University. International Agricultural Economics Study 17 (July).

Edwards, Clark. 1988. Real prices received by farmers keep falling. *Choices* (fourth quarter):22–23.

Elias, Victor J. 1985. *Government expenditures on agriculture and agricultural growth in Latin America*. Washington, D.C.: International Food Policy Research Institute. IFPRI Research Report 50.

Elliott, Kathleen. 1978. Editorial. *Lancet* ii:300.

Erlich, P., and A. Erlich. 1991. *Healing the planet.* Reading, Mass.: Addison-Wesley.

Evelth, P. G., and J. M. Tanner. 1967. *Worldwide variation in human growth.* Cambridge: Cambridge U. Press.

Evenson, Robert E. 1981. Benefits and obstacles to appropriate agricultural technology. *Annals of the American Academy of Political and Social Science* 458:54–67, as quoted in *Agricultural development in the third world*, ed. Carl K. Eicher and John M. Staatz, 348–361. Baltimore: Johns Hopkins University Press, 1984.

Evenson, R. E., and P. M. Flores. 1978. Social returns to rice research. In *Economic consequences of the new rice technology*, ed. R. Barker and Y. Hayami, 243–265. Los Banos, Philippines: International Rice Research Institute.

Family Health International. 1997. Internet page available at http://www.fhi.org/fp/fpfaq/index.html

FAO (Food and Agriculture Organization of the United Nations). 1974. *FAO/WHO handbook on human nutritional requirements.* Rome: FAO Nutritional Studies No. 28.

———. 1989. *Food Outlook* (May).

———. 1991. *Food balance sheets, 1984–86 average.* Rome: FAO.

———. 1994. *Body mass index: A measure of chronic energy deficiency in adults.* Rome: FAO.

———. 1996a. World Food Summit (WFS) Technical Background Papers, nos. 1–15. Rome: FAO, UN. Available at http://www.fao.org/wfs/final/e/list-e.htm

———. 1996b. *Fact sheet on water and food security.* Rome: FAO. Available at http://www.fao.org/wfs/fs/e/WatIrr-e.htm

———. 1996c. *Sixth world food survey.* Rome: FAO.

———. 1996d. Special feature: The cereals sector outlook to 2010 seen from mid-1996. *Food Outlook* 5/6 (May/June):8. Available at http://www.fao.org/WAICENT/faoinfo/economic/giews/english/fo/fo9606/fo960607.htm

———. 1997. Factfile. *Contribution of greenhouse gases to global warming.* Available at http://www.fao.org/NEWS/FACTFILE/FF9715–E.HTM

Fass, Simon M. 1982. Water and politics: The process of meeting a basic need in Haiti. *Development and Change.* London and Beverly Hills: Sage 13:347–364.

Feacham, R. G., and M. A. Koblinsky. 1983. Interventions for the control of diarrhoeal diseases among young children: Measles immunization. *Bulletin of the World Health Organization* 61(4):641–652.

———. 1984. Interventions for the control of diarrhoeal diseases among young children: Promotion of breast-feeding. *Bulletin of the World Health Organization* 62(2):271–291.

Fei, John C. H., and Gustav Ranis. 1964. *Development of the labor surplus economy: Theory and policy.* New Haven: Yale University Press.

FIAN (FoodFirst Information and Action Network). 1997. *Twelve misconceptions about the right to food.* Available at http://www.fian.org/miscon.htm.

Finch, V. C., and O. E. Baker. 1971. *See* U.S. Department of Agriculture. 1917.

Fishstein, Paul. 1985. Pre and post green revolution income distribution in a North Indian village. Master's thesis, University of Maryland.

Fogel, Robert W. 1994. Economic growth, population theory, and physiology: The bearing of long-term processes on the making of economic policy. *American Economic Review* 84, no. 3 (June):369–395.

Food for the Hungry Homepage. 1998. Available at http://www.fh.org/

Foster, Phillips. 1972. *Introduction to environmental science.* Homewood, Ill.: Richard D. Irwin.

————. 1978. See U.S. Department of State 1978.

————. 1991. Malnutrition, starvation, and death. In *Horrendous death, health and well-being*, ed. Dan Leviton, 205–218. New York: Hemisphere.

Foster, Phillips, and Herbert Steiner. 1964. *The structure of Algerian socialized agriculture.* College Park: University of Maryland. Ag. Expt. Station MP No. 527.

Frejka, Thomas. 1973. The prospects for a stationary world population. *Scientific American* 228 (March):15.

Frisancho, A. Roberto. 1981. New norms of upper limb fat and muscle areas for the assessment of nutritional status. *American Journal of Clinical Nutrition* 34:2540–2545.

————. 1989. *Anthropometric standards for the evaluation of nutritional status of children and adults.* Ann Arbor: U. of Michigan Press.

Galler, Janina R. 1986. Malnutrition—A neglected cause of learning failure. *Journal of Postgraduate Medicine* 80 (October):225–230.

Galway, Katrina, et. al. 1987. *Child survival: Risks and the road to health.* Columbia, Md.: Westinghouse Institute for Resource Development. Demographic Data for Development Project.

Garcia, Marito, and Per Pinstrup-Andersen. 1987. *The pilot food price subsidy scheme in the Philippines: Its impact on income, food consumption, and nutritional status.* Washington, D.C.: International Food Policy Research Institute. IFPRI Research Report 61.

Gardner, Bruce L. 1979. *Optimal stockpiling of grain.* Lexington: Heath.

————. 1987. *The economics of agricultural policies.* New York: Macmillan.

Gardner, Gary. 1996. *Shrinking fields: Cropland loss in a world of eight billion.* Washington, D.C.: WorldWatch Institute.

George, P. S. 1988. Costs and benefits of food subsidies in India. In *Food subsidies in developing countries*, ed. Per Pinstrup-Andersen, 229–241. Baltimore: Johns Hopkins.

Gershwin, M. Eric, et al. 1985. *Nutrition and immunity.* New York: Academic Press.

Gilmore, Richard, and Barbara Huddleston. 1983. The food security challenge. *Food Policy* 8 (February):31–45.

Glewwe, Paul, Hanan Jacoby, and Elizabeth King. 1996. An economic model of nutrition and learning: Evidence from longitudinal data. Washington, D.C.: World Bank, Policy Research Department.

Godwin, William. 1793. Political justice. In *A reprint of the essay on "Property,"* ed. H. S. Salt. London: Allen & Unwin. 1949.

Goldenberg, R. L., et al. 1995. The effect of zinc supplementation on pregnancy outcome. *Journal of the American Medical Association* 274, no. 6 (August 9):463–468.

Gómez, F., R. Galvan, S. Frank, R. Chavez, and J. Vazquez. 1956. Mortality in third degree malnutrition. *Journal of Tropical Pediatrics* 2:77+.

González-Vega, Claudio. 1983. Arguments for interest rate reform. In *Rural financial markets in developing countries: Their use and abuse*, ed. J. D. von Pischke, et al., 365–372. Baltimore: Johns Hopkins Press.

Goodall, Roger M. 1984. CDD Information Papers No. 1 and 2, New York: UNICEF (United Nations Children's Fund) (June).

Gopalan, C. 1986. Vitamin A deficiency and child mortality. *Nutrition Foundation of India Bulletin (NFI Bulletin).* Vol. 7, No. 3.

————. 1970. Some recent studies in the nutrition research laboratories: Hyderabad. *Journal of Clinical Nutrition* (January):35–53.

Gopalan, C., and K. S. Rao. 1979. Nutrient needs. In *Human nutrition: A comprehensive treatise. Vol. 2, Nutrition and growth.*, ed. D. Jelliffe and E. Jelliffe. New York: Plenum Press, 1979.

Graham, K. K., et al. 1994. Pharmacologic evaluation of megestrol acetate oral suspension in cachectic AIDS patient. *Journal of Acquired Immune Deficiency Syndromes* 7, no. 6:580–585.

Grapentine, Liz. 1998. The official page of breastfeeding propaganda. Available at http://members.aol.com/cgrapentin/brstfeed.html

Gray, Cheryl W. 1982. *Food consumption parameters for Brazil and their application to food policy.* Washington, D.C.: International Food Policy Research Institute. IFPRI Research Report 32.

Griffiths, Marcia. 1985. *Growth monitoring of preschool children: Practical considerations for primary health care projects.* Geneva: World Federation of Public Health Associations.

Griliches, Zvi. 1958. Research costs and social returns: Hybrid corn and related innovations. *Journal of Political Economy* 66:419–431.

Guggenheim, Karl Y. 1981. *Nutrition and nutritional diseases, The evolution of concepts.* Lexington, Mass.: Heath.

Gupta, Arun, and Jon E. Rohide. 1993. Economic value of breast-feeding in India. *Economic and Political Weekly* 28, no. 26:1390.

Haggblade, Steven, and Peter Hazell. 1989. Agricultural technology and farm-nonfarm growth linkages. *Agricultural Economics: The Journal of the International Association of Agricultural Economists* 3:345–364.

Hancock, G. 1985. *Ethiopia: The challenge of hunger.* London: Victor Gollancz.

Harberger, Arnold. 1983. Basic needs versus distributional weights in social cost-benefit analysis. *Economic Development and Cultural Change* 32, no. 3:455–474.

Harlan, Jack R. 1975. *Crops and man.* Madison: American Society of Agronomy.

Haub, Carl. 1987. Understanding population projections. *Population Bulletin* 42, no. 4.

Hayami, Yujiro, and Robert Herdt. 1977. Market price effects of technological change on income distribution in semisubsistence agriculture. *American Journal of Agricultural Economics* 69:245–256.

Heilbroner, Robert L. 1953. *The worldly philosophers.* New York: Simon and Schuster.

Herbert, Sandra. 1971. Darwin, Malthus and selection. *Journal of History of Biology* 4:209–217.

Herdt, Robert W. 1970. A disaggregate approach to aggregate supply. *American Journal of Agricultural Economics* 52:512–520.

———. 1983. Mechanization of rice production in developing Asian countries. In *Consequences of small-farm mechanization,* 1–13. Manila: International Rice Research Institute.

Herdt, Robert W., and Jock R. Anderson. 1987. The contribution of the CGIAR Centers to world agricultural research. In *Policy for agricultural research,* ed. Vernon W. Ruttan and Carl E. Pray, 39–64. Boulder: Westview.

Herdt, Robert W., and John W. Mellor. 1964. The contrasting response of rice to nitrogen—India and United States. *Journal of Farm Economics* 46:150–160.

Herring, Ronald J. 1983. *Land to the tiller: The political economy of agrarian reform in South Asia.* New Haven: Yale University Press.

Hicks, L. E., R. A. Langham, and J. Takenaka. 1992. Cognitive and social measures following early nutritional supplementation: A sibling study. *American Journal of Public Health* 72.

Ho, T. J. [1984]. Economic status and nutrition in East Java. TMs. Washington, D.C.: World Bank Working Paper. Unpublished data from The East Java Nutrition Study sponsored by the University of Airlangga, Surabaya, the Provincial Health Services of East Java and the Royal Tropical Institute of Amsterdam.

Hopkins, Raymond F. 1988. Political calculations in subsidizing food. In *Food subsidies in developing countries*, ed. Per Pinstrup-Andersen, 107–125. Baltimore: Johns Hopkins.

Hossain, Mahabub. 1988a. *Credit for alleviation of rural poverty: The Grameen Bank in Bangladesh*. Washington, D.C.: International Food Policy Research Institute. IFPRI Research Report 65.

————. 1988b. *Nature and impact of the green revolution in Bangladesh*. Washington, D.C.: International Food Policy Research Institute. IFPRI Research Report 67.

Huang, Kuo W. 1985. *U.S. demand for food: A complete system of price and income effects*. Washington D.C.: USDA Tech. Bul. No. 1714.

Huddleston, Barbara. 1984a. *Briefs*. New York.: CARE.

————. 1984b. *Closing the cereals gap with trade and food aid*. Washington, D.C.: International Food Policy Research Institute. IFPRI Research Report 43.

Hull, T. H. 1978. Where credit is due: Policy implications of the recent rapid fertility decline in Bali. TMs. Paper presented at the annual meeting of the Population Association of America, Atlanta.

Hull, T. H., et al. 1977. Indonesia's family planning story: Success and challenge. *Population Bulletin* 32, no. 6.

Hutabarat, Pos M. Proyeksi distribusi konsumsi kalorie menurut kelompok-kelompok pendapatan di Indonesia tahun 1990. [Projections of the distribution of caloric consumption by income groups in Indonesia in 1990.] Master's thesis, Bogor Agricultural University Agricultural School.

Ibe, A. C., and L. F. Awosika. 1991. Sea level rise impact on African coastal zones. In *A change in the weather: African perspectives on climate change*, eds. S. H. Omide and C. Juma 105–112. Nairobi, Kenya: African Centre for Technology Studies.

Indonesia Oleh Direktorat Gizi Departemen Kesehatan R.I. 1979. *Daftar Komposisi Bahan Makanan*. Jakarta: Bhratara Karya Askara.

International Labor Organization (ILO). 1987. *Yearbook of Labor Statistics 1987*. Geneva: International Labor Office of the ILO.

————. 1988. *I. L. O. Information* Geneva: International Labor Office of the ILO. 16, no. 3 (August).

International Rice Research Institute (IRRI). 1989. Azolla helps organic farmer earn more. Manila: International Food Policy Research Institute. *The IRRI Reporter* (June).

Imam, Izzedin I. 1979. *Peasant perceptions: Famine*. Dacca, Bangaladesh: Bangladesh Rural Advancement Committee (July). In *People centered development— Contributions toward theory and planning frameworks*, ed. David C. Korten and Rudi Klauss, 152–155. West Hartford, Conn.: Kumarian Press, 1984.

ISRIC and UNEP. 1991. *World map of the status of human-induced soil degradation* (by L. R. Oldeman, R. T. A. Hakkeling, and W. G. Sombroek). Global Assessment of soil degradation, 2d ed. Niarobi: Wageningen.

Jackson, Tony, with Deborah Eade. 1982. *Against the grain: The dilemma of project food aid*. Oxford: OXFAM.

James, W. P. T., and E. C. Schofield. 1990. Human energy requirements: A manual for planner and nutritionists. Oxford: Oxford University Press.

Jamison, Dean T., et al., eds. 1993. *Disease control priorities in developing countries.* New York: Oxford University Press for the World Bank.

Jelliffe, D. B. 1966. *The assessment of the nutritional status of the community.* Geneva: WHO Monograph Series No. 53.

Johnson, Stanley R., Zuhair A. Hassan, and Richard D. Green. 1984. *Demand systems estimation methods and applicaitons.* Ames: Iowa State University Press.

Joy, Leonard. 1973. Food and nutrition planning. *Journal of Agricultural Economics* 24:166–197.

Judd, M. Ann, James K. Boyce, and Robert E. Evenson. 1987. Investment in agricultural research and extension. In *Policy for Agricultural Research,* ed. Vernon Ruttan and Carl E. Pray, 7–38. Boulder: Westview.

Kakwani, Nanak 1987. Lorenz curve. In *The new Palgrave: A dictionary of economics,* vol. 3., ed. John Eatwell, et al., 243–244. New York, Stockton Press.

Kamrin, M. n.d. Environmental "hormones" pesticide information project. Michigan State University. Available at http://ace.ace.orst.edu/info/extoxnet/tics/env-horm.txt

Karim, Rezaul, Manjur Majid, and F. James Levinson. 1984. The Bangladesh sorghum experiment. *Food Policy* 5:61–63.

Kates, Robert W., et al. 1988. *The hunger report: 1988.* Providence: Brown University, World Hunger Program.

Kates, Robert. 1997. Ending hunger: Current status and future prospects. *Consequences* 2, no. 2. Available at http://gcrio.gcrio.org/CONSEQUENCES/vol2no2/article1.html

Keilmann, A. A., and C. McCord. 1978. Weight-for-age as an index of death in children. *The Lancet* (June):1247–1250.

Kendall, H. W., and D. Pimentel. 1994. Constraints on the expansion of the global food supply. *Ambio* 23:198–205.

Kennedy, Eileen T. 1989. *The effects of sugar cane production on food security, health and nutrition in Kenya: A longitudinal study.* Washington, D.C.: International Food Policy Research Institute. Research Report No. 78.

Kennedy, Eileen T., and Bruce Cogill. 1987. *Income and nutritional effects of the commercialization of agriculture in southwestern Kenya.* Washington, D.C.: International Food Policy Research Institute. IFPRI Research Report 63.

Kennedy, Eileen T., and Odin Knudsen. 1985. A review of supplementary feeding programmes and recommendations on their design. In *Nutrition and development,* ed. Margaret Biswas and Per Pinstrup-Andersen, 77–96. Oxford: Oxford University Press.

Kennedy, Eileen T., P. Pinstrup-Andersen, et al. 1983. *Nutrition-related policies and programs: Past performance and research needs.* Washington, D.C.: International Food Policy Research Institute (February).

Kenya Ministry of Planning and National Development. 1984. *Kenya contraceptive prevalence survey.* Nairobi: Central Bureau of Statistics.

Keys, Ancel, et al. 1950. *The biology of human starvation.* Minneapolis: University of Minnesota Press.

Kostermans, Kees. 1994. *Assessing the quality of anthropometric data: Background and illustrated guidelines for survey managers.* Washington, D.C.: World Bank.

Krick, Jackie. 1988. Using the Z score as a descriptor of discrete changes in growth. *Nutritional Support Services* 6, no. 8 (August).

Krueger, Anne, Maurice Schiff, and Alberto Valdes. 1991. *The political economy of agricultural pricing policy.* Baltimore, Md.: Johns Hopkins University Press for the World Bank.

Kuznets, Simon. 1955. Economic growth and income inequality. *American Economic Review* 65:1–28.

Lancet editorial. 1995. Health effects of sanctions on Iraq. *Lancet* 346, no. 8988 (December 2):1439.

Landman, Lynn. 1983. China's one-child families—Girls need not apply. *RF Illustrated*. New York: The Rockefeller Foundation (December): 8–9.

Lappe, Frances Moore. 1971. *Diet for a small planet*. New York.: Balantine.

Lappe, Francis Moore, and Joseph Collins. 1977. *Food first*. Boston: Houghton Mifflin.

Lashof, D., and D. Tirpak. 1990. Policy options for stabilizing global climate. U.S. Environmental Protection Agency report. New York: Hemisphere.

Latham, Michael C. 1984. International nutrition problems and policies. In *World food issues,* ed. Matthew Drosdoff, 55–64. Ithaca: Cornell University, Center for the Analysis of World Food Issues, Program in International Agriculture.

Leclercq, Vincent. 1988. *Conditions et limites de l'insertion du Bresil dans les echanges mondiaux du soja.* Montpellier, France: INRA.

Lee, John E., and Gary C. Taylor. 1986. Agricultural research: Who pays and who benefits? *Research for Tomorrow, 1986 Yearbook of Agriculture,* 14–21. Washington, D.C.: United States Department of Agriculture.

Lee, Richard. B. 1968. What hunters do for a living, or how to make out on scarce resources. In *Symposium on man the hunter,* ed. R. B. Lee and Irven DeVore, 30–48. Chicago: Aldine.

Lele, Uma. J. [1989]. Overall flows of official development assistance to the MADIA countries. In *Aid to African agriculture: Lessons from two decades of donor experience,* ed. Uma Lele. World Bank discussion paper, undated. (The discussion papers reflect only the views of their authors and should not be attributed to any other people or institutions.)

Lele, Uma J., and Arthur Goldsmith. 1989. The development of national agricultural research capacity: India's experience with the Rockefeller Foundation and its significance for Africa. *Economic Development and Cultural Change* 37:305–343.

Lele, Uma J., Bill H. Kinsey, and Antonia O. Obeya. 1989. Building agricultural research capacity in Africa: Policy lessons from the Madia countries. Unpublished working paper presented for the Joint TAC/CGIAR Center Directors Meeting, Rome, 1989.

Levine, R. E., et al. 1990. *Breastfeeding saves lives: An estimate of breastfeeding related infant survival.* Bethesda, Md.: Center to Prevent Childhood Malnutrition.

Levinger, Beryl. 1994. *Nutrition, health and education for all.* New York: United Nations Development Programme.

———. 1995. Critical transitions: Human capacity development across the lifespan. Available at http://www.edc.org/INT/HCD/

Lewis, W. Arthur. 1954. Economic development with unlimited supplies of labor. *The Manchester School of Economic and Social Studies* (May):139–191.

Li, R., et al. 1994. Functional consequences of iron supplementation in iron-deficient female cotton mill workers in Beijing, China. *American Journal of Clinical Nutrition* 59, no. 4 (April):908–913.

Lipton, Michael. 1977. *Why poor people stay poor: Urban bias in world development.* Cambridge: Harvard University Press.

Lipton, Michael, with Richard Longhurst. 1990. *New seeds and poor people.* Baltimore: Johns Hopkins.

Lorenz, Max C. 1905. Methods of measuring the concentration of wealth. *Publications of the American Statistical Association* 9:209–219.

Mabbs-Zeno, C. C. 1987. *Where, if anywhere, is famine becoming more likely.* College Park, Md.: World Academy of Development and Cooperation (21 ISSN 0882-3235). Also available as an unpublished manuscript from ERS, USDA, Washington, D.C. 20005

Malthus, T. R. 1803–1826. *An essay on the principle of population or a view of its past and present effects on human happiness with an inquiry into our prospects respecting the future removal or mitigation of the evils which it occasions* (first edition 1803, sixth and last 1826). London: Ward, 1890.

Mamarbachi, D., et al. 1980. Observations on nutritional marasmus in a newly rich nation. *Ecology of Food and Nutrition* 9:43–54.

Mann, Charles. 1997. Reseeding the green revolution. *Science* 277 (August 22): 1038–1043.

Martorell, Reynaldo. 1980. The impact of ordinary illnesses on the dietary intakes of malnourished children. *American Journal of Clinical Nutrition* 33:345–350.

———. 1988. Seminar at U. of Md. Nut. Dept. 12/12/88.

———. 1989. Body size, adaptation and function. *Human Organization* 48:15–20.

Masoro, E. J., B. P. Yu, and H. A. Bertrand. 1982. Action of food restriction in delaying the aging process (longevity/metabolic rate/lifetime caloric expenditure/life prolongation). *Proceedings, National Academy of Science* 79:4239–4241.

Maxwell, Simon J. 1978a. Food aid, food for work and public works. Brighton, England: University of Sussex. Institute of Development Studies, Discussion Paper 127 (March).

———. 1978b. Food aid for supplementary feeding programmes: An analysis. *Food Policy* 3:289–298.

Maxwell, Simon J., and H. W. Singer. 1979. Food aid to developing countries: A survey. *World Development* 7:225–247.

Mayer, Jean. 1976. The dimensions of human hunger. In *Food and agriculture*, 14–23. San Francisco: Freeman.

Mazumdar, D. 1965. Size of farm and productivity: A problem of Indian peasant agriculture. *Economica* 32 (May):161–173.

———. 1975. The theory of sharecropping with labor market dualism. *Economica* 42 (August):261–271.

McFarland, William E., et al. 1974. *Demos, demographic-economic models of society—A computerized learning system.* Santa Barbara: General Electric Tempo.

McGuire, Judy S. 1988. *Malnutrition—Opportunities and challenges for A.I.D.,* Resources for the Future, Washington, D.C. 20036 (November).

McKigney, John, and Hamish Munro, ed. 1976. *Nutrient requirements in adolescence.* Cambridge: MIT Press.

McLaughlin, M. 1984. Interfaith Action for Economic Justice (publisher unknown), p. 3.

Meier, G. 1979. Family planning in the banjars of Bali. *International Family Planning Perspectives* 5:63–66.

Mellor, John W. 1984. Food price policy and income distribution in low-income countries. In *Agricultural development in the third world*, ed. Carl K. Eicher and John M. Staatz. Baltimore, Md.: Johns Hopkins University Press.

———. 1985a. *Agricultural change and rural poverty.* Washington, D.C.: International Food Policy Research Institute. Food Policy Statement No. 3.

———. 1985b. *The role of government and new agricultural technologies.* Washington, D.C., International Food Policy Research Institute. Food Policy Statement No. 4.

————. 1986a. *The new global context for agricultural research: Implications for policy.* Washington, D.C.: International Food Policy Research Institute. Food Policy Statement No. 6.

————. 1986b. Dealing with the uncertainty of growing food imbalances: International structures and national policies. In Proceedings nineteenth international conference of agricultural economists, 191–198. Brookfield, Vt.: Grower.

————. 1988. Global food balances and food security. *World Development* 16:997–1011.

Mellor, John W., and Bruce F. Johnston. 1984. The world food equation: Interrelations among development, employment, and food consumption. *Journal of Economic Literature* 22:531–574.

Merrick, Thomas W., et al. 1986. World population in transition. *Population Bulletin* 41:1986.

Miller, Gay Y., Joseph Rosenblatt, and Leroy Hushak. 1988. The effects of supply shifts on producer's surplus. *American Journal of Agricultural Economics* 70:886–891.

Mincer, Jacob. 1976. Unemployment effects of minimum wages. *Journal of Political Economy* 84, no. 4, part 2 (August):87–104.

Mintz, Sidney W. 1989. Food and culture: An anthropological view. In *Completing the food chain: Strategies for combating hunger and malnutrition,* ed. Paula M. Hirschoff and Neil G. Kolter, 114–121. Washington, D.C.: Smithsonian.

Mitchell, Donald O., Merlinda D. Ingco, and Ronald C. Duncan. 1997. *The world food outlook.* Cambridge: Cambridge University Press.

Monto, A. S., and J. W. Koopman. 1980. The Tecumseh study XI, occurrence of acute enteric illness in the community. *American Journal of Epidemiology* 112:323–333.

Mundlak, Yair, Donald Larson, and Al Crego. Agricultural development: Issues, evidence, and consequences. World Bank, International Economics Department, Washington, D.C.

Myers, Robert G. 1988. *Programming for early child development and growth.* Paris: Unesco-Unicef Cooperative Program (June).

————. *The twelve who survive: Strengthening programmes of early childhood development in the third world.* London: Routledge (forthcoming).

Nakajima, Hiroshi. 1989. World health statistics annual. Geneva: WHO.

Naiken, L. 1988. Comparison of the FAO and World Bank methodology for estimating the incidence of undernutrition. *FAO Quarterly Bulletin of Statistics* 1, no. 3:iii–v.

National Science and Technology Council. n.d. *Biotechnology for the 21st century: New horizons.* Available at http://www.nal.usda.gov/bic/bio21/tablco.html

Neue, H. 1993. Methane emission from rice fields: Wetland rice fields may make a major contribution to global warming. *BioScience* 43, no. 7:466–473.

Newbery, D., and J. Stiglitz. 1981. *The theory of commodity price stabilization: A study in the economics of risk.* Oxford: Clarendon.

Overpeck, M., H. Hoffman, and K. Prager. 1992. The lowest birth-weight infants and the US infant mortality rate: NCHS 1983 linked birth/infant death data. *American Journal of Public Health* 82, no. 3:441–444.

Notestein, Frank W. 1945. Population—The long view. In *Food for the world,* ed. Theodore W. Schultz. Chicago: U. of Chicago Press.

Oram, Peter. 1995. *The potential of tehchnology to meet world food needs in 2020.* IFPRI 2020 Briefing Paper #13. Washington, D.C.: International Food Policy Research Institute.

Paglin, M. 1974. The measurement and trend of inequality: A basic revision. *American Economic Review* 65:598–609.

Parizokova, Jana. 1977. *Body fat and physical fitness*. The Hague: Martinus Nijhoff, B. V./Medical Division.

Pardey, Philip G., IFPRI, and Julian M. Alston. 1995. Revamping agricultural R&D. *IFPRI 2020 Briefing Paper #24*. Washington, D.C.: International Food Policy Research Institute.

Park, Robert Ezra. 1934. Forward. In *Shadow of the plantation*, ed. Charles Spurgen. Chicago: University of Chicago Press.

Parry, M. L., A. R. Magalhaes, and N. H. Nih. 1992. *The potential socio-economic effects of climate change: A summary of three regional assessments*. Nairobi, Kenya: United Nations Environment Programme (UNEP).

Payne, Philip R. 1985. The nature of malnutrition. In *Nutrition and development*, ed. Margaret Biswas and P. Pinstrup-Andersen. Oxford: Oxford University Press.

Pelletier, D. L., E. A. Frongillo Jr., and J. P. Habicht. 1993. Epidemiologic evidence for a potentiating effect of malnutrition on child mortality. *American Journal of Public Health* 83 (August):1130–1133.

———. 1995. The effects of malnutrition on child mortality in developing countries. *Bulletin of the World Health Organization* 73, no. 4:443–448

Pellett, Peter L. 1977. Marasmus in a newly rich urbanized society. *Ecology of Food and Nutrition* 6:53–56.

———. 1987. Problems and pitfalls in the assessment of nutritional status. In *Food and evolution: Toward a theory of food habits*, ed. Marvin Harris and Erick B. Ross, 163–179. Philadelphia: Temple University Press.

Pelto, Gretl H. 1987. Cognitive performance and intake in preschoolers. Chapter 30 in *Cognitive performance and intake in preschoolers*, ed. Lindsay H. Allen, Adolfo Chavez, and Gretl H. Pelto. Mexico, DF: University of Connictcut and Instituto Nacional de la Nutricion, Final report, C.R.S.R. on food intake and human factors, Mexico Project.

Penning de Vries, F. W. T. , H. Van Keulen, R. Rabbinge, and J. C. Luyten. 1995. *Biophysical limits to global food production*. IFPRI 2020 Brief 18 (May). Washington, D.C.: International Food Policy Research Institute.

Perisse, J., F. Sizaret, and P. Francoise. 1969. The effect of income on the structure of the diet. *FAO Nutrition Newsletter* 7 (July-September):2.

Peterson, Willis L. 1979. International farm prices and the social cost of cheap food policies. *American Journal of Agricultural Economics* 61 (February): 12–21.

Pfeifer, Karen. 1985. *Agrarian reform under state capitalism in Algeria*. Boulder: Westview Press.

Philippines Ministry of Agriculture. 1981a. *Food consumption and nutrition*. Memo to Agricultural Minister Tanco. Manila: National Agricultural Policy Staff (September 8).

———. 1981b. *National agricultural policy staff memo*. Manila: National Agricultural Policy Staff (September 8).

———. [1983] *National consumption patterns for major foods, 1977–1982*. Manila: Special Studies Division, Economic Research and Statistics Directorate, National Food Authority.

Philippines National Economic Development Authority. 1983. 1987–88 Integrated survey of households (ISH), as quoted in *1983 economic and social indicators*, p. 157. Manila: National Economic Development Authority.

Philippines National Science and Technology Authority. 1983. Manila: FNRI Publication no. 82–ET-10 (February).

———. 1984. *Second nationwide nutrition survey: Philippines, 1982*. Manila: Food and Nutrition Research Institute (October).

Philippines Journal of Nutrition. 1971. 24:161.

Philippines Ministry of Agriculture. 1981. *Seasonal price indices of selected agricultural commodities*. Manila: National Policy Staff Paper: 81–2, Ministry of Agriculture.

Phillips, Marshall, and Albert Baetz, eds. 1980. *Diet and resistance to disease*. New York: Plenum Press.

Phipps, Tim T. 1984. Land prices and farm-based returns. *American Journal of Agricultural Economics* 66 (November):422–429.

Pike, Ruth L, and Myrtle Brown. 1984. *Nutrition: An integrated approach*. New York: John Wiley.

Pimentel, D. 1993. Climate changes and food supply. Forum for Applied Research and Public Policy 8, no 4:54–60. Available at http://www.ciesin.org/docs/004-138/004-138.html

Pimentel, David, and Mario Giampietro. 1994. Food, land, population and the U.S. economy. Washington, D.C.: Carrying Capacity Network.

Pimentel, D., et al. 1994. Natural resources and an optimum human population. *Population and Environment* 15:347–369.

———. 1995. Environmental and economic costs of soil erosion and conservation benefits. *Science* 267:1117–1123.

———. 1996. Impact of population growth on food supplies and environmnet. Presented at AAAS annual meeting, February 9, in Baltimore.

Pinstrup-Andersen, Per, et al. 1976. The impact of increasing food supply on human nutrition: Implications for commodity priorities in agricultural research and policy. *American Journal of Agricultural Economics* 58:137–138.

Pinstrup-Andersen, Per, and Elizabeth Caicedo. 1978. The potential impact of changes in income distribution on food demand and human nutrition. *American Journal of Agricultural Economics* 60 (August):402–415.

Pinstrup-Andersen, Per, and Peter Hazell. 1985. The impact of the green revolution and prospects for the future. *Food Reviews International* 1, no. 1:11. (Also available from IFPRI as a reprint.)

Pinstrup-Anderson, Per, David Nygaard, and Annu Ratta. 1995. The right to food: Widely acknowledged and poorly protected. IFPRI 2020 Briefing Paper #22. Washington, D.C.: International Food Policy Research Institute.

Pinstrup-Andersen, P., R. Pandya-Lorch, and M. Rosegrant. 1998. *The world food situation: Recent developments, emerging issues, and long-term prospects*. Washington, D.C.: International Food Policy Research Institute.

Pollitt, E., K. Gorman, P. Engle, R. Martorell, and J. Rivera. 1993. Early supplementary feeding and cognition. *Monographs of the Society for Research in Child Development* 58, no. 235(7).

Population Information Program. 1985. Fertility and family planning surveys. *Population Reports*. Baltimore: Johns Hopkins University, Series M, No. 8 (September-October).

Population Reference Bureau. 1970. *1965 World population data sheet*. Washington D.C.: Population Reference Bureau.

———. 1987. *1987 World population data sheet*. Washington D.C.: Population Reference Bureau.

Posner, R. A. 1986. *Economic analysis of the law*, 3d ed. Boston: Little, Brown.

Postel, Sandra. 1997. Dividing the waters. *Technology Review* (July). Available at http://web.mit.edu/techreview/www/articles/apr97/toc.html

————, G. C. Daily, and P. R. Erlich. 1996. Human appropriation of renewable fresh water. *Science* 271:785–788.

Prentice, A. M., G. R. Goldberg, and Ann Prentice. 1994. Body mass index and lactation performance. *European Journal of Clinical Nutrition* 48, supp. 3 (November):S78.

Pullum, Thomas W. 1983. Correlates of family-size desires. In *Determinants of fertility in developing countries, vol. 1, supply and demand for children*, ed. Rudolfo A. Bulatao et al., 334–386. New York: Academic Press.

Quandt, Sara A. 1987. Methods for determining dietary intake. In *Nutritional anthropology*, ed. Francis E. Johnson, 67–84. New York: Alan R. Liss.

Ramalingaswami, Vulimiri, Urban Jonsson, and John Rohde. 1996. Commentary: The Asian enigma. In *The progress of nations*. Washington, D.C.: United Nations International Children's Fund.

Ranade, C. G., and R. W. Herdt. 1978. Shares of farm earnings from rice production. In *Economic consequences of the new rice technology*, ed. R. Barker and Y. Hayami, 87–104. Los Banos, Philippines: International Rice Research Institute.

Rangarajan, C. 1982. *Agricultural growth and industrial performance in India.* Washington, D.C.: International Food Policy Research Institute. IFPRI Research Report 33.

Rask, Norman. 1986. Economic development and the dynamics of food needs. Unpublished paper delivered at College Park, U. of Md. Global Development Conference (September).

Ravallion, Martin. 1997. Famines and economics. *Journal of Economic Literature* 35 (September):1205–1242.

Ray, Anandarup. 1986. Trade and pricing policies in world agriculture. *Finance and Development* 23 (September):2–5.

Repetto, Robert. 1985. *Paying the price: Pesticide subsidies in developing countries.* Washington, D.C.: World Resources Institute. Research Report No. 2 (December).

Reuters Information Service. 1996. *Tension in Jordan's Karak after bread riots* (August 16). Available at http://www.nando.net/newsroom/ntn/world/081696/world7_23344.html.

Reutlinger, Schlomo. 1983. Policy implications of research on energy intake and activity levels with reference to the debate on the energy adequacy of existing diets in developing countries. Washington, D.C.: World Bank. Agriculture and Rural Development Department Research Unit Discussion Paper 7.

————. 1985. Food security and poverty in LDCs. *Finance and Development* 22 (December):7–11.

Reutlinger, Schlomo, et al. 1986. *Poverty and hunger—Issues and options for food security in developing countries.* Washington D.C.: World Bank.

Reutlinger, Shlomo, and Marcelo Selowsky. 1976. *Malnutrition and poverty: Magnitude and policy options.* Washington D.C.: World Bank, Staff Occasional Paper No. 23.

Rivera, Juan, and Reynaldo Martorell. 1988. Nutrition, infection, and growth, Part I: Effects of infection on growth. *Clinical Nutrition* 7:156–162.

————. 1988. Nutrition, infection, and growth, Part II: Effects of malnutrition on infection and general conclusions. *Clinical Nutrition* 7:163–167.

Roberts, D. F. 1953. Body weight, race and climate. *American Journal of Physical Anthropology* 11:533–558.

Rogers, Beatrice Lorge. 1988a. Design and implementation considerations for consumer-oriented food subsidies. In *Food subsidies in developing countries*, ed. Per Pinstrup-Andersen, 127–146. Baltimore: Johns Hopkins University Press.

———. 1988b. *Economic perspectives on combating hunger.* Presentation at the Second Annual World Food Prize Celebration. Washington, D.C., Smithsonian, September 30. An edited version of this paper is available in *Completing the food chain: Strategies for combating hunger and malnutrition,* ed. Paula M. Hirschoff and Neil G. Kolter, 122–126. Washington, D.C.: Smithsonian, 1989.

———. 1988c. Pakistan's ration system: Distribution of costs and benefits. In *Food subsidies in developing countries,* ed. Per Pinstrup-Andersen, 242–252. Baltimore: Johns Hopkins University Press.

Rose, Stephen, and David Fasentast. 1988. *Family incomes in the 1980's.* Washington, D.C.: Economic Policy Institute. Working Paper No. 103 (November).

Rosegrant, Mark W.. 1986. Irrigation with equity in Southeast Asia. Washington, D.C.: International Food Policy Research Institute. *IFPRI Report* 8 (January): 1, 4.

Rosenzweig, C., M. L. Parry, G. Fischer, and K. Frohberg. 1993. Climate change and world food supply. Research Report No. 3. Oxford: Oxford University, Environmental Change Unit.

Rosenzweig, C., and M. L. Parry. 1994. Potential impact of climate change on world food supply. *Nature* 367, no. 6459.

Rosenzweig, Cynthia, and Daniel Hillel. 1995. Potential impacts of climate change on agriculture and food supply. *Consquences* (summer).

Rountree, John. 1985. Computations done at the University of Mryland from data provided by the Egyption Ministry of Agriculture, the Central Agency for Public Mobilization and Statistics and the Ministry of Supply.

Rustein, Shea O. 1984. Infant and child mortality: Levels, trends and demographic differentials. Table 14 in *World Fertility Survey Comparative Studies No. 45, Revised Edition.* Voorburg, Netherlands: International Statistical Institute.

Ryan, James G. 1977. *Human nutritional needs and crop breeding objectives in the Indian Semi-Arid Tropics.* Huderabad, India: International Crops Research Institute for the Semi-Arid Tropics (ICRISAT).

Sahlins, Marshall. 1968. Notes on the original affluent society. In *Man the hunter,* ed. R. B. Lee and I. DeVore, 85–89. Chicago: Aldine.

Sahn, David E., and Neville Edirisinghe. Politics of food policy in Sri Lanka: From basic human needs to an increased market orientation, Chapter 3 in *The political rconomy of food and nutrition policy,* ed., Per Pinstrup-Andersen. In process.

Sahn, David E., ed. 1989. *Seasonal variability in third world agriculture—The consequences for food security.* Baltimore: Johns Hopkins, 1989.

Salaff, Janet W., and Arline Wong. 1983. *Incentives and disincentives in population policies.* Washington, D.C.: Draper World Population Fund Report, No. 12 (August).

Samuels, B. 1986. Infant mortality and low birth weight among minority groups in the United States: A review of the literature. In *Report of the Secretary's Task Force on Black and Minority Health, Vol. 4: Infant mortality and low birth weight.* Washington, D.C.: U.S. Department of Health and Human Services.

Sandburg, Carl. 1936. *The people, yes.* New York: Harcourt, Brace and Co.

Santos-Villaneuva, P. 1966. The value of rural roads. In *Selected readings to accompany getting agriculture moving,* ed. Raymond E. Borton, 775–795. New York: Agricultural Development Council.

Sazawal, S., et al. 1995. Zinc supplementation in young children with acute diarrhea in India. *New England Journal of Medicine* 333, no. 13 (September): 839–844.

Scandizzo, Pasquale L., and Colin Bruce. 1980. *Methodologies for measuring agricultural price intervention effects.* Washington, D.C.: World Bank. Staff Working Paper 394 (June).

Scandizzo, Pasquale L., and I. Tsakok. 1985. Food price policies and nutrition in developing countries. In *Nutrition and development,* ed. Margaret Biswas and Per Pinstrup-Andersen, 60–76. Oxford: Oxford University Press.

Scherr, Sara J., and Satya Yadav. 1997. Land degradation in the developing world: Issues and policy options for 2020. IFPRI 2020 Brief no. 44 (June). Washington, D.C.: International Food Policy Resarch Institute.

Schiff, Maurice, and Alberto Valdés. 1995. The plundering of agriculture in developing countries. *Finance & Development* (March). Washington, D.C.:World Bank.

Schroeder D. G., and K. H. Brown. 1994. Nutritional status as a predictor of child survival: Summarizing the association and quantifying its global impact. *Bulletin of the World Health Organization* 72, no. 4:569–579.

Schuh, G. Edward. 1988. Some issues associated with exchange rate realignments in developing countries. In *Macroeconomics, agriculture, and exchange rates,* ed. Philip L. Paarlberg and Robert G. Chambers, 231–240. Boulder: Westview Press.

Schultz, Theodore W. 1979. *The economics of research and agricultural productivity.* Arlington, Va.: International Agricultural Development Services Occasional Paper. As quoted in *Agricultural development in the third world,* ed. Carl K. Eicher and John M. Staatz, 335–347. Baltimore: Johns Hopkins University Press, 1984.

Scobie, Grant M., 1983. *Food subsidies in Egypt: Their impact on foreign exchange and trade.* Washington D.C.: International Food Policy Reserach Institute, IFPRI Research Report No. 40 (August).

Scobie, Grant M. and Rafael Posada T. 1984. The impact of technical change on income distribution: The case of rice in Colombia. In *Agricultural development in the third world,* ed. Carl K. Eicher and John M. Staatz, 378–388. Baltimore: Johns Hopkins University Press.

Scrimshaw, Nevin S. 1988. Completing the food chain: From production to consumption. Remarks presented at the Scond Annual World Food Price Celebration. Washington, D.C., Smithsonian, September 30. An edited version of this paper is available in *Completing the food chain: Strategies for combating hunger and malnutrition,* ed. Paula M. Hirschoff and Neil G. Kolter, 1–17. Washington, D.C.: Smithsonian, 1989.

Scrimshaw, Nevin S., and Vernon R. Young. 1976. The requirements of human nutrition. In *Food and agriculture,* 26–40. San Francisco: Freeman.

Scrimshaw, Nevin S., Carl Taylor, and John Gordon. 1968. *Interactions of nutrition and infection.* Geneva: World Health Organization.

Scrimshaw, Susan. 1978. Infant mortality and behavior in the regulation of family size. *Population and Development Review* 4:383–403.

Scrimshaw, Susan. 1984. Infanticide in human populations: Societal and individual concerns. In *Infanticide: Comparative and evolutionary perspectives,* ed. Glen Hausfater and Sarah B. Hardy, 439–462. New York: Aldine.

Seckler, David. 1982. "Small but healthy": A basic hypothesis in the theory, measurement and policy of malnutrition. In *Newer concepts in nutrition and their implications for policy,* ed. P. V. Kukhtame, 127–137. Pune, India: Maharastra Association for the Cultivation of Science Research Institute, Law College Road.

Semba, R. D., et al. 1994. Maternal vitamin A deficiency and mother-to-child transmission of HIV-1. *Lancet* 343, no. 8913 (June 25):1593–1597.

Sen, Amartya K. 1964. Size of holdings and productivity. *Economic and Political Weekly* (February).

————. 1966. Peasants and dualism with or without surplus labor. *Journal of Political Economy* 74:425–450.

————. 1973. *On economic inequality.* London: Oxford University Press.

————. 1981. *Poverty and famines: An essay on entitlement and deprivation.* Oxford: Clarendon Press.

Senauer, Benjamin, et al. 1988. Determinants of the intrahousehold allocation of food in the rural Philippines. *American Journal of Agricultural Economics* 70:170–180.

Shakir, A. 1975. The surveillance of protein-calorie malnutrition by simple and economic means (a report to UNICEF). *Journal of Tropical Pediatrics and Environmental Child Health* 21:69–85.

Shekar, Meera. 1991. *The Tamil Nadu Integrated Nutrition Project: A review of the project with special emphasis on the monitoring and information system.* Working Paper No. 14. Cornell Food and Nutrition Policy Program, Ithaca, N.Y.

Sherman, Adria R. 1986. Alterations in immunity related to nutritional status. *Nutrition Today* (July/August):7–13.

Sicat, Gerardo P. 1983. Toward a flexible interest rate policy, or losing interest in the usury law. In *Rural financial markets in developing countries: Their use and abuse,* ed. J. D. Von Pische, et al., 373–386. Baltimore: Johns Hopkins Press.

Simmons, George B., and Robert J. Lapham. 1987. The determinants of family planning program effectiveness. In *Organizing for effective family planning programs,* ed. Lampham and Simmons, 683–706. Washington, D.C.: National Academy Press.

Simon, Julian L. 1986. *Theory of population and economic growth.* New York: Blackwell.

————. 1996. *The ultimate resource.* Princeton, N.J.: Princeton University Press. Available at http://www.inform.umd.edu/EdRes/Colleges/BMGT/Faculty/JSimon/Ultimate_Resource/

Sinaga, R. S., and B. M. Sinaga. 1978. Comments on shares of farm earnings from rice production. In *Economic consequences of the new rice technology,* ed. R. Barker and Y. Hayami, 105–109. Los Banos, Philippines: International Rice Research Institute.

Smale, Melinda. 1997. The green revolution and wheat genetic diversity: Some unfounded assumptions. *World Development* 25, no. 8:1257–1269.

Snyder, J. D., and M. H. Merson. 1982. The magnitude of the global problem of acute diarrhoeal disease: A review of active surveillance data. *Bulletin of the World Health Organization* 60:605–613.

Soliman, Ibrahim, and Shahla Shapouri. 1984. See U.S. Department of Agriculture. 1984.

Sommer, Alfred, et al. 1986. Impact of vitamin A supplementation on childhood mortality—A randomized controlled community trial. *Lancet* (May 24):1169–1173.

Sperduto, R. D., et al. 1993. The Linxian cataract studies. Two nutrition intervention trials. *Archives of Ophthalmology* 830, no. 111:1246–1253.

Spurr, G. B., M. Barac-Nieto, and M. G. Maksud. 1976. See U.S. Department of State 1976.

Stackman, E. C., Richard Bradfield, and Paul C. Mangelsdorf. 1967. *Campaigns against hunger.* Boston: Bellknap Press of Harvard University Press.

Stanbury, John, ed. 1994. *The damaged brain of iodine deficiency: Cognitive, behavioral, neuromotor, educative aspects.* Port Washington, N.Y.: Cognizant Communication Corp.

Steindl, Josef. 1987. Pareto Distribution. In *The new Palgrave: A dictionary of economics,* vol 3., ed. John Eatwell et al., 809–810. New York: Stockton Press.

Stephenson, Lani S., M. C. Latham, and A. Jansen. 1983. *A comparison of growth standards: Similarities between NCHS, Harvard, Denver and privileged African children and differences with Kenyan rural children.* Ithaca: Cornell International Nutrition Monograph Series No. 12.

Stevens, Robert D., and Cathy L. Jabara. 1988. *Agricultural development principles: Economic theory and empirical evidence.* Baltimore: Johns Hopkins University Press.

Stiglitz, Joseph E. 1986. *Economics of the public sector.* New York: Norton.

Stone, Bruce. 1985. *Fertilizer pricing policy and foodgrain production strategy.* Washington, D.C.: International Food Policy Research Institute. *IFPRI Report* 7 (May):1, 4.

Strauss, John, and Duncan Thomas. 1998. Health, nutrition, and economic development. *Journal of Economic Literature* 36:766–818.

Streeten, Paul. 1987. *What price food? Agricultural price policies in developing countries.* London: MacMillan.

Stuart, H., and S. Stevenson. 1950. Physical growth and development. In W. Nelson, ed., *Textbook of pediatrics,* 5th edition. Philadelphia: Saunders.

Susser, E., et al. 1996. Schizophrenia after prenatal famine: Further evidence. *Archives of general psychiatry* 53, no. 1 (January):25–31.

Sutton, John. 1989. See U.S. Department of Agriculture 1989a.

Tang, A. M., et al. 1993. Dietary micronutrient intake and risk of progression to acquired immunodeficiency syndrome (AIDS) in human immunodeficiency virus type 1 (HIV-1)-infected homosexual men. *American Journal of Epidemiology* 138, no. 11 (December 1):937–951.

Tanner, J. M. 1977. Human growth and constitution. In *Human biology—An introduction to human evolution, variation, growth and ecology,* by G. A. Harrison, et al., 301–385. Oxford: Oxford University Press.

Tanner, J., R. Whitehouse, and M. Takaishi. 1966. Standards from birth to maturity for height, height velocity and weight velocity: British children I. *Archives of Disease in Childhood* 41:454+.

Timmer, C. Peter. 1984. Choice of technique in rice milling on Java. In *Agricultural development in the third world,* ed. Carl K. Eicher and John M. Staatz, 278–288. Baltimore: Johns Hopkins University Press.

Timmer, C. Peter, Walter P. Falcon, and Scott R. Pearson. 1983. *Food policy analysis.* Baltimore: Johns Hopkins University Press.

Tinker, Anne, et al. 1994. *Women's health and nutrition: Making a difference.* Washington, D.C.: World Bank.

Todaro, Michael P. 1980. Internal migration in developing countries: A survey. In *Population and economic change in developing countries,* ed. Richard A. Easterlin, 361–402. Chicago: University of Chicago Press.

Traub, James. 1988. Into the mouths of babes. *New York Times Magazine.* (July 24), 18.

Tupasi, T. E. 1985. Nutritional and acute respiratory infection. In *Acute respiratory infections in childhood, Proceedings of an international workshop,* ed. R. Douglas and E. Kerby-Eaton. Adelaide, Australia: University of Adelaide.

UNICEF (United Nations International Children's Fund). 1982. *News* 113:9.

———. 1987. *ORT and much more—Developing whole CDD programmes.* CF/PD/PRO-1987-001, Memo to all field offices, January 15.

———. 1988. *State of the world's children, 1988.* New York: Oxford University Press.

———. 1996. *Progress of nations.* New York: United Nations. Available at http://www.unicef.org/pon96/

Urban, Francis, and Arthur J. Dommen. 1989. See U.S. Department of Agriculture 1989b.

United Nations. 1991. *World population prospects 1990.* New York: United Nations. Population Study No. 120, Department of International Economic and Social Affairs.

UNEP (United Nations Environment Programme). 1990. *The impacts of climate change on agriculture.* United Nations Environment Programme Information Unit for Climate Change (IUCC) Fact Sheet 101. Nairobi, Kenya: United Nations Environment Programme (UNEP).

UN, FAO. 1996. Backgrounder on plant genetic resources and plant breeding. Rome: FAO. Available at http://www.fao.org/FOCUS/e/96/06/02-e.htm

UN, Population Information Network (POPIN). 1995. Population and land degradation. Vol. 2 of *Population and the environment: A review of issues and concepts for population programmes staff.* New York: United Nations.

U.S. Bureau of Census. 1961. *Historical statistics of the U.S. from colonial times to 1956.* Washington, D.C.: Bureau of Census.

———. 1987. *Statistical abstract of the United States: 1988.* Washington, D.C.: Bureau of Census.

U.S. Congress. 1974. *National nutrition policy study—1974: Hearings before the Select Committee on Nutrition and Human Needs, Part 3—Nutrition and Special Groups.* 93rd Cong., Washington, D.C.: Government Printing Office.

U.S. Congress, Office of Technology Assessment. 1986. *Technology, public policy, and the changing structure of American agriculture.* Washington, D.C.: Government Printing Office. OTA-F-285.

U.S. Department of Agriculture (USDA). 1917. *Geography of the world's agriculture,* by V. C. Finch and O. E. Baker, Office of Farm Management. Washington D.C.

———. 1963. *Composition of foods, raw, processed, prepared.* Washington D.C.: Agricultural Handbook No. 8.

———. 1970. *Feed Situation Report* (November).

———. 1984. *The impact of wheat price policy change on nutritional status in Egypt,* by Soliman, Ibrahim and Shahla Shapouri. Washington, D.C.: United Stated Department of Agriculture, ERS, International Economics Division (February).

———. 1985. *U.S. demand for food: A complete system of price and income effects,* by Kuw W. Huang. Washington, D.C.: USDA Tech. Bul. 1714.

———. 1988. *World food needs and availabilities, 1988/89: Summer.* Washington, D.C.: USDA, ERS (August).

———. 1989a. Environmental degradation and agriculture, by John Sutton. Washington, D.C.: USDA/ERS *World Agriculture Situation and Outlook Report.* WAS-55 (June): 35–41.

———. 1989b. *World agriculture,* by Francis Urban and Arthur J. Dommen. Washington, D.C.: USDA (June).

———. 1990. *U.S. government concessional exports, commodity by country and fiscal year.* Washington, D.C.: Unpublished data base. Washington, D.C.

———. 1991. *Food cost reviews.* Washington, D.C.: United Sates Department of Agriculture.

———. 1998. *Agricultural baseline projections to 2007.* Washington D.C.: United States Department of Agriculture. Available at http://www.econ.ag.gov/Briefing/baseline/index98.htm

400   *References*

U.S. Department of Health, Education and Welfare. 1976. NCHS Growth Charts. *Monthly Vital Statistics Report* 25, no. 3, Supp. (HRA) 76–1120. Rockville, Md.: National Center for Health Statistics, Resources Administration (June).
———. 1979. *Weight by height and age for adults 18–74 years: United States, 1971–74.* Hyattsville, Md.: Public Health Service, Office of Health Research, Statistics and Technology, National Center for Health Statistics (NCHS), Vital and Health Statistics, Data from the National Health Survey, Series 11, Number 208.
U.S. Department of Health and Human Resources. 1981. *Height and weight of adults ages 18–74 years by socioeconomic and geographic variables, United States.* Hyattsville, Md.: National Center for Health Statistics, DHHS Publication No. (PHS) 81–1674. Data from the National Health Survey, Series 11, No. 224 (August).
U.S. Department of Health and Human Services. 1987. *Anthropometric reference data and prevalence of overweight, United States, 1976–80.* Hyattsville, Md., National Center for Health Statistics, DHHS Publication No. (PHS) 87–1688 (October).
———. 1988. *The Surgeon General's report on nutriton and health, 1988.* Washington, D.C.: Public Health Service Publication No. 88–50210.
U.S. Department of State. 1976. *Clinical and subclinical malnutrition and their influence on the capacity to do work,* by G. B. Spurr, M. Barac-Nieto, and M. G. Maksud. Washington D.C.: State Department, Project AID/CSD 2943, Final Report.
———. 1978. *Agricultural policies and rural malnutrition,* by Phillips Foster. Washington, D.C.: State Department, USAID Economics and Sector Planning Division, Office of Agriculture, Technical Assistance Bureau, Occasional Paper No. 8.
———. 1986a. *Development and spread of high yielding rice varieties in developing countries,* by Dana G. Dalrymple. Washington, D.C.: Agency for Internatonal Development.
———. 1986b. *Development and spread of high yielding wheat varieties in developing countries,* by Dana G. Dalrymple. Washington, D.C.: Agency for Internatonal Development.
U.S. Federal Reserve System. Board of Governors. 1989. *Balance sheets for the U.S. economy, 1949–88.* Washington, D.C. (October).
U.S. National Academy of Sciences. 1974. *Recommendeed dietary allowances.* Washington, D.C.: National Academy of Sciences.
U.S. White House, Council of Economic Advisers. 1989. *Economic indicators.* Washington, D.C.: The White House (December).
U.S. White House, President's Science Advisory Committee. 1967. *The world food problem, Volumes II and III, Report of the panel on the world food supply.* Washington, D.C.: The White House.
University of California Food Task Force. 1974. *A hungry world: The challenge to agriculture, summary report.* Berkeley: Division of Agriculural Sciences.
Uvin , Peter. 1993. State of world hunger. In *The hunger report 1993.* New York: Gordon and Breach.
Vergara, Benito S. 1979. *A farmer's primer on growing rice.* Los Banos, Philippines: International Rice Research Institute.
Von Braun, Joachim, and Eileen Kennedy. 1986. *Commercialization of subsistence agriculture: Income and nutritional effects in developing countries.* Washington, D.C.: International Food Policy Research Institute, Working Paper on Commercialization of Agriculture and Nutrition, No. 1.

————, eds. 1994. *Agricultural commercialization, economic development, and nutrition.* Baltimore: Published for the International Food Policy Research Institute by Johns Hopkins University Press.

Von Braun, Joachim, et al. 1989. *Nontraditional export crops in Guatemala: Effects on production, income, and nutrition.* Washington, D.C.: International Food Policy Research Institute, IFPRI Research Report 73.

Walinsky, Louis. 1962. *Economic development in Burma, 1951–1960.* New York: Twentieth Century Fund.

Walker, Alexander, and Harry Stein. 1985. Growth of third world children. Chapter 20 in *Dietry fibre, fibre-depleted foods and disease,* ed. H. Trowell et al., 331–344. London: Academic Press.

Waterlow, J., R. Buzina, W. Keller, J. Lane, M. Nichaman, and J. Tanner. 1977. The presentation and use of height and weight data for comparing the nutritional status of groups of children under the age of ten years. *Bulletin of WHO* 55:489–498.

Weiner, J. S. 1977. Nutritional ecology. In *Human biology—An introduction to human evolution, variation, growth and ecology,* by A. G. Harrison et al., 400–423. Oxford: Oxford University Press.

Whitney, Eleanor N., and Eva Hamilton. 1977. *Understanding nutrition.* St. Paul: West.

WHO (World Health Organization). 1985a. *Energy and protein requirements, Report of a joint FAO/WHO/UNU expert consultation.* Geneva: WHO, Technical Report Series 724.

————. 1985b. *Fourth programme report for control of diarrheal diseases 1983–1984.* Geneva: WHO, Program for Control of Diarrheal Diseases.

————. 1985c. *The management of diarrhoea and use of oral rehydration therapy.* Geneva: World Health Organization/UNICEF.

————. 1989. *Report on world health.* Washington D.C.: WHO Regional Office for the Americas. Press release, September 25.

————. 1995a. *Physical status: The use and interpretation of anthropometry.* Report of a WHO Expert Committee. WHO Technical Report Series No. 854. Geneva: WHO.

————. 1995b. *World health report 1995: Bridging the gaps.* Geneva: WHO.

————. 1996a. *Investing in health research and development: Ad hoc committee on health research relating to future intervention options.* New York: United Nations.

————. 1996b. *State of the world's vaccines and immunization.* New York: United Nations. Available at http://www.who.ch/gpv/tEnglish/avail/sowvi.htm

————. 1996c. *World health report, 1996.* Geneva: WHO.

————. 1997. *World health report, 1997.* Geneva: WHO.

WHO and UN. 1997. Micronutrient and trace element deficiencies: General information. Available at http://www.who.org/nut/micr/micrgen.htm

Winick, M., K. Meyer, and R. Harris. 1973. Malnutrition and environmental enrichment by early adoption. *Science* 190 (December):1173–1175.

Winter, Roger P. 1988. In Sudan, both sides use food as a weapon. *Washington Post,* November 19:A25.

Wittwer, Sylvan. 1995. *Food, climate, and carbon dioxide: The global environment and world food production.* New York: Lewis Publishers.

World Bank. 1975. *Land reform sector policy paper.* (May).

————. various years. *World development report.* New York: Oxford University Press.

————. 1994b. Enriching lives: Overcoming vitamin and mineral malnutrtion in developing countries. Washington, D.C.: World Bank.

————. 1997. Does better nutrition improve academic achievement? Yes. *World Bank Policy and Research Bulletin* 8, no. 2 (April-June).

World Bank and UNDP (United Nations Development Program). 1990. *A proposal for an internationally supported programme to enhance research in irrigation and drainage technology in developing countries.* Vol. 2. Washington, D.C.: World Bank and UNDP.

World Food Council. 1988. *The global state of hunger and malnutrition, 1988 report.* Nicosia: Secretariat, World Food Council (May).

World Food Program. 1989. *Food aid works.* Rome: FAO, World Food Program.

World Resources Institute. 1997. *World resources 1996/96: The urban environment.* Washington, D.C.: World Resources Institute. Availabe at http://www.wri.org/wr-96–97

WorldWatch Institute. 1996. WorldWatch Institute urges World Bank and FAO to overhaul misleading food supply projections, press release (May 1), Washington, D.C.

Ying, Yvonne. 1996. *Poverty and inequality in China.* Washington, D.C.: World Bank. Available at http://www.worldbank.org/html/prddr/trans/ja96/art2.htm

Zaidi, S., and M. C. Fawzi. 1995. Health of Baghdad's children [letter], *Lancet* 346, no. 8988 (December 2):1485.

☐ Index

Acute undernutrition, defined, 38
Afghanistan, undernutrition in, 84
Africa: agricultural research and, 339–341;
  agricultural workforce in, 192, 193T;
  average calorie requirements in, 172–173;
  life expectancy in, 111; potential
  agricultural land in, 184, 185
Africa, sub-Saharan: contraceptive use in,
  265; diet in, 26; fertilizer use in, 188,
  189; undernutrition in, 77, 87
Agricultural chemicals, environmental
  hazards of, 212, 213, 214
Agricultural experiment stations, payoffs to
  research in, 337, 338T
Agricultural extension services, 342–343
Agricultural labor: in Africa and Asia, 192,
  193T; marginal product of labor and,
  192–194; population growth and,
  191–192, 195–196; wages, Third World,
  194
Agricultural land: available and potential,
  184–186; degradation of, 185, 186–188,
  211–213; global warming and, 218;
  irrigated, 186–187, 218, 323–324;
  taxation on, 276–277. *See also* Land
  reform
Agricultural machinery, worldwide use of,
  18, 189–191
Agricultural production/productivity, 144;
  and degradation of land and water,
  211–214; economic policy and, 280–281,
  285–289; environmental concerns in, 204,
  211–220; and food supply and demand, 7;
  future prospects, 214–215; and global
  warming, 217–220; and land reform, 273;
  livestock production vs. grain production

and, 350; output subsidies and, 320–323;
  overvalued domestic currency and,
  309–311; ozone layer depletion and, 220;
  price elasticities and, 132–134; and
  purchasing power, 132–134; subsidies,
  324–327; sustainable methods in,
  215–216, 343. *See also* Agricultural
  labor; Crop production; Food
  production
Agricultural research: on crop varieties, 336;
  on crop yields, 196–209; government
  sponsorship of, 338; and household food
  production, 98; modern-day challenges to,
  339; subsidies, 336–341. *See also*
  Technological improvements
Agroforestry, 341
Aid, food, 293–294; famine and, 296–302;
  major donors/recipients, 10–11. *See also*
  Food subsidies
AIDS (acquired immunodeficiency
  syndrome): future populations and, 112;
  mother-child transmission of, 48; vitamin
  consumption and, 17
Algeria, land reform in, 271, 274
Angola, undernutrition in, 84
Anthropometric assessment, 59–65; defined,
  59
Aquaculture, 215–216
Argentina, pricing policies in, 308–309
Asia: agricultural workforce in, 192, 193T;
  average fertilizer use in, 188–189; fertility
  rates in, 111; food supplies and seasonal
  nutrition in, 83–84; South, potential
  agricultural land in, 184; undernutrition
  in, 77
Attention deficit disorder (ADD), 53

403

☐ About the Book

This long-awaited second edition of The World Food Problem incorporates an up-to-date description of the state of world food supply and demand, as well as an assessment of prospects for the future. Recognizing that millions of people in the less-developed countries continue to go hungry, while there is more than enough food in the world to feed them, the authors tackle the question of why and what can be done about it.

Added features of the new edition include a section on food and the environment, a discussion of prospects for continued growth in agricultural productivity, and reports of recent research conducted by international organizations (e.g., the World Bank and FAO), NGOs such as the World Watch Institute, and individual scholars and practitioners.

Integrating knowledge from many disciplines (agronomy, economics, nutrition, anthropology, demography, geography, health science, and public policy analysis), this highly readable and comprehensive text provides a combination of information and explanation designed specifically to be used in the undergraduate classroom.

Phillips Foster is professor emeritus of agricultural and resource economics and **Howard D. Leathers** is associate professor of agricultural and resource economics at the University of Maryland, College Park.